JAMES COWLES PRICHARD'S ANTHROPOLOGY: REMAKING THE SCIENCE OF MAN IN EARLY NINETEENTH-CENTURY BRITAIN

THE WELLCOME INSTITUTE SERIES IN THE HISTORY OF MEDICINE

Forthcoming Titles

Drugs On Trial:
Experimental Pharmacology and Therapeutic Innovation
in the Eighteenth Century
Andreas-Holger Maehle

Surgery, Skin and Syphilis
Daniel Turner's London (1667-1741)
Philip K. Wilson

Academic enquiries regarding the series should be addressed
to the editors C. J. Lawrence, V. Nutton, and Roy Porter at
the Wellcome Institute for the History of Medicine,
183 Euston Road, London NW1 2BE, UK

JAMES COWLES PRICHARD'S ANTHROPOLOGY:
REMAKING THE SCIENCE OF MAN IN EARLY NINETEENTH-CENTURY BRITAIN

H. F. Augstein

Amsterdam – Atlanta, GA 1999

First published in 1999
by Editions Rodopi B. V., Amsterdam – Atlanta, GA 1999.

H.F. Augstein © 1999

Design and Typesetting by Alex Mayor, the Wellcome Trust.
Printed and bound in The Netherlands by Editions Rodopi B. V.,
Amsterdam – Atlanta, GA 1999.

British Library Cataloguing in Publication Data
A catalogue record for this book is available from the British Library
ISBN 90-420-0404-5 (Paper)
ISBN 90-420-0414-2 (Bound)

James Cowles Prichard's Anthropology:
Remaking the Science of Man in Early
Nineteenth-Century Britain –
Amsterdam – Atlanta, GA:
Rodopi. – ill. ·
(Clio Medica 52 / ISSN 0045-7183;
The Wellcome Institute Series in the History of Medicine)

Front cover:
"Monkey"
Print published 1st Oct. 1806, by James Curndee, London.
All other illustrations in this book are reproduced by courtesy
of the Wellcome Institute Library, London.

© Editions Rodopi B. V., Amsterdam – Atlanta, GA 1999

Printed in The Netherlands

Contents

Acknowledgements

Though James Cowles Prichard of Bristol lived a rather sedentary life, he had an illustrious fictional predecessor: Captain William Prichard, according to Jonathan Swift "the master of the Antelope, who was making a voyage to the South Sea", setting sail from Bristol 4 May, 1699, taking Lemuel Gulliver towards foreign shores. Researching the story of this book was not quite so adventurous a naval exploration, but at times it was no less exotic, if not wayward in its direction. I should like to express my gratitude to all those who have generously helped me steer my course during the last years. First, I owe my thanks to those who have assisted me in piling up the material and coming to terms with it: Michael Biddiss, Bill Bynum, Chris Lawrence, Michael Neve and Bernd Weisbrod who all gave me much good and stimulating advice. Then, my gratitude is due to those who encouraged me to cut down to size what I had written, in particular John Burrow and Sander Gilman. The staff of the Wellcome Institute Library in London, the Bristol Record Office, the Bristol Central Library and the Special Collections Department of Edinburgh University Library have been exceedingly welcoming. I am particularly grateful to everybody working at the old North Library which was something of a home from home to me. Special thanks are due to Caroline Overy of the Wellcome Institute, London, who out of sheer kindness came to my rescue whenever I was at a loss concerning obscure authors or unknown references. Finally, I should like to thank a man who dislikes dedications: my husband. Thanks to him, I enjoyed the time while working on this book.

"Civilization comes from what men call greed."
Plantagenet Palliser
in Anthony Trollope's *The Way We Live Now*

Introduction

The farthest the Bristol doctor James Cowles Prichard ever got away from home were visits to Paris and Switzerland. His mind, however, was widely travelled. In his spare hours, mostly between five and eight in the morning, Prichard studied descriptions of aboriginal populations all over the world, perusing countless volumes of travel literature, anatomical observations and linguistic tracts, contemplating how mankind had spread over the globe in those almost six thousand years between the creation of Adam and Eve and his own birth in 1786.

He was born into an age when Britain was vigorously expanding, and at the same time defending, her colonial Empire. Within a certain latitude, and subject to individual initiative, scientific explorations followed suit. At the turn of the nineteenth century, Joseph Banks (1743-1820), the naturalist and influential president of the Royal Society, was at the centre of British natural history, organizing "a vast network of botanical activity", including voyages of discovery and the foundation of Kew Gardens.[1] While it is debatable to what extent British explorations of the eighteenth century followed the commercial interests,[2] the colonial system was fervently attacked on moral grounds: Britons supporting the liberation war of the American colonies and abolitionists fighting slavery. Many dissenting denominations took up causes of philanthropy such as the Greek freedom movement, the newly-founded nation of ex-slaves in Liberia and the protection of those native peoples who were exploited and deprived of their living in the name of British trade.

The history of Western scientific progress, to which Prichard contributed his share, goes hand in hand with the history of secularization, in which the quest for scientific impartiality gradually consigned Biblical "truths" to the realm of cultural anachronisms. The more the notion of *truth* became dissociated from piety, the greater grew the void which many nineteenth-century thinkers tried to fill with home-brewed ideas. Some poetic minds, including certain German idealists, fed the notion of God into the machinery of the world: for them God existed insofar as the world existed, He was continuous Becoming. For others, science, the very motor and aim of secularization, was imbued with theological overtones. The age was replete with prophets who were not prepared to accept that the changes they were witnessing must ultimately render the world spiritually emptier than it had been during the age of God's unchallenged reign. Carlyle, Comte, Renan and many other sages tried to rescue metaphysics in what they perceived as a disenchanted world.[3] In Britain the emphasis on common sense led many philosophically complex ideas to be habitually dismissed as "fanciful". But if nineteenth-century Britain opened itself to continental philosophy only by degrees, the same did not apply to the life sciences.

At the time, various new speculations on species change were put forward, Immanuel Kant developing the concept of the "germ", and Erasmus Darwin theorizing the transformation of one species into another. Around the turn of the nineteenth century similar tenets by Jean-Baptiste de Lamarck made their way across the Channel. The tranquil notion of a fnite Creation, embodied in the concept of the Chain of Being, gave way to dynamic theories of change and fluidity.[4] Hitherto the world had been stable and intelligible; now it became, in the words of George Eliot's Mr Tulliver, "an uncommon puzzling thing", being subjected to blind forces whose purposes seemed impenetrable. The very existence of natural laws was traditionally considered to exemplify divine Providence. But once it was found that the known laws could not explain all natural phenomena, the foundations of natural theology were shaken. Orthodox defenders of religion felt increasingly besieged, their position being threatened from the very quarter which was the pride of the age: the sciences.[5] Faced with the challenge, British opinion resorted to traditionalism. Age-old concepts of natural theology were thriving well into the 1830s, when the will of the Earl of Bridgewater ensured that reputable scientists would seek out evidence for Christianity in the natural world – exerting themselves as dutifully as Archdeacon Paley a generation previously.[6] The famous *Bridgewater Treatises*, published between 1833 and 1837, aimed to reconcile religious and scientific truth. Scholarly clergymen and ordained academics occupied themselves with natural analogies between divine and worldly spheres. Their enemy was described by Christian Carl Josias von Bunsen, the Prussian ambassador in London, as the shallow "Trinity" of utilitarianism "in which Washington is the Father, Franklin the Son, Steam the Pneuma; and, further, Lafayette the

John, Robespierre the Paul, and Napoleon the Mahomet!"[7]

If large sections of the British intellectual community combined forces in upholding the old metaphyics, few came close to the achievements of Dr Prichard. In his own day a scientist of great breadth and much renown, he single-handedly charted the waters of the pre-Victorian human sciences. Philology, anthropology, mythology, Biblical criticism, the philosophy of the human mind, comparative anatomy, physiology, and practical medicine: Prichard mastered subjects so diverse that his learning may be called truly universal. In terms of output, diligence, and scholarship he was the paladin of all those who aimed to bolster a Christian science of man. While nowadays Prichard is regarded as "a leading student" of his field,[8] in a semantically less scrupulous age he was revered as "the founder of the English branch of the sciences of anthropology and ethnology".[9] From his M. D. dissertation in 1808 until his death, he strove to prove that the Scriptures gave the correct account of what he termed "the natural history of man".[10] Saint Augustine had deplored a lack of interest in man's moral nature; Prichard held that the same was true for man's "physical nature" as well.[11] His *Researches into the Physical History of Man* (1813) aimed to fill that gap. Just as the naturalist investigated the vegetable and animal realm, paying due tribute to the manifold forms extant in various geographical provinces, he argued that "human tribes" also had to be studied assiduously. From the 1830s he subsumed the particular thrust of his researches under the name "ethnology", which he conceived as a historical discipline that probed into the comparative development of human populations. When he introduced it in 1836, he defined it as a method to determine "as to Identity and Diversity of Species". Ethnology was not proudly presented as "a new science", it slipped in as a humble method, comprising "a survey of the different races of men, an investigation of their physical history, the ethnography, as it is termed, of every tribe of the human family".[12] It was only in the 1840s when Prichard perceived the need to push the image of his new discipline amongst members of the British Association for the Advancement of Science, that he made big words about ethnology, maintaining that it was a historical science which did for mankind what geology did for the rest of the natural realm.[13]

The *Researches* have an interesting publishing history: Prichard wrote and rewrote the same book again and again, it grew in extent, it grew in learning; but all editions, as well as the abbreviated spin-off, *The Natural History of Man* (1843), served the purpose of welcoming the prodigal son of scientific scepticism back into the house of faith. Prichard's world was open to scientific scrutiny, yet enlivened by philanthropic zeal, and preserved a harmonious balance between the physical and the moral spheres endowed by the Creator. He was a staunch monogenist, believing that all mankind was one and thence accountable to the same God, and that, therefore, nobody had the right to enslave or to kill another human being.[14] For the same reason he dismissed the Chain of Being: all human varieties holding the same station in Creation, there were no "lesser" humans to fill the gap between civilized white men and apes.[15] Prichard's aversion to the various tendencies which to him embodied the dangers of the age – materialist physiology, physical determinism, sensationalism, and the praise of reason at the expense of faith – crystallized in his fight against polygenism. As he feared more for religion than for his brain-child ethnology, his research programme, as one may call it, was intended to use science to prove religion as it was laid down in the Scriptures. In that respect he was following the dictates of evidential theology. At the same time, however, he felt that accomplishing this goal was not enough: in the end, Christianity hinged on faith – a sentiment which in his eyes could be traced in all peoples across the globe: this impression, in turn, inspired him to one of his most extraordinary ideas: as early as the 1830s he advocated the notion that comparative psychology was the ultimate goal of all ethnological endeavours.

Psychology seemed to provide a key to the inner secrets of the soul – the last refuge of the inborn knowledge (or the "inner light" as Prichard's Quaker parents would have called it) of the Deity. Seeing the world through Prichard's eyes and by the ardent glimmer of the inner light, we will encounter many analogical relations permeating his thought. Some of these he devised himself, others crept in, as it were, behind his back. Some were instances of the assumption, backed by natural theology, that nature was suffused by providential principles. Others arose from the fact that his scholarship followed a single overarching goal dictated by his pious morality.

Cultural, intellectual, and religious chaos dominated the world into which Prichard was born. With the French Revolution traditional social ties seemed to be dissolving. As industrialization gathered momentum, there were growing perceptions of class struggle, hence the great fear that the "French disease", the revolutionary spirit, might be contagious. The ideology of liberty was equated by many with a "materialism" whose influences made themselves felt in all areas of life. As the comfortable analogy between God the Father of Creation and the monarch as father of the nation broke up, the natural theology tradition was cast into doubt. And, if anything, the spirit of unease was growing. "The period 1815 to 1840", Dwight Culler has reminded us, "was a dark one in English history, with the economic collapse following the Napoleonic wars, the oppressiveness of the Tory reaction, the agitations surrounding the Catholic emancipation and the first Reform Bill, the hopes and fears of the Revolution of 1830, the Bristol riots and rick-burning, the fearful suffering of the poor".[16] Britons reacted in various ways to the challenges of the new disorder: some turned into political Radicals who believed that social change had to be reflected in political reform. Liberal utilitarian theory attempted to play down the influences of central government, stressing the ordering principles inherent to the operation of market mechanisms. Idealist conservatives strove to safeguard the old world, stressing the qualities of ancestral values which appeared all the more virtuous as their evocation was no longer disturbed by social reality. While these conservatives found consolation in the past, others commended a retreat into inner values. Instead of focusing on material gains, better living standards and political participation, a return to morality was recommended. Inward ethical nobility was extolled over superficial wealth and social status. German Romantic Idealism accompanied a new religious piety. In Britain, the Evangelical movement[17] set out to safeguard Christianity and morality.

Prichard, too, sympathized with Evangelicalism. He was deeply sceptical towards anything new: his inability to identify with reform revealed his deep conservatism, mitigated only by his philanthropical opposition to slavery. His monogenism reflected his desire to return to a paternalistic world order where all members were responsible to each other, the lower classes owing deference to their superiors, while these in turn had to provide for those in need. Even though he never spelt it out, this was the notion on which his concept of the relationship between the human varieties was modelled. He argued incessantly against polygenists and materialists of all shades and denominations. The species unity of mankind, guaranteeing the validity of Prichard's Christian outlook, could be proved only through intimate knowledge of all human varieties. Hence his intense preoccupation with ethnological investigations.

Ethnology and anthropology were the fields in which the new taste for theories of race expressed itself. To Prichard they appeared perhaps the greatest scientific blunder – indeed the greatest scientific sin – of his time: theories of race implied the notion of original diversity, that is, polygenism. If, by contrast, monogenism were true then there was no foundation for theories of race. But Prichard lived to see that this link was broken: lip-service was paid to notions of common ancestry, but nevertheless, race became a cardinal tenet of anthropological theorizing.[18] While this development reached its height after the breakthrough of Darwinism, it visibly gained ground before mid-century. An erstwhile representative of British restoration science, Prichard fell out with his times, increasingly believing that all his efforts had been in vain.

He lived through a transitional epoch. Born under the *ancien régime*, he passed his childhood during the era of the French Revolution, witnessing the turmoils of the Anglo-French wars and the subsequent rise of a new European order. Having been educated by those whose outlook had been formed during the eighteenth century, he found his views challenged by younger generations. His life straddled the old and the new. The overriding characteristic of the latter was, in his view, a tendency towards materialism, by which he understood not just materialism *à la française* but also British utilitarianism, which served as the philosophical legitimation for economic and colonial expansion. Opposing these views, he advocated a strict distinction between the realm of the soul and that of the body. This dualism referred to the analogous distinction between the realm of man and nature on the one hand, and the kingdom of God, on the other. The latter was supreme: in all his works Prichard buttressed the idea that men had the duty to heed the demands of the invisible moral part of their cosmos. That, too, was part of his notion of psychology.

During his lifetime he exerted great influence over his peers and those younger scholars who trod in his footsteps. While French, German and American ethnologists were split between monogenist and polygenist doctrines, Prichard's personal influence ensured that until the 1840s British ethnology was dominated by monogenism.[19] Of course, he did not so much guide as articulate the predominant sentiments of his age. If we look at beliefs across Europe we find that early nineteenth-century France polygenism was a product of *Idéologue* philosophy. It exerted some influence on German thinkers. In post-revolutionary Britain, by contrast, enmity towards French philosophy was great, hence it was not until the 1820s and 1830s that polygenist views became popular in Britain, mainly through the influence of a new generation of French scholars – historians and physiologists who had discarded the cultural universalism of their Enlightenment forebears.[20] Prichard perceived that, despite all his efforts, pockets of resistance to his ideas were developing. Shortly after his death, British ethnological opinion on the question of monogenesis was as divided as in other countries. If his attempts to hold on to what we have called a Christian science of man are characteristic of British social values at the beginning of the nineteenth century, the swift eclipse of his fame, which set in no sooner than he had died in 1848, illustrates the rapid changes society was going through at the time. It was only in the 1880s and 1890s when British ethnology was paying tribute to its forefathers, that Prichard's efforts were, once again, evoked. Although not many ethnologists professed to have learned from him, E. B. Tylor and his contemporaries continued asking the same questions Prichard had dealt with.

Attempting to shake materialism by its philistine lapels, Prichard was not so much a stone relic in the Victorian cabinet of antiquities as a prophet of a special kind: he had a vision of the old order. What this vision was about, how it exploited modern scientific insights, and where its most powerful enemies were located, form the subject of this book. Not a biography – the scarcity of personal information precluding such a venture[21] – the narrative sketches the landscape of Prichard's mind.[22] As he was the model of a bookish man, it will do him justice if we concentrate on the texts he read and on those he wrote – seventeen volumes and numerous articles.[23] He is often cited in modern scholarship by authors who do not appear to have wider knowledge of his full writings and intentions. Hopefully, this book will help to give Prichard his due. It will examine issues such as his famous "invention" of a disease called "moral insanity", his usage of psychology as anthropological category, his vindication of Hebrew as a God-given institution, his insistence that the history of languages was a key to the history of the human species, and the ways in which his ethnological research interest survived his own fame. Following up his theoretical allegiances and aversions, his sources and how he used them, we shall survey several fields of European theorizing between the 1750s and the late nineteenth century, evoking a world-view which contrasts starkly with the concerns of the present age. A central place will be given to the topic of racial theory. In the second half of the nineteenth century concepts of racial evolution and degeneration, and the dangers of racial mixture, were employed to account for the character of peoples and individuals alike. In conjunction with the notion of the "survival of the fittest" and widespread social paranoia, racial theories justified the extirpation of "bad stocks", furthering theories of degeneration. One of the key questions we shall address is how Prichard's concepts should be ranged within the history of racial theory and the history of anthropology: his explicit anti-racialism[24] distinguished him from the type of theorizing prevalent from the 1840s. Indeed, had his views of human nature survived, world history would have taken a very different course.

In the first chapter, Prichard's biography will be delineated as well as his role and situation as a doctor. One aspect of his medical practice was his expertise in insanity. He gained lasting fame as the "inventor" of a new nosological category, "moral insanity". The origins of this concept and its anthropological implications will be demonstrated in the second chapter. Having thus outlined Prichard's philosophy of the human mind we shall turn to his *magnum opus*, the *Researches*. The third chapter will explain his proofs of monogenesis, discussing concepts of analogy, animal hybridity, and the distribution of plants, animals and mankind across the globe. While this chapter is dedicated to probing into Prichard's theorizing of natural similarity, the fourth chapter will deal with his explanations of variety: to sustain monogenism he was obliged to establish why human populations looked different from each other. The fourth chapter will also tackle the question of whether Prichard's views changed from the first to the second and third editions of the *Researches*. As we shall see, his religious commitments ensured that his theories of man were remarkably consistent over the years. In the fifth chapter we shall examine his ethnology, addressing Prichard's views of human development as well as his attitude towards budding racial theories. Two central aspects of his ethnology will be mentioned separately, namely, his theories of philology and mythology which will be discussed in the last two chapters. This table of contents reflects to a certain extent the fields of Prichard's publishing activities. In line with early modern notions of philosophical hierarchy, we shall also, so to speak, ascend from the earth-bound field of medicine and physiology towards the purely mental sphere of religious mythologies, thus ending with a subject which was of deep concern to later generations of British ethnologists. Prichard was not given to contemplate beauty. Yet in one sense his mental cosmos was exceedingly well proportioned – it was a universe where everything grew out of an alliteration: monotheism and monogenesis.

Introduction

Notes

David Philip Miller, "Introduction". In *Visions of Empire. Voyages, Botany, and Representation of Nature*, ed. David Philip Miller, Peter Hanns Reill (Cambridge: Cambridge University Press, 1996), pp. 1-18, see p. 5.

For the rather extensive debate on the question to what extent science and colonialism were correlated, see: David Mackay, *In the Wake of Cook: Exploration, Science & Empire, 1780-1801* (London: Croom Helm, 1985); *idem*, "Agents of Empire: The Banksian Collectors and Evaluation of New Lands". In *Visions of Empire*, ed. David Philip Miller *et al.*, pp. 38-57. See also Simon Schaffer, "Visions of Empire: Afterword". In *ibid.*, pp. 335-52, see note 3 on p. 348.

Cf., e.g., Jeffrey Paul von Arx, *Progress and Pessimism. Religion, Politics, and History in Late Nineteenth Century Britain* (Cambridge, Mass.: Harvard University Press, 1985); Peter Allan Dale, *The Victorian Critic and the Idea of History* (Cambridge, Mass.: Harvard University Press, 1977).

W. F. Bynum, "The Great Chain of Being After Forty Years: An Appraisal". *History of Science* 13 (1975): 1-28.

Cf. John Hedley Brooke, *Science and Religion. Some Historical Perspectives* (Cambridge: Cambridge University Press, 1991); Pietro Corsi, *Science and Religion: Baden Powell and the Anglican Debate 1800-1860* (Cambridge: Cambridge University Press, 1988), chs 12 and 15. For secularization see Owen Chadwick, *The Secularization of the European Mind in the Nineteenth Century* (Cambridge: Cambridge University Press, 1975). According to Cannon, Turner, and Young, the relationship between science and religion became difficult not in the first but in the second half of the century. See Susan F. Cannon, "The Cambridge Network". In *idem, Science in Culture: The Early Victorian Period* (New York: Dawson and Science History Publications, 1978), pp. 29-71; Frank M. Turner, *Between Science and Religion: The Reaction to Scientific Naturalism in Late Victorian England* (New Haven, London: Yale University Press, 1974); *idem*, "The Victorian Conflict Between Science and Religion: A Professional Dimension". *Isis* 69 (1978): 356-76; Robert M. Young, *Darwin's Metaphor: Nature's Place in Victorian Culture* (Cambridge: Cambridge University Press, 1985). Yeo, by contrast, holds that the position of science was not uncontested. See Richard Yeo, *Defining Science: William Whewell, Natural Knowledge, and Public Debate in Early Victorian Britain* (Cambridge: Cambridge University Press, 1993).

6   For the Bridgewater Treatises, see Jonathan R. Topham, "Beyond the 'Common Context': The Production and Reading of the Bridgewater Treatises". *Isis* 89 (1998): 233-52.

7   *A Memoir of Baron Bunsen*, ed. Frances Bunsen, 2 vols (London: Longmans, Green, and Co, 1868), 1:390. The bulk of the *Memoir* consists of Bunsen's letters. For the prevalence of utilitarian doctrines in nineteenth-century science see Hans Aarsleff, *The Study of Language in England, 1780-1860* (Minneapolis: University of Minnesota Press, 1983 (1967)); Charles Coulston Gillispie, *Genesis and Geology. A Study in the Relations of Scientific Thought, Natural Theology, and Social Opinion in Great Britain, 1790-1850* (Cambridge, Mass.: Harvard University Press, 1969 (1951)), pp. 30-39.

8   Nancy Stepan, "Biology and Degeneration: Races and Proper Places". In *Degeneration. The Dark Side of Progress*, ed. J. Edward Chamberlin, Sander L. Gilman (New York: Columbia University Press, 1985), pp. 97-120, see p. 106.

9   See the entry for Prichard in *Encyclopaedia Britannica*, ed. Hugh Chisholm, 11. ed., 29 vols (Cambridge: Cambridge University Press, 1911), vol. 22. He himself employed both terms only from the 1830s. This is in line with Stagl's observation that the "*éthnos*-terms" came into French and English usage only from around 1820. See Justin Stagl, *A History of Curiosity. The Theory of Travel 1550-1800* (Chur: Harwood Academic Publishers, 1995), pp. 233-51.

10   In Prichard's understanding the term "man" designated the whole of mankind. In this book words like "mankind", "humanity", and "men" occur interchangeably and in accordance with Prichard's usage.

11   Prichard, *Researches into the Physical History of Mankind*, 3rd ed., 5 vols (London: Sherwood, Gilbert, Piper, 1836-47), 1: v. Prichard had derived the idea from Johann Friedrich Blumenbach. Cf. Nicholas Hudson, "From 'Nation' to 'Race': The Origin of Racial Classification in Eighteenth-Century Thought". *Eighteenth-Century Studies* 29 (1996): 247-64, p. 252. For the implications of natural history for the study of man see Christopher Fox, Roy Porter, Robert Wokler, eds., *Inventing Human Science. Eighteenth-Century Domains* (Berkeley: University of California Press, 1995); Jacques Roger, *Les sciences de la vie dans la pensée française du XVIIIe siècle* (Paris: Armand Colin, 1963); Robert Wokler, "From *l'homme physique* to *l'homme moral* and back: Towards a History of Enlightenment Anthropology". *History of the Human Sciences* 6 (1993): 121-38; P. B. Wood, "The Natural History of Man in the Scottish Enlightenment". *History of Science* 28 (1990): 89-123.

12   Prichard, *Researches*, 3rd ed., vol. 1, pp. 109-10.

13 *Idem*, "On the Relations of Ethnology to Other Branches of Knowledge" (Anniversary Address delivered at the Anniversary Meeting, 22. 6. 1847, of the Ethnological Society). *Journal of the Ethnological Society of London* 1 (1848): 301-29, p. 303. His emphasis on the historical side of ethnology notwithstanding, Prichard was not greatly interested in archaeological history. Besides, Jacques Boucher de Perthes's *Antiquités Celtiques et Antédiluvienne* appeared only in 1847 – too late for Prichard to engage with its central idea that there were human remains dating from before the Flood. Cf. Glyn Daniel, *The Origins and Growth of Archaeology* (Harmondsworth: Penguin, 1967), p. 59. Cf. also *idem, The Idea of Prehistory* (Harmondsworth: Penguin, 1964 (1962)).

14 For Prichard's views of slavery and colonialism see Chapter 5 below. For his rejection of capital punishment see Prichard, *A Treatise on Insanity, and Other Disorders Affecting the Mind* (London: Sherwood, 1835), p. 399.

15 This has been pointed out by William F. Bynum, "Time's Noblest Offspring: The Problem of Man in the British Natural Historical Sciences, 1800-1863" (Ph.D. diss., University of Cambridge, 1974), p. 70.

16 A. Dwight Culler, *The Victorian Mirror of History* (New Haven, London: Yale University Press, 1985), p. 78.

17 Whenever I refer to a particular wing of the Established Church, the word "Evangelical" will be spelt with a capital letter; when it refers to evangelical tendencies the term will be used like any other adjective.

18 See, e.g., "Physical History of Mankind". *Prospective Review* 3 (1847): 355-69, p. 357.

19 See John Burrow, *Evolution and Society. A Study in Victorian Social Theory* (Cambridge: Cambridge University Press, 1966), p. 124.

20 Cf. Chapter 6 below. Powerful American theories of racial inequality were to develop only from the 1830s.

21 I have been informed by Dr Neve that Mr John Crump has been planning for some years to publish a biography of Prichard, based upon unpublished manuscript material in his possession. My attempts to make contact with Mr Crump have been to no avail.

22 This is the first monograph dealing with Prichard. So far his thinking has been explained best by Bynum, "Time's Noblest Offspring", esp. pp. 74-117; George W. Stocking Jr, "From Chronology to Ethnology. James Cowles Prichard and British Anthropology. 1800-1850". Introduction to James Cowles Prichard, *Researches into the Physical History of Man*, 1813. Reprint, ed. George W. Stocking Jr (Chicago: University of Chicago Press, 1973), pp. ix-cx. Hereafter references to

the *Researches* will be made by quoting: *Researches*, number of edition, volume number. It should be noted, however, that in the 2nd and 3rd editions Prichard substituted "Mankind" for "Man".

23   Most of Prichard's publications will be discussed here, though not all of them. For further information, including a bibliography of Prichard's texts, see my "James C. Prichard's Views of Mankind. An Anthropologist Between the Enlightenment and the Victorian Age" (Ph.D. diss., University College London, 1996).

24   The earliest usage of the term "racialism", recorded in the *OED*, is from 1901. See *The Oxford English Dictionary*, ed. J. A. Simpson, E. S. C. Weiner, 2nd ed., 20 vols (Oxford: Clarendon Press, 1989), vol. 13. Strictly speaking, its use with reference to Prichard's times is anachronistic. In this book it is employed to denote a system of racial theories and in conformity with the definition given in Graham Richards, *"Race", Racism and Psychology. Towards a Reflexive History* (London: Routledge, 1997), p. xi.

1

The Life of James Cowles Prichard

In the eighteenth century Bristol was a thriving port, bustling with merchants and sailors of all nationalities. It counted among one of Britain's five biggest cities, contributed substantially to the national output of brass and iron, and was the British end of the Atlantic slave trade. After the turn of the century, however, Bristol's economy slowly but steadily declined. By 1800 the population had risen to 85 000, while its mercantile power was relatively stagnant.[1] Between 1800 and 1820 several riots broke out among the hunger-stricken paupers.[2] Bristol's merchants upheld their status on several fronts, fending off the demonstrations of the lower classes, trying to assert themselves against the landed aristocracy of the surrounding shires, and striving to keep up with fashionable London as well as the centres of erudition, Oxford and Cambridge. They consciously created what may be called a "public sphere", setting up clubs and learned societies, fostering the arts and sciences as a gentlemanly pursuit which united the bourgeois community across political and theological differences. By virtue of their scientific culture, the bourgeois citizenry of Bristol aligned themselves around common goals and a common identity. As Michael Neve has pointed out, "scientific culture in early nineteenth century Bristol was markedly non-utilitarian, and conservative".[3]

For a long time Bristol had been one of the strongholds of the Society of Friends. Economically promising, the city lured many a Quaker to settle down there. One of them was the merchant Thomas Prichard (1765-1843); his wife Mary, born Leys, was Welsh. Coming from Ross in Herefordshire, the Prichards moved to Bristol in 1793.[4] Thomas Prichard already had ties to the city: he owned shares in the iron business of the local Harford family.[5] From 1782 and well into the 1790s he was one of the subscribers to the Bristol Infirmary.[6] This subscription was part of the philanthropic duty he owed to God and his country. It was not his idea that his eldest son should spend almost thirty years of his life as a physician to the Infirmary.

Born on 11 February 1786, James Cowles was the eldest of four children.[7] (His middle name derived from the wife of his grandfather, Ann Cowles.) When he had become an ethnologist of renown, it was said that he had an "inbred" propensity for learning. His friend and colleague John Addington Symonds (1807-71) told the story of James, the little boy who, strolling around the colourful area of Bristol's harbour, liked "to talk with foreigners, who arrived at that port, in their own tongues. On one occasion he accosted a Greek sailor in Romaic, and the man was so delighted that he caught the boy-linguist in his arms and kissed him heartily".[8] If Prichard had a talent for languages, his education furthered the natural inclination. After the early death of his wife, Thomas Prichard retired from his business and, in 1800, moved his family back to Ross. Henceforth his children were taught solely by private tutors, the greatest emphasis being put on languages, namely, French, Latin and Greek.

Thomas Prichard intended James to follow him into the iron trade. He wanted his son to "retain the primitive simplicity & orthodoxy of genuine quakerism which he feared the study of medicine would contaminate".[9] But James objected to the plan, wishing to become a man of science instead. His father's protestations cannot have been too severe, for in 1802 James started on a string of medical apprenticeships. From September 1804 he attended medical lectures at a school attached to St Thomas's Hospital in London. In 1805 he entered the University of Edinburgh, taking his M. D. degree in 1808. For his dissertation subject he chose what was to become his life-long preoccupation: an investigation into the origin of the varieties of man.

To complete his education Prichard elected to spend some time at Cambridge and Oxford. These universities not being open to students of dissenting denominations, Prichard might have thought that they were well worth a mass: in 1808 he left the Quaker sect and embraced the Anglican faith. Subsequently he entered Trinity College, Cambridge, as a Gentleman Commoner – his father must have paid a substantial amount of money to enable him to assume such a privileged position. If the son, in turn, was to uphold many of the moral principles dearest to his father, including the doctrine of monogenesis,[10] this may have been due to a feeling of filial obligation.[11]

Judging from his doctoral dissertation and his contributions to the student society at Edinburgh Prichard must have been an ambitious youth. Yet ambition was only one driving motive. It was, perhaps, compounded by a life-long need to justify his desire for study. His relationship with Quakerism was surely of a difficult nature. His friend, the Quaker doctor Thomas Hodgkin (1798-

1866), later surmised that Prichard converted "on the grounds of conviction". Possibly it went with the wish to attend England's most prestigious universities. Predictably, Hodgkin "never learned ... the doctrinal points which occasioned his separation".[12] It is, in fact, quite likely that his Edinburgh training had spoiled Prichard for Quakerism. When the seventh edition of the *Encyclopaedia Britannica* appeared in 1830, a Bristol Quaker journal reviewed it very negatively, regretting most of all "that we perceive ... the peculiarities of what has been not inaptly termed 'Scotch Philosophy'".[13] This rift over the appreciation of Scottish philosophy may have been decisive: while Quakers tended to reject it, Prichard was greatly influenced by Thomas Reid, Dugald Stewart and other Scottish philosophers.

In some people's eyes the Enlightenment had become a scapegoat for all that went amiss in the nineteenth century, but Prichard's attitude towards it was more complex. On the one hand he adopted its approach to the natural history of man, on the other, and insofar as he identified the Enlightenment with materialism, he castigated it. Prichard entertained a Romantic disgust with Enlightenment materialism and shared in the Romantic sorrow over the loss of a unified world-view in which the one and the many, reason and feeling, God and science had been united.[14]

Edinburgh University

Until the 1840s most Bristol doctors learned their trade at Edinburgh University.[15] It not only admitted dissenters but was also cheaper than Oxbridge colleges. Edinburgh provided Prichard with a sound eighteenth-century education and an introduction to Continental learning. In the extramural schools in particular, the ideas of the great Göttingen anatomist Johann Friedrich Blumenbach (1752-1840) and of the leading French physiologists, Georges Cuvier (1769-1832), Etienne Geoffroy de Saint-Hilaire (1772-1844), and Jean-Baptiste de Lamarck (1744-1829) were being discussed soon after they had been published on the Continent.[16]

Student societies gave the young academics the opportunity to put their growing erudition to the test. Most prominent among medical students was the Royal Medical Society of Edinburgh, convening fortnightly on Saturday evenings.[17] Prichard was a member, and so were some of those young men who remained his friends in later life, including John Bishop Estlin (1785-1855), his future brother-in-law.[18] Here students could mix with University professors in an atmosphere more casual than that of the lecture

3

room. The Society awarded a "diploma" to all students who had presented a Question and a Dissertation. Estlin tried to rehabilitate necessitarianism.[19] Another student questioned Blumenbach's concept of a vital principle.[20] Prichard wrote, for a session in Spring 1807, some fifty pages on the varieties of the human species, presenting a short version of his later M. D. dissertation.[21]

Although Prichard did not generally refer to his former tutors by name, the influence of Dugald Stewart's moral philosophy is clearly discernible.[22] The common-sense philosophy of Thomas Reid and Stewart, with its concept of innate faculties, challenged Locke's model of the mind as a tabula rasa to be inscribed through the impressions a human being received after birth. Since Etienne de Condillac (1714-80) had appropriated Locke for a theory of sensationalism and Hume had used him to support scepticism, Locke's philosophy had become problematic.[23] Reid's and Stewart's innatism attempted to establish a counter-model against Hume's and Condillac's alleged materialism, one which supported the moral doctrines of Christianity and of natural theology, in particular.

Advocating "an inductive science of mind",[24] Stewart lectured on almost everything pertaining to what nowadays is called the moral and social sciences. Not least thanks to him, the philosophy of the human mind was considered the paramount and most noble subject of study a scholar could deal with. An echo of this opinion is found in Prichard's first book on the subject of mental alienation, where he stated that his discussion of insanity was "an inquiry which is of itself equally important in its relation to the philosophy of the human mind".[25]

Medicine at Edinburgh was, in Lisa Rosner's words, "a literary activity".[26] This fitted with Prichard's personal taste. He also had a predilection for languages. By the time he graduated from Edinburgh he had sound Latin, Greek, and French. It was not uncommon for students of medicine to learn German as well, which Prichard did between 1816 and 1819.[27] In subsequent years he also made himself familiar with Sanskrit, Hebrew, Arabic, and the Celtic languages.[28] Henry Alford, a student pupil at the Bristol Infirmary, observed him conversing with foreign patients in "French, German, and especially Welsh ... It was said that he had talked Hebrew with a Jew".[29]

While virtually all Professors at Edinburgh University subscribed to natural theology, it was understood that references to Providence and the Scriptures had to be avoided as far as possible. Scientific pursuits in Edinburgh were carried out according to what were depicted as Baconian and Newtonian principles, while it was taken for granted that the final principles of life were inscrutable to human

4

reason. As Prichard put it at the Royal Medical Society: if problems seemed to be insoluble they should not be referred to God but left "for the attempts of future inquirers".[30] It is easy to imagine that this was exactly the attitude his father had wanted to save him from when pressing his son to enter the iron trade. In later life James Prichard often complained about being accused of insufficient Scripturalism. The reviews of his books, however, do not bear out this impression. His complaints may have reflected his own scruples rather more than those of his peers. Prichard felt intimidated by the fact that medicine was reproached by some for giving rise to "scepticism and irreligion".[31] Though the times brought a steady stream of conversions from the Society of Friends, leaving the network of the Quaker sect was not an easy thing to do.

Quakerism

In the early nineteenth century the Quakers were split into two factions: there were the strict "Quietists" who trusted only the "light within" and lived in retreat from the business of the world. And there were the more open-minded "gay" Quakers. While relying on the word of the Bible, they were not averse to questioning its meaning to gain greater understanding: Biblical scholarship and even Biblical criticism were part and parcel of their spiritual life. As Evangelicalism gained ground it was embraced by many "gay" Quakers.[32] Although they might not have admitted it, they could agree on many theological matters with other religious dissenters. According to Elisabeth Isichei, "a Quaker evangelical felt himself closer to a non-Quaker evangelical than to a quietist from his own church".[33]

If Prichard discarded Quaker customs (known as their "peculiarity") such as addressing other people as "thou" and "thee", that did not thereby extinguish the Quaker light in himself. Aligning himself to the evangelical wing of the Anglican church, he retained the spiritual elements of the creed. The outward "peculiarity" of the Quakers was, so to speak, a matter of appearance only, comparable to bodily integuments such as hair and skin colour which – as we will see – Prichard was to discount as meaningful criteria for the classification of mankind. In that respect the Quaker and the evangelical traditions were at one. Both "spurned nominal Christianity that allegedly involved the outward forms without the inner experience confirming the presence of real Christian faith".[34] In a scientifically acceptable form, both the doctrine of original sin and the Quaker notion of the "inner light" were to permeate Prichard's anthropology as well as his notions of the human mind.

After a year at Trinity College, Cambridge, Prichard went to St John's College, Oxford. Not feeling comfortable there, he swiftly moved within Oxford to Trinity College where he took the gown of a Gentleman Commoner and stayed until 1810.[35] Finally, he returned to Bristol and set up in medical practice while sharing in another practice run by his colleague Dr King. On 28 February 1811 he married the sister of a friend from his Edinburgh days. Anna Maria Estlin was the daughter of the Unitarian minister John Prior Estlin and the sister of John Bishop Estlin, Prichard's friend, who established an Eye Dispensary in Bristol. Anna Maria was a good match, as the Estlins were one of Bristol's most prominent families. The couple were to have ten children, (three daughters and seven sons), of whom eight survived to adulthood.[36]

Prichard and his brother-in-law stood at opposite ends of the cultural-political outlook of the Bristol bourgeoisie. In the parliamentary polls Estlin voted regularly for the liberal representatives while Prichard preferred conservative candidates.[37] He inhabited a complex conceptual world. There was the religious sphere which was horizontally organized, all men being equal in the eyes of God; and there was the world of men which was vertically structured, consisting of hierarchies whose existence – as the French Revolution had proved – was vital for political coherence as well as the future of religion.[38] Due to the particular solidarity of the Bristol bourgeoisie, matters of politics rarely got in the way of good relations. This did not change in the early 1830s when Bristol was debating the Reform Bill. Prichard rejected the social and moral assumptions behind the Bill, adhering to an old-style society of "Christian patriarchy" which he felt to be "under threat from the bourgeois utilitarianism" that engineered the Poor Law reforms to which he objected as well. Commenting on the medical system established under its rules, he said in 1840, at the first meeting of the Bristol branch of the Provincial Medical Association:

> I am not called upon to consider the results of this proceeding in regard to the unfortunate beings committed to our care, or to contrast the liberality of former generations which made provision for the cure of souls and for the support of an apostolical church, by the patriarchal gift of tenths, with the sordid penury of the present age, which confides the infirm bodies of the poor to hands whose principal qualification for that trust is greediness to undertake what they cannot, on the conditions offered, faithfully perform.[39]

The subject gave Prichard the opportunity to lambast "a so-called utilitarian age whose scarcely disguised principle is to crush out of existence or drive out from the table of nature those who have not the strength and energy to scramble for their places".[40] This abhorrence of "utilitarianism" was characteristic of the older Prichard. In his youth, while he was anxiously building up his career, he had other matters on his mind.

In 1811 he became a physician to Saint Peter's Hospital, a combined poor house and lunatic asylum.[41] He remained in his position at the Hospital until 1832.[42] Early on he tried to become a physician to the Infirmary, yet his entry into the higher echelons of Bristol's tight-knit medical body was not easy.[43] The physicians to the Infirmary were elected by the subscribers. Prichard got in only at his third attempt, in 1816. Traditionally, hospital physicians would not receive any remuneration, yet their cooptation to prestigious institutions brought on a steady stream of well-off private patients. In 1813 he had brought out an extended version of his M. D. dissertation, *Researches into the Physical History of Man*. It was well received by the press, yet failed to procure him much support for his entry into the Infirmary. For that purpose it was vital to participate in municipal affairs, give lectures, become a member of the right clubs, know the right people. Prichard did what he could and finally succeeded.

Prichard's Medicine

Working for the Bristol Infirmary was prestigious, albeit not because of the *clientèle*. Well-to-do people relied on private medical services, hospitals were only for the poor. Like Saint Peter's, the Infirmary was overcrowded, two patients usually having to share one bed.[44] The regulations were strict, the treatment sometimes more feared than the disease, particularly so by those patients who were assigned to Dr Prichard: first of all, there was his predilection for bleeding. It drove one man to poetry:

> Dr. Prichard do appear.
> With his attendance & his care,
> He fills his patients full of sorrow
> – You must be bled to day & cupped tomorrow.[45]

Christian Carl Josias von Bunsen (1791-1860), the scholar, liberal theologian and Prussian diplomat in London, was very impressed by Prichard's learning when he met him in 1838 at a Welsh festival in Llanover, the Eisteddfod of the Cymreigyddion y Fenni (the Welsh Association of Abergavenny).[46] Feeling somewhat ill, Bunsen invited

Prichard to exert his medical expertise. The result was that, the next day, he felt "not up to any resolution, first owing to having taken Dr. P.'s prescription".[47] If the doctor had little compunction about administering rough treatments to mortal flesh, he did not restrict his care to his patients alone, applying the lancet to his own veins whenever he suffered from a severe headache.[48]

But there was another type of cure which appeared savage to some of his contemporaries.[49] Nicknamed by others the "Tomahawk practice", commonly known as trepanning, Prichard introduced it as a "peculiar mode of counter-irritation in all those forms of cerebral disease which are accompanied by coma, stupor, or diminished sensibility, excluding those which are attended with excitement". The doctor would make an incision into the scalp, fill the wound with peas and have it suppurate for a few weeks, or even months, in order to restore the balance of liquids to the vascular system of the brain.[50] The cure was certainly apt to remind every patient of his faculty of sensibility. Alford, the student pupil at the Infirmary, later remembered Prichard's medical approach as "heroic": "counter-irritation in every form he pushed to an extreme degree".[51]

Prichard's medical views were consciously conservative: in terms of medical theory he did not believe that there had been much progress since the age of Sydenham. In an address he delivered to the Provincial Medical and Surgical Association in 1835 he gave an overview of the history of medicine. Ostensibly historical, it was an enthusiastic manifesto against the fever theory of William Cullen (1710-90) and all versions of a doctrine of a *vis medicatrix* or a vital principle. Cullen's pathology, standard teaching at Edinburgh University, had threatened the end of dualism.[52] Since Prichard strongly believed in dualism he rejected the theories of the Edinburgh Professor of the Theory of Physic and those of his successors, including the rival "Brunonian" system of John Brown, that seemed, to him, to deny the dichotomy between body and mind. Humoralism, though "inadequate and conjectural", was a sounder basis of medical knowledge than these modern "speculations, which may be said to have divided between them, as votaries, the last generation of physicians", Prichard remarked in 1835.[53]

The doctor's admission as physician to the Infirmary was the main hurdle on his career path. When he was finally elected in 1816 he quickly established his reputation as a worthy member of Bristol's great and good. Among the many clubs he joined and the committees he sat on, one is particularly important. In 1822 the

Bristol Institution for the Advancement of Science was set up. It included the Philosophical and Literary Society whose occupations ranged from geology to philology, from the interpretation of engravings on ancient stones to deliberations about the advantages of literal translations of the Bible. Sometimes the Society invited controversial speakers, for example in 1827 the phrenologist Johann Caspar Spurzheim. On one memorable evening in 1825 the members of the Society assisted at the opening of an Egyptian mummy which the Chamberlain of the city had brought home from an excursion to Egypt.[54]

Prichard swiftly assumed a central position; by the 1830s he was, together with the Anglican clergyman and amateur geologist William Daniel Conybeare (1787-1857), a leading spirit in the Society. Conybeare was Prichard's friend, yet his antithesis in many respects: he was a Whig, Prichard was a Tory; Conybeare was short-tempered and "perfectly content laughing at his own jokes",[55] Prichard was shy and quiet. Yet the two got on well with each other, they could converse on aspects of Christian revelation and moral corruption. Prichard shared in Conybeare's views of geology, and when he published a book on Celtic languages he dedicated it to Conybeare. Other members of the Society were to include the Dean of Bristol the Revd Henry Beeke, the printer John M. Gutch, the German-born J. S. Miller who was the curator of the Institution, the eminent, albeit eccentric, surgeon Richard Smith, John Bishop Estlin, and the Revd Lant Carpenter as well as his son, the physician William Benjamin Carpenter. In 1827 the Institution had over 300 members.[56]

By the mid-twenties Prichard's reputation was established, the fact being sealed by his election into the Royal Society of London in 1827, following the publication, in 1826, of the second edition of his *opus vitae*, the *Researches into the Physical History of Mankind*. He had a crowded schedule. In addition to his private practice, and his obligations at Saint Peter's Hospital and the Infirmary, he gave medical lectures at the Infirmary and literary lectures at the Philosophical and Literary Society where he also held various posts. Between 1826 and 1828 he acted as a medical visitor to Gloucestershire madhouses. In 1829, the year of Catholic emancipation, he was one of the protagonists behind the plan to set up a college to offer "classical and scientific education" to religious dissenters.[57] Bristol College was hailed as another manifestation of that "progressive conservatism" that had already brought forward the Institution and a number of new churches.[58] The school thrived for a number of years, Prichard's sons attended it as well as Walter

9

Bagehot, its most illustrious pupil and Prichard's nephew on the Estlin side of the family.[59]

While Prichard was restlessly scurrying between private patients, hospitals, learned societies and attendance at church, he wrote one book after another. In 1819 he published a volume on Egyptian mythology, in 1822 one on madness, and in 1826 the second edition of his *Researches*. In 1829 he brought out a refutation of the vital principle and in 1831 the outcome of his researches on the origin of the Celtic language. He was a regular contributor to journals of medical and general interest, wrote articles for scientific dictionaries, published two more books on insanity (1835 and 1842), the five volumes of the third edition of the *Researches* (1836-47), and then their abridgement, *The Natural History of Man* (1843).

In the 1830s, Prichard's activities expanded further: he was Pro-Director of the Bristol Institution, a Vice-President of The Bristol Established Church Society and Book Association, and a member of the Bristol Auxiliary Temperance Society. He was involved in the attempt to set up a Statistical Society. In 1834 he co-founded the Bristol District Branch of the Provincial Medical and Surgical Association which had been set up two years previously. At the fourth meeting of the Association in 1835, Prichard was elected into the Council of the Association. In 1837 he was elected President of the Bristol Medical Library Society.[60] In 1837, 1838 and 1840 he was sitting on the governing board of Bristol College.[61] As if all that were not enough, he suggested, in 1840, the establishment of an independent medical school.[62] One organization in which he was most actively involved, was the British Association for the Advancement of Science, set up in 1831 on the example of a similar body in Germany.[63]

His financial position was never threatened, yet he had to work to support his growing family: "here I am fully engaged in my medical practice on which I am mainly dependent", he wrote when declining an invitation to come to London to see a tribesman of the African Mandingos about whom he had written many a page – surely he must have been keen to see a Mandingo at last! As he had a large family, however, "of course all other matters must be very subordinate".[64] What he referred to as his "scribbling habit which custom has rendered" the outlet "of an in-born propensity", was done in the early morning hours before his life as a doctor began.[65] It was common for a doctor to have a private practice and work at a hospital at the same time. Prichard followed both occupations until 1843 when he resigned from the Infirmary. His private practice was said to be "large".[66] In 1837 he bought by auction, for £1800, a spacious house, known as the Red Lodge, which he had been renting.[67] All in all, he was living comfortably, without, however, being well-off.

Personal Disposition

We must assume that the bulk of Prichard's correspondence has been lost. Since he did not leave any diaries or personal accounts it is difficult to reconstruct even the most rudimentary features of his personal life. A few characteristics, however, were so remarkable that his contemporaries did not fail to note them. Most prominently among them was his deep shyness: the older he grew, the quieter Prichard appeared.

In his youth, by contrast, he certainly was not the embodiment of humility and calmness. No contemporary evidence survives as to his attitudes towards the French Revolution and the subsequent descent into war; we know, however, that in 1815, as a 29 year-old, he enrolled as a volunteer to defend his country against Napoleon's impending invasion, confident that his riding practice had turned him into "a tolerable good Match for a Frenchman".[68] In those years Prichard was a member of the Wernerian Society. He had been elected at the suggestion of Robert Jameson (1774-1854), at the time the dominant naturalist in Edinburgh.[69] The Society supported the "Neptunist" theory of a universal Deluge, rejecting the rival claim of the "Vulcanists" who privileged fire as a geological agent. It was flattering for Prichard to be accepted in the midst of members as famous as the mineralogist Richard Kirwan and the biogeographer Robert Brown. The energy he could not spend fighting the French hordes was invested on behalf of Wernerian geology; a defence of Werner's theory, published in Thomas Thomson's *Annals of Philosophy*,[70] sparked a heated debate with an anonymous reader who was theologically even more orthodox than the Wernerians.[71]

In 1824 Prichard chaired a committee collecting £7000 to assist the Greeks in their war against the Turks that had broken out in 1822. The money was "expended in such articles as were judged best adapted to the wants of the Greeks", including printing-presses, with Greek and Roman types, a compass, surgical and mathematical instruments, as well as medicines (it seems that the Greeks were expected to defend themselves against "the ferocious tyranny of their barbaric oppressors" through superior scholarship).[72] Apart from his readiness to fight Napoleon, it was the only occasion on record when he supported an explicit political cause beyond the hustings. In both cases, however, he acted as a patriot and in unison with British sentiment.

In private company Prichard seemed to flourish. When he was about fifty years old an American visitor described him as "a short compact, close-made man, with bluish gray eyes, large and prominent features, and expression uncommonly mild, open, and benevolent". He appeared "cheerful, sociable, frank, easy and unpretending in his discourse and manners".[73] In public, however, he was rather ill at ease. When he addressed the Provincial Medical and Surgical Association in 1835, a contribution to the *Lancet* characterized his speech as "exceedingly long. Of the first portion, hardly an entire sentence crossed the table to the right or left".[74] This incidence was typical: Prichard was ardent of mind, and resolute in the pursuit of his medical duties, yet in person he was barely audible. His Bristol colleague, the doctor John Addington Symonds, described Prichard's voice as "rather weak and low, but very distinct in articulation. His manners and deportment ... were simple and unaffected; – and in general company he evidently spoke with effort or even reluctance, unless upon subjects of business or of scientific and literary interest".[75] Similar problems arose for his readers: "my manuscripts generally puzzle printers", Prichard confessed; and it was not easy for the public to follow the thread of his thoughts through the mass of details.[76]

When the British Association was looking for a president for the Bristol meeting in 1836 they contemplated Prichard and Conybeare. In the end Lord Lansdown was elected. The other two were given the position of vice-president, "Conybeare and Prichard being either too *excitable* or too tame", as John Phillips, the local secretary of the BAAS in Yorkshire, put it in a letter to William Vernon Harcourt, the vice-president of the Association.[77] But the influential Harcourt had already had the same thought: "I should have proposed Conybeare but do not think he would get decently through the dinners and Prichard is too quiet."[78] Much as his reticence was appreciated – "like all great men he was wonderfully humble", wrote the philologist Max Müller[79] – it was a hindrance for somebody wishing to become a man of consequence. At the same time, he did not fail to impress: "Dr P.", Bunsen wrote, "is an admirable man; his great work is beyond all my expectations. But nothing is worth as much as himself, his fine tone of mind, his admirable activity, and healthy system of employment".[80] Bunsen was in a position to judge: sent to London, in 1838, to promote the "protestant union" between Prussia and Britain, the politically liberal envoy counted illustrious contemporaries among his friends and associates, most of them being "Broad Churchman", like himself: the historians Thomas Arnold and

Connop Thirlwall, the natural philosopher William Whewell, the Cambridge classicist Julius Hare, the philologists F. A. Rosen, John Kemble and Benjamin Thorpe.[81] Bunsen, the foreigner, lived at the centre; compared to such a man Prichard spent his life in seclusion. Bunsen and Prichard's mutual esteem is indicative not just of shared values – an emphasis on the religious shaping of human history, the preoccupation with historical development revealed in the history of languages – but also of those many scholarly links which unified the erudite strata of various countries.

Given that Bristol was out of the way of national scientific debates, Prichard's reticent disposition had at least one advantage. He derived his knowledge from books. If he regretted living in a provincial town it was because it impeded his access to great libraries. A man like the physiologist William Benjamin Carpenter, by contrast, was desperate to partake in live debates. He felt, in Adrian Desmond's words, "hopelessly isolated in Bristol".[82] "Living as I do", Carpenter lamented, "so completely out of the way of knowing what is being done in Science, except through the ordinary Journals, I am always uncertain if I am really working to any advantage."[83]

Prichard was content in Bristol as long as he obtained the publications he required and which he solicited from booksellers in and beyond Britain as well as from generous benefactors who were happy to lend him what he needed. His library was deemed to be "excellent".[84] His bookishness had the side-effect that his knowledge of Continental learning was at least as great as that of British science – to the extent that he was accused of neglecting the achievements of British medicine.[85] Living with and surrounded by books, Henry Alford recalled, "he generally wore a large, loose overcoat, with roomy side-pockets, large enough to hold a quarto or small folio case-book; and he generally carried other books with him on the seat of his carriage".[86] Like Carpenter, Prichard was aware that he was living "out of the world, in association with almost none except patients and apothecaries".[87]

He tried, though without success, to get professorial status at the Bristol Institution.[88] He wanted to leave the medical profession, but the opportunity never presented itself. In 1842 he attempted to secure the Regius Professorship of History at Oxford, vacated at the recent death of Thomas Arnold. At the suggestion of his friend Conybeare and the renowned geologist William Buckland, he recommended himself in a letter to Prime Minister Robert Peel.[89] But the chair went to the rather insignificant classicist John Cramer: despite all his publications Prichard was not considered enough of a national scientific celebrity to deserve the gratification of a post at Oxford. Again, in 1845 he endeavoured to solicit a chair of linguistics at the Oxford Taylorian Institution. Seeking Buckland's support he wrote: "I have often read papers or lectures on ethnological subjects containing general views of philology, which have been well received by large audiences at the Bristol Institution and think I could lecture on philology ... well enough for the purposes of the new appointment."[90] But once more his hopes were dashed. Instead, he accepted the invitation to become a Commissioner on Lord Shaftesbury's Lunacy Commission, which was deemed "an honourable and comparatively lucrative appointment".[91] The latter factor was especially important as his last child had been born in 1831. There was still a family to support. In 1845 Prichard moved to London. He was said to loathe the new job which involved arduous travels across the country.[92] After three years of inspecting psychiatric institutions he caught a fever and died, reportedly of pericarditis, on 22 December 1848, aged 63.[93]

In his obituary address Symonds said that "although Dr. Prichard appears to have applied himself with zeal to the practice of his profession ... his favourite study evidently absorbed much of his attention".[94] Indeed, Prichard's national and international honours were bestowed upon him for his achievements in the field of ethnology. He was a corresponding member of many international institutions, in France, America, Russia and Italy,[95] as well as becoming a Fellow of the Royal Society. In 1835 he received an honorary doctorate from Oxford University; this was conferred upon him at the occasion of the Oxford meeting of the Provincial Medical and Surgical Association – "Dr. Prichard appeared rather pained than elated by all the flattering notice that fell upon him", Symonds remarked, "and was obviously relieved to turn attention from topics so personal to him by reading his Retrospective Address".[96]

Piety, hard work, intellectual profundity, and an aversion to flippancy prevented Prichard from keeping the company of illustrious artists and philosophical speculators. Among his correspondents were scholars like the American ethnologist Charles Pickering,[97] the Göttingen physiologist Rudolph Wagner,[98] and the German Johann Friedrich Blumenbach, whom Prichard was pleased to call his "venerable friend".[99] In addition to English dignitaries, Prichard met Alexander von Humboldt, as well as Christian Carl Josias von Bunsen ("a most enlightened and learned man") and the promising philologist Max Müller who came to London in 1846, having already established a reputation as an excellent philologist.[100]

Although some of these acquaintances – such as that between Prichard and Bunsen – entailed notions of mutual scholarly, if not spiritual, understanding, they were subject to the casualness dictated by the distance of character, social standing, and the geographical space between London and Bristol. Even among Prichard's fellow countrymen it is difficult to single out truly intimate friendships. Apart from Conybeare, the mathematician Francis Newman and his relatives, there were the Quakers Dr Thomas Hancock and Dr Thomas Hodgkin whom Prichard genuinely valued. He and Hodgkin exchanged skulls of their specimen collections, and collaborated in gathering ethnographic data and supporting philanthropic causes.[101] Despite his frequent appearance in chairing committees, he was personally a reserved man. His learning and his kindness were highly valued. Yet if we follow Symonds's characterization it is rather difficult to imagine Prichard at the centre of sophisticated intellectual conversation. For the doctor was not only shy, but also somewhat dry:

> Fancy and imagination were not prominent faculties in Dr. Prichard. He was never at a loss for a suitable illustration to enrich his style, which was affluent as well as terse and vigorous. Yet there was not that conscious enjoyment in the pursuit of analogies and likenesses, which belongs to men in whom the faculties I have adverted to are strongly marked. And, correspondently with this, I think that he had no decided aesthetical tendency, no such sensibility to the beautiful as would lead him to dwell on the enjoyments of poetry and the fine arts.[102]

There is, indeed, no sign that Prichard read contemporary literature or poetry, no sign that he contemplated beauty. Symonds's description of his style was kind: Prichard's sentences were rather cautious than terse. It is unlikely that he was well read when entering Edinburgh University. And subsequent years did not incite the desire to become a man of the world. His judgement was not informed by aesthetic opinions but by moral views. In conjunction with his much-praised benevolence, his indifference to many topics which engaged his times speaks of an underlying naïvety. He "has so much modesty, artlessness, and child-like simplicity about him", Hodgkin wrote, "that no one would be prepared to say, upon slight acquaintance, that he was anything more than an ordinary, sensible, well-disposed man".[103] Prichard's "provincial" abstention from social festivities gave him the opportunity to display the solid learning which became the basis of his reputation. And the stern morality of the man who dominated British ethnology in the early decades of the century ensured that the discipline rose as a thoroughly Protestant endeavour.

Notes

1 For the history of Bristol see the compilation of John Latimer, *The Annals of Bristol*, 3 vols, 1887-1902 (Bath: Kingsmead Reprints, 1970), vol. 3. For modern accounts see Graham Bush, *Bristol and its Municipal Government, 1820-1850* (Bristol: printed for the Record Society, 1976); Bryan Little, *The City and County of Bristol. A Study in Atlantic Civilisation* (London: Werner Laurie, 1954); Michael Neve, "Natural Philosophy, Medicine and the Culture of Science in Provincial England: The Case of Bristol, 1780-1850, and Bath, 1750-1820" (Ph.D. diss., University College London, 1984).

2 Cf. J. M. Harrison, "The Crowd of Bristol 1790-1835" (Ph.D. diss., University of Cambridge, 1983).

3 Neve, "Science in Provincial England", p. 128. The city had also a strong anti-slavery movement, see Peter Marshall, *Bristol and the Abolition of Slavery* (Bristol: printed for the Historical Association, 1973).

4 Richard Smith, "Manuscript Memoirs". MS. 35893 (36) k. i., Bristol Public Record Office, pp. 504-5. Unless otherwise stated all citations refer to the same volume. Smith was a senior colleague of Prichard and not a little eccentric. As if possessed by a Hegelian desire of acquiring power over people by knowing them, he collected newspaper clippings, letters, and all kinds of information concerning Bristol's medical establishment. In Prichard's case he even urged J. B. Cross, a former teacher of Greek in Thomas Prichard's household, to provide him with some information on Prichard's *vita*. See Cross's reply from 13 July 1831 in Smith, "Manuscript Memoirs", p. 504.

5 Isabel Southall, *Memorials of the Prichards of Almeley and Their Descendants* (Birmingham, 1901), p. 39.

6 "A List of Subscribers and Donations to Bristol Infirmary 1761-1805". MS. 35893 (21), Bristol Public Record Office. Thomas Prichard figures as a subscriber almost without interruption from 1782 to 1795.

7 For Prichard's biography see the details in my forthcoming entry in the *New DNB*, as well as Richard Cull, "Short Biographical Notice of the Author". In Prichard, *The Natural History of Man*, 4th edn, 2 vols, ed. Edwin Norris (London: Baillière, 1855), vol. 1, pp. xxi-xxiv; Thomas Hodgkin, "Biographical Notice of Dr. Prichard". *British Foreign and Medical Review* 27 (1849): 550-59; Denis Leigh, "James Cowles Prichard, M. D., 1786-1848". *Proceedings of the Royal Society*

of Medicine 48 (1955): 586-90; Neve, "Science in Provincial
England"; Herbert Odom, "Prichard, James Cowles". In *Dictionary
of Scientific Biography*, ed. Charles Coulston Gillispie, 14 vols (New
York: Charles Scribner's Sons, 1970-76), 11: 136-38; George W.
Stocking Jr, "From Chronology to Ethnology"; John Addington
Symonds, *Some Account of the Life, Writings, and Character of the
Late James Cowles Prichard* (Bristol: Evans & Abbott, 1849); D.
Hack Tuke, *Prichard and Symonds in Especial Relation to Mental
Science with Chapters on Moral Insanity* (London: Churchill, 1891),
pp. 65-100. All of these accounts are based mainly on Richard
Smith's "Manuscript Memoirs" and Southall's *Memorials*.
Symonds, *Some Account*, p. 7. Romaic is the vernacular language of
modern Greece.
Smith, "Manuscript Memoirs", p. 504.
Thomas Hodgkin, "Obituary of Dr. Prichard". *Journal of the
Ethnological Society of London* 2 (1848-50): 182-207, esp. p. 186.
Indeed, a contemporary explained Prichard's adherence to
monogenism as a duty owed to his father. See Hodgkin, "Obituary
of Dr. Prichard", p. 186.
Hodgkin, "Biographical Notice", p. 553.
The Friends' Monthly Magazine 1, no. XII, tenth month (1831): 704-9,
p. 704.
On the spirit of materialism and the Romantic reaction see Robert
E. Schofield, *Mechanism and Materialism: British Natural Philosophy
in an Age of Reason* (Princeton: Princeton University Press, 1970);
Andrew Cunningham, Nicholas Jardine, eds, *Romanticism and the
Sciences* (Cambridge: Cambridge University Press, 1990). For the
impact of Idealist philosophy on transcendental anatomy see Philip
F. Rehbock, *The Philosophical Naturalists. Themes in Early
Nineteenth-Century British Biology* (Madison: The University of
Wisconsin Press, 1983).
Neve, "Science in Provincial England", p. 268.
For Edinburgh University and the extramural schools see L. S.
Jacyna, *Philosophic Whigs. Medicine, Science and Citizenship in
Edinburgh, 1789-1848* (London, New York: Routledge, 1994);
Christopher Lawrence, "The Edinburgh Medical School and the
End of the 'Old Thing' 1790-1830". *History of Universities* 7 (1988):
259-86. For its politics see also Jack B. Morrell, "Professors Robison
and Playfair, and the Theophobia Gallica: Natural Philosophy,
Religion and Politics in Edinburgh, 1789-1815". *Notes and Records
of the Royal Society of London* 26 (1971): 43-63. For its medical
faculty see Lisa Rosner, *Medical Education in the Age of Improvement.*

Edinburgh Students and Apprentices, 1760-1826 (Edinburgh: Edinburgh University Press, 1991). For the Royal Infirmary of Edinburgh see Guenter B. Risse, *Hospital Life in Enlightenment Scotland* (Cambridge: Cambridge University Press, 1986). For medical theory at Edinburgh see Michael Barfoot, "James Gregory (1753-1821) and Scottish Scientific Metaphysics. 1750-1800" (Ph.D. diss., University of Edinburgh, 1983); Christopher John Lawrence, "Medicine as Culture: Edinburgh and the Scottish Enlightenment" (Ph.D. diss., University College London, 1984); Richard Olson, *Scottish Philosophy and British Physics 1750-1880. A Study in the Foundations of the Victorian Scientific Style* (Princeton: Princeton University Press, 1975).

17 Rosner, *Medical Education*, pp. 119-28.

18 "Obituary of John Bishop Estlin". *Bristol Mirror*, 16 June 1855.

19 John B. Estlin, "On Philosophical Necessity". In "Records of the Royal Medical Society of Edinburgh" 57 (1807-08): 387-418, Archives of the Royal Medical Society of Edinburgh.

20 J. Thatcher, "What is the Most Plausible Theory of Generation?" In *ibid.* 56 (1806-07): 250-65.

21 Prichard, "Of the Varieties of the Human Race". In *ibid.*, 58 (1807-8): 87-134.

22 He attended Stewart's course on Moral Philosophy, see the Matriculation Indexes. MS. Da 35, Edinburgh University Library, Special Collections. Prichard referred to Stewart in his *Researches*, 1st ed., p. ii.

23 This subject will be discussed in Chapter 2.

24 Biancamaria Fontana, *Rethinking the Politics of Commercial Society: the Edinburgh Review 1802-1832* (Cambridge: Cambridge University Press, 1985), p. 84.

25 Prichard, *A Treatise on Diseases of the Nervous System, Part the First: Comprising Convulsive and Maniacal Affections* (London: Thomas and George Underwood, 1822), p. 8.

26 Rosner, *Medical Education*, p. 121.

27 To practice his skills he published a translation, in collaboration with his medical teacher William Tothill, of Johannes von Müller, *An Universal History in Twenty-Four Books*, 3 vols (London: Longman, Hurt, Rees, Orme, and Brown, 1818). For the collaboration with Tothill see Symonds, *Some Account*, p. 46. The *Universal History* was reprinted in 1834 and again in 1840.

28 Cull, "Short Biographical Notice", p. xxiii. It is doubtful, however, whether he had fluent German: when corresponding with Rudolph Wagner, the Göttingen editor of his *Researches*, he wrote in French.

See Prichard's letter to Rudolph Wagner, 30 April 1841. MS. R.
Wagner 6, Nachlaß Rudolph Wagner, Göttinger
Universitätsbibliothek, Manuskriptabteilung.

29 Henry Alford, "The Bristol Infirmary in My Student Days, 1822-
1828". *Bristol Medico-Chirurgical Journal* 8 (1890): 165-91, p. 176.

30 Prichard, "Of the Varieties of the Human Race", p. 89.

31 Prichard, "An Address, Delivered at the Third Anniversary Meeting
of the Provincial Medical and Surgical Association, July 23rd, 1835".
The Transactions of the Provincial Medical and Surgical Association, 4
(1836), 1-54, p. 53. The text was also printed separately (Worcester:
Tymbs and Deighton, 1835).

32 For analyses of evangelicalism see Ian Bradley, *The Call to Seriousness:
the Evangelical Impact on the Victorians* (London: Cape, 1976); Boyd
Hilton, *The Age of Atonement. The Influence of Evangelicalism on
Social and Economic Thought, 1785-1865*, 2d ed. (Oxford: Oxford
University Press, 1991 (1988)).

33 This account of the Quakers follows Elisabeth Isichei, *Victorian
Quakers* (London: Oxford University Press, 1970), ch. 1, quotation
from p. 11. See also B. W. Young, *Religion and Enlightenment in
Eighteenth-Century England. Theological Debate from Locke to Burke*
(Oxford: Clarendon Press, 1998), p. 61; Arthur Raistrick, *Quakers in
Science and Industry* (London: Bannisdale Press, 1950).

34 Frank M. Turner, "The Crisis of Faith and the Faith that was Lost".
In *idem, Contesting Cultural Authority. Essays in Victorian Intellectual
Life* (Cambridge: Cambridge University Press, 1993), pp. 73-100,
quotation from p. 78.

35 Unfortunately we do not know anything about Prichard's stay at
either of these universities.

36 There being hardly any information on Prichard's private life, we do
not know anything about his wife. The fate of his children is equally
obscure. The oldest son, James Cowles, became a minister (he died
in 1848). Among the others were: another minister (Constantine
Estlin, born 1820), a post-master at Merton College, Oxford (Albert
Hermann, born 1831), a soldier and author on India (Iltutus
Thomas, born 1825), and a son called Theodore who committed
suicide (cf. Neve, "Science in Provincial England", p. 334).
Prichard's third son, Augustin (born 1818), took over his father's
practice in the 1840s.

37 Prichard voted in 1812, 1832, 1837, and 1841. In 1830 and 1835
he did not participate in the Bristol polls. See *The Bristol Poll, being
a List of the Householders, Freeholders, and Freemen, who voted at the
General Election for Members to Serve in Parliament, for the City and*

County of Bristol, published in Bristol following the general elections of 1812, 1820, 1830, 1832, 1835, 1837, 1841, by three different publishers: J. Mills, Philip Rose, J. Wansbrough.

38 The conservative bent of Anglicanism has been emphasized, e.g., by Turner, "Cultural Apostasy and the Foundations of Victorian Intellectual Life". In *idem, Contesting Cultural Authority,* pp. 38-72, esp. p. 46.

39 See Richard Smith, "Manuscript Memoirs", p. 622. Quoted in Neve, "Science in Provincial England", p. 289. In 1832 Prichard voted against the supporters of the Reform Bill; see *The Bristol Poll* (Bristol: J. Wansbrough, 1833).

40 *Ibid.* For the debate on the Poor Laws see J. R. Poynter, *Society and Pauperism. English Ideas on Poor Relief, 1795-1834* (London: Routledge, 1969).

41 Prichard, *A History of the Epidemic Fever, Which Prevailed in Bristol, During the Years 1817, 1818, and 1819; Founded on Reports of St. Peter's Hospital and the Bristol Infirmary* (London: John and Arthur Arch, 1820), p. 88. On 21 November 1817 Prichard published an open letter in *Felix Farley's Bristol Journal,* warning of the epidemic. His letter was discounted as irresponsible scare-mongering by James Johnson, the Deputy-Governor of St Peter's Hospital. Cf. the newspaper-clippings in Smith, "Manuscript Memoirs", p. 538.

42 His resignation took effect in July 1832. See *ibid.,* p. 540.

43 For the Infirmary see Alford, "The Bristol Infirmary"; Munro Smith, *A History of the Bristol Royal Infirmary* (Bristol: J. W. Arrowsmith, 1917). For Bristol medicine see also Neve, "Orthodoxy and Fringe: Medicine in Late Georgian Bristol". In *Medical Fringe and Medical Orthodoxy 1750-1850,* ed. W. F. Bynum, Roy Porter (London: Croom Helm, 1987), pp. 40-55.

44 Smith, *The Bristol Royal Infirmary,* p. 198.

45 Smith, "Manuscript Memoirs", p. 512.

46 *Memoir of Baron Bunsen,* 1: 472.

47 *Ibid.,* 1: 478.

48 See D. Hack Tuke's entry on Prichard in *Dictionary of National Biography,* ed. Leslie Stephen, Sidney Lee, 63 vols (London: Smith, Elder & Co., 1885-1900), vol. 46.

49 See Prichard's rejoinder to the allegation of unnecessary cruelty: "A Clinical Lecture Delivered to the Pupils of the Bristol Infirmary". *London Medical Gazette* n.s., 1 (1840-41): 8-13, p. 12.

50 "Abstract of the Proceedings of the Medical Section of the Meeting of the British Association for the Advancement of Science held at Bristol, in August, 1836". *British and Foreign Medical Review* 2

(1836): 594-601, p. 596.

51 Alford, "The Bristol Infirmary", p. 177.

52 Lawrence, "Medicine as Culture", p. 429.

53 Prichard, "An Address, Delivered at the Third Anniversary Meeting of the Provincial Medical and Surgical Association, July 23d 1835", p. 3. His admiration for Blumenbach was not diminished by the latter's adherence to vitalism.

54 See the first entry of "Abstracts of Papers, & c Read Before the Philosophical & Literary Society Annexed to the Bristol Institution. Beginning with the Paper Read at the Evening Meeting on 6th January 1825". Compiled by the Philosophical and Literary Society. MS. B 12361, Bristol Central Library; see also Richard Smith, "Manuscript Memoirs", pp. 644-46. For a more detailed account of the event see Chapter 8, below.

55 According to Nicolaas Rupke, *The Great Chain of History. William Buckland and the English School of Geology (1814-1849)* (Oxford: Clarendon Press, 1983), p. 10.

56 Bristol Institution, *Proceedings of the Annual Meeting, Held February 8, 1827* (Bristol: J. Mills, 1827), pp. 5-8. Coleridge was made an honorary member in 1823 but did not appear to have any interest in events at the Society.

57 *Prospectus of a College for Classical and Scientific Education, to be Established in or near the City of Bristol,* s.l., s.d. MS. B 23363, Bristol Central Library.

58 Quoted from Neve, "Science in Provincial England", p. 200.

59 The American president Woodrow Wilson is said to have referred Bagehot's views of society to Prichard's teachings; see Nancy Stepan, "Biology and Degeneration: Races and Proper Places", p. 186.

60 Smith, "Manuscript Memoirs", pp. 520, 624, 626.

61 See the "List of the Council and Shareholders of the Bristol College". *Ibid.*, pp. 674, 678; the list covers only the period 1837-1840 from 1837 to 1839 Prichard sat on the College's council.

62 Neve, "Science in Provincial England", p. 204.

63 Its model was the Gesellschaft Deutscher Naturforscher und Ärzte. See Jack B. Morrell, Arnold Thackray, *Gentlemen of Science. Early Years of the British Association for the Advancement of Science* (Oxford: Clarendon Press, 1981), p. 44.

64 Letter to Washington, August 1838, Prichard Papers, Royal Geographical Society.

65 Letter to Thomas Hodgkin, 23 June 1838. Mss. Brit. Emp, S.18, press mark C. 122/51, Hodgkin Papers, Rhodes House Oxford.

66 Symonds, *Some Account*, p. 8.

67   See the contract. MS. 5535 (50), Bristol Public Record Office.

68   See Prichard's letter to John Rose Hale, 6 April 1815. MS. 15385
     (f.3), National Library, Edinburgh.

69   See the entry for 13 March 1813 of the "Wernerian Society
     Minutes". Vol. 1, Edinburgh, 1808. MS. Dc. 2.55-56, Edinburgh
     University Library. As happened so often, Prichard's name was taken
     down as "Pritchard". By 1835 he was no longer a member. See *ibid.*,
     vol. 2 (1830).

70   Prichard, "Remarks on the Older Floetz Strata of England". *Annals
     of Philosophy* 6 (1815): 20-26.

71   F. E...s [sic], Andrew Horn, Prichard, "On the Cosmogony of
     Moses". *The Philosophical Magazine* 46 (1815): 285-92; 47 (1816):
     9-11, 110-17, 241-43, 258-63, 339-44, 346-48, 431-34; 48 (1816):
     18-22, 111-17, 201, 276-78, 300. For the Wernerian outlook see
     Roy Porter, *The Making of Geology. Earth Science in Britain 1660-
     1815* (Cambridge: Cambridge University Press, 1977), p. 154.

72   See the newspaper clipping in Smith, "Manuscript Memoirs",
     p. 572.

73   Southall, *Memorials*, p. 43.

74   "Meeting of the Provincial Medical Association, 3. Anniversary
     Meeting, Oxford, July 23, 1835". *Lancet*, Pt. 2 (1834-35): 553.

75   Symonds, *Some Account*, p. 50.

76   Letter to Washington, 18 April 1839, Prichard Papers, Royal
     Geographical Society.

77   See his letter to William Vernon Harcourt, the vice-president of the
     BAAS, 5 August 1836. In *Gentlemen of Science. Early Correspondence
     of the British Association for the Advancement of Science*, ed. Jack
     Morrell, Arnold Thackray (London: Royal Historical Society, 1984),
     p. 234 (original emphasis).

78   See Harcourt's letter to James David Forbes, 1 October 1835. In
     Early Correspondence, p. 219.

79   Max Müller, *My Autobiography. A Fragment* (London: Longmans *et
     al.*, 1901), p. 205.

80   *Memoir of Baron Bunsen*, 1: 478.

81   Robert Preyer, "Bunsen and the Anglo-American Literary
     Community in Rome". In *Der gelehrte Diplomat. Zum Wirken
     Christian Carl Josias Bunsens*, ed. Erich Geldbach (Leiden: E. J. Brill,
     1980), pp. 35-44.

82   Adrian Desmond, *Archetypes and Ancestors. Palaeontology in Victorian
     London 1850-1875* (London: Blond and Briggs, 1982), p. 16.

83   Letter of W. B. Carpenter to R. Owen, 23 September 1842. Cited in
     Desmond, *Archetypes and Ancestors*, p. 16.

84 *Memoir of Baron Bunsen*, 1: 477.
85 "Prichard's Retrospect Address". *Transactions of the Provincial Medical and Surgical Association* 4 (1837): 159-60.
86 Alford, "The Bristol Infirmary", p. 176.
87 See Prichard's letter to Thomas Hodgkin, 23 June 1838.
88 Neve, "Science in Provincial England", p. 204.
89 See Buckland's letter to Whewell, 22 July 1842. Cited in Rupke, *The Great Chain of History*, p. 202. See also Prichard's letter to Peel, December 1842. MS. 40512. f. 93, Peel Papers, vol. 3411, British Library, Manuscript Dept.
90 Prichard's letter to Buckland, 8 March 1845. MS. BU. 241 111, Royal Society of London. Bunsen, too, believed that Prichard would be the right choice for a "linguistic professorship of a comparative ethnographical character". See *Memoir of Baron Bunsen*, 2: 105. These plans, however, came to nothing.
91 Symonds, *Some Account*, p. 9. Nicholas Hervey, "The Lunacy Commission 1845-60, with Special Reference to the Implementation of Policy in Kent and Surrey" (Ph.D. diss., Bristol University, 1987). References to Prichard are on pp. 95, 109, 142, 146-47. According to Hodgkin, "Biographical Notice", p. 559, Prichard earned £1800 per year. Bunsen believed that his personal intervention had secured Prichard the position. See *Memoir of Baron Bunsen*, 2: 33.
92 Hervey, "The Lunacy Commission", p. 146.
93 Cull, "Short Biographical Notice", p. xxiv.
94 *Ibid.*, p. xxiii.
95 MS. 16082, Bristol Public Record Office.
96 Symonds, *Some Account*, pp. 10-11.
97 See Prichard's letter to Washington, 3 April 1840, Prichard Papers, Royal Geographical Society.
98 Wagner published a translation of the third edition of Prichard's *Researches*. The project was conceived unbeknownst to Prichard who was elated when he learned about it, see his letter to Wagner, 30 April 1841.
99 See Prichard's letter to Washington, 23 May 1840, Prichard Papers, Royal Geographical Society.
100 *Ibid.*, Prichard's letter to Washington, 3 April 1840.
101 Amalie M. Kass, Edward H. Kass, *Perfecting the World. The Life and Times of Dr. Thomas Hodgkin 1798-1866* (Boston: Harcourt Brace Jovanovich, 1988), p. 260.
102 Symonds, *Some Account*, p. 48.
103 Hodgkin, "Biographical Notice", p. 558.

2

Moral Insanity:
A Medical Theory of the Corruption of Human Nature

Although the term "anthropology" derives from antiquity, it was only in the latter half of the eighteenth century that it came into common usage. Immanuel Kant (1724-1804), Ernst Platner (1744-1818), a doctor of philosophy as well as medicine, and other Germans employed it to refer to combined research into the body, the mind, and their interrelations.[1] Prichard's Edinburgh education had familiarized him with a similar approach towards the phenomena of mind and body, although it was not until the 1830s that he adopted Continental terminology, talking about matters "anthropological" and "ethnological".

Prichard's medical occupations and his interest in the natural history of mankind mutually informed each other so that his deliberations on the workings of the mind went hand in hand with his anthropological ideas. In this chapter we shall examine to what extent he, in his capacity as a "mad-doctor", considered a certain kind of insanity as forming part of what may be called the anthropological condition, and how far his understanding of this condition depended on religious beliefs. His was an attempt to conceptualize madness, its physical manifestations, its material and moral causes, without compromising those parts of the human mind that, in his view, belonged to the realm of the immaterial soul rather than to the sphere of base corporality. The role of the brain in madness stood at the centre of Prichard's deliberations: while he was convinced that madness had something to do with the conformation of the brain, he yet repudiated all those theories which overemphasized its role at the expense of the immaterial or transcendental which Prichard regarded as a reality in its own right. He turned from a steadfast follower of the Lockean definition of mental derangement with its emphasis on human rationality into a philosopher attempting to account for feelings of existential alienation and despair.[2] In the following pages we shall probe the strategies he chose to support his changing opinions between the 1820s and the 1830s. Prichard's mature theories of madness drew on three different approaches: first, the writings of the doctor Thomas Hancock who dealt with the notion of human instincts; second, the doctrines by France's most famous alienists, Philippe Pinel and J. E. D. Esquirol; and third, German notions of madness, in particular those of the so-called somatists. But before these issues can be discussed, we must juxtapose Prichard's early notions of madness against his 1830s concept of "moral insanity" which was to gain him lasting fame.

The Limits of Locke's Rational "Delusion": Diseases of the Passions

In Britain in the second half of the eighteenth century, insanity was widely explained within the Lockean philosophical framework of enlightened rationality: delusions or illusions led human reason into error.[3] By the beginning of the nineteenth century, in the wake of the French Revolution and in the midst of the transformations which the industrial revolution was bringing about, new theories of insanity emerged. First developed on the Continent, they soon made their way to Britain. Prichard was one of those who attempted to rechart the traditional understanding of madness. This appeared necessary to him because his observations of mental unsoundness seemed incompatible with older nosological descriptions. Madness had become as unfathomable as the epoch itself appeared to many.

Increasingly, cases of insanity came to attention in which patients did not seem to dwell in some delusive state. Rather they displayed deep sullenness, unmitigated fury, or utter shamelessness, a propensity to theft, or pyromania, seemingly without either purpose or motivation. One of the constructs used to explain the evidence was Prichard's new concept of moral insanity. On the surface it accounted for a changed perception of insanity; on a deeper level, however, moral insanity was expressive of Prichard's religious views as well as his ideas about the human constitution, and it was his response to the problems inherent in the rise of capitalist society.

Moral insanity referred to a derangement of those mental faculties which presided over man's emotive framework as well as his moral faculty. Prichard first put the notion forward in 1833, in an article in *The Cyclopaedia of Practical Medicine*.[4] In his *Treatise on Insanity*, a survey published in 1835 and dedicated to Esquirol whom he had visited in 1831 at his hospital at Ivry near Paris, he gave an account of the state of medical thinking on madness, inscribing moral insanity into nosology and embedding the doctrine in his medical philosophy.[5] As a doctor to St Peter's Hospital, part of which served as lunatic asylum, Prichard had had ample opportunity to observe the workings of defective minds. In elaborating the concept, he presented a number of case studies, some of which he had solicited from other doctors, to back up his theory. One of these was the case of "a gentleman", provided by his Bristol colleague, John Addington Symonds: "in his social relations he had become fickle, suspicious, and irascible; he was reckless in his expenditure, and uncertain in his projects, while his general behaviour was such as to impress almost every one who came in contact with him". But, Symonds reported, there was no "evidence that he entertained any belief in things morally or physically impossible, or in opposition to the general opinion of mankind". The gentleman

> had suffered a severe concussion of the brain, and since his recovery had conducted himself more extravagantly than ever. He advertised for sale property which he knew to be entailed; after a little increase of income by the death of a near relative, he commenced great alterations in his residence, and before they were finished suddenly left his family, together with a large establishment, under the care of a youth, his son, who was provided with no other means of supplying the wants of the household than a power of attorney for collecting rents.

The man had inflicted "so great injury" to the property of his family "that it became a very desirable object to enforce some restraint upon his actions".[6] Communications like this seemed to Prichard to warrant the name and theory of moral insanity.

Prichard defined it as a form of "madness consisting in a morbid perversion of the natural feelings, affections, inclinations, temper, habits, moral dispositions, and natural impulses, without any remarkable disorder or defect of the intellect or knowing and reasoning faculties, and particularly without any insane illusion or hallucination". People suffering from this mental disorder displayed, he wrote, "eccentricity of conduct, singular and absurd habits" combined with "a wayward and intractable temper, with a decay of social affections, an aversion to the nearest relatives and friends formerly beloved, – in short, with a change in the moral character of the individual".[7] It could best be diagnosed by those who knew the afflicted well and were hence able to note that they, literally, no longer were quite themselves. In pinpointing actions that were out of character as the main indication of mental illness Prichard was treading on rather new ground. The structure of his thinking on moral insanity was highly complicated and of a lengthy evolution. It must be explained stage by stage. For during its development

Prichard had encountered several medical and physiological theories, and although, in some cases, he was hostile to the underlying philosophies he was able to bend them to his own purposes.

Neither the sources of the concept, nor its social and philosophical implications have been adequately described. It has been pointed out that Paris alienists, namely Philippe Pinel (1746-1826) and Jean Etienne Dominique Esquirol (1772-1840), inspired Prichard, and that his thinking was grounded in Scottish Enlightenment philosophy.[8] These explanations, however, do not suffice: they reiterate what Prichard himself acknowledged.[9] But his own testimony as to the sources of the concept was not complete. The issue appears confused, especially when we consider that Pinel applied his notion of "manie sans délire" only to cases of raving madness – a thing which Prichard himself considered as mistaken.[10] Moreover Esquirol was himself to deny the connection between his own concepts and that of Prichard's "moral insanity".[11] Finally, there were other alienists who had in mind a type of insanity that was not accompanied by an impairment of the reasoning faculties. These were those German doctors who intellectually gathered around a specialist magazine called *Zeitschrift für psychische Ärzte* and propounded a somatic theory, tracing the sources of mental alienation in bodily ailments. As we shall see, their theories complemented the tenets of Pinel and Esquirol. And where French thought did not agree with Prichard's own notions and observations, the Germans came very near it. He knew their publications, in some cases he even cherished their sagacity. Yet he did not acknowledge the connection between their ideas and his own, at least not during the 1830s when he formulated his theory of moral insanity. One guiding question of this chapter is why Prichard was so reticent regarding those German concepts.

Moral insanity is probably the most complex of Prichard's theories. By retracing his route to the idea, we shall see that it also served to reflect his despondency over the decline of religion in a materialist age. Yet this was not merely the disillusioned response of a cultural pessimist. By explaining madness within the framework of humoralism as a bodily constitution, Prichard dispensed with the idea that reason was the supreme arbiter of humanity. He showed madness to be part of the human condition.

The Phrenological Trap

At the outset of his reflections on the mental mechanisms inherent to insanity, Prichard had a rather clear-cut notion of who his adversaries were: being a dualist who believed in the independence of the soul from bodily functions, he defied the pretensions of the phrenologists who claimed to have found the physiological key to the human psyche.[12] Between 1810 and 1819, Franz Joseph Gall and his collaborator Johann Caspar Spurzheim published five big volumes on the anatomy and functions of the brain, asserting that all mental differences among humans were due to organic differences in the brain. In this multi-volume insult to Prichard's worldview, Gall and Spurzheim divided the cortex into numerous distinct "organs", each of which was responsible for a particular mental faculty. Summing up his system, Gall wrote "that the moral and intellectual world of man begins where the brain begins, and that it ends where the brain ends".[13] If the Austrian doctor did not mean to deny the existence of the soul, this was nevertheless the conclusion which his opponents drew. Prichard, too, took phrenology for yet another head of the materialist hydra. Although he respected Spurzheim as an anatomist, he used the first opportunity to reject his (and Gall's) dubious doctrine. "I must take the liberty of doubting altogether that part of his system which refers to cranioscopy", Prichard wrote in his first book on lunacy, *A Treatise on Diseases of the Nervous System* (1822).[14]

Seeking to disparage phrenology, he claimed that there were a number of mental faculties whose operations were above madness: they simply could not be deranged. The *Treatise on Diseases of the Nervous System* was in many respects a conventional account of insanity, devised along the lines of the Lockean notion that a madman had lost his wits, but not his soul.[15] Apart from establishing its author's authority as alienist, it fulfilled two purposes. First, Prichard used it to refute the popular, non-medical idea that the soul or mind itself could be diseased. Second, he employed it to defend religion against materialists, most prominently the phrenologists, who located all mental faculties in the brain and appeared to reduce the soul to a function of the brain. Against both these notions Prichard pitted the idea that insanity consisted in a faulty transmission of data from the brain into the mind. Madness, in other words, arose from some organic malfunctioning either in the brain or in the nervous system more generally. The brain was not the organ of mind but the intermediary between the body and the immaterial reasoning powers which were "*in no wise* involved in the calamity".[16] But owing to some mechanico-chemical disorder in the nervous system the mind took for "memory" what in fact was merely "reverie", so that its reasoning operations subsequently went amiss.[17]

Prichard distinguished between those faculties – memory,

29

perception, dreaming – that depended on organic stimuli, and those faculties – passions, emotions, and moral as well as rational judgement – whose workings operated entirely independent of any physical cause: "as the organized structure acts upon the mind, in the case of sensation and perception", he claimed, "so, in the instance of the passions, the primary operations of the mind react upon the body".[18] His distinction between "affections of the soul, or immaterial principle" and organically determined sensations was a medical expression of his moral dualism. From this it followed that the phrenological pretensions were ill-grounded: if there were mental faculties that could not be referred to the material fabric of the brain, what point was there in elaborately locating them in the cranial hemisphere?

As time went on, however, this argument ran into an increasing array of problems: during the 1820s, a rising number of pathological anatomists attributed insanity to lesions of specific parts of the brain. The results of experimental physiologists, who manipulated the brain structures in animals, made it more and more difficult to deny that mental functions were dependent on the cerebral structure.[19] Moreover, it was not clear how the bodily functions and those of the mind were related.

A solution was found by the early 1830s. Now, Prichard discussed insanity within a theoretical framework which hitherto had played merely a subordinate role: by relating humoralism to the notion of instincts, he took a step towards shifting the debate on insanity from its focus on the possible role of the brain to an appreciation of the entire bodily disposition.[20] In doing so, he pursued a train of thought begun in the 1820s, though, in his 1822 *Treatise*, humoralism featured less prominently than it did in later publications; and the role of the instincts had not then been appreciated.

In the last chapter we saw that, in 1835, Prichard came out as an old-fashioned humoralist in medical theory; the same preference turns up in his work on madness. In his 1833 article on "Insanity" he counted "temperament" among the causes of insanity. Generally speaking, a constitution "predisposing to violent passions also predisposes to madness".[21] (The tranquillity of his own temper might have conditioned Prichard to regard any exuberance in behaviour as a first step on the road towards mental disorder.) In the same article, he introduced moral insanity. Within the framework of this concept and also of time-honoured humoralism madness was considered to be a problem of both the intellect and the emotions. That was a great novelty, the necessary prerequisite for the doctrine of moral insanity.

Gone were the times when Prichard had thought that insanity consisted exclusively in delusioned reasoning. He himself noted his departure from Lockeanism: in *A Treatise on Insanity* (1835) he dismissed Locke's theory as "by far too limited".[22] The formula "reasoning correctly from erroneous premises" was applicable to certain forms of insanity only, namely to all those in which the understanding was out of order. But there existed another type of madness to which Locke's definition did not apply, namely the perversion of emotive faculties such as the sense of self-preservation or natural affection for one's relatives.

In 1822, Prichard had stipulated that these faculties, together with the power of reasoning, were beyond physical illness since they were innate attributes of the immaterial mind.[23] In 1835, they were still faculties of the mind of an immaterial nature, but, he declared, they could be impaired.[24] Empirical observation played a large role in his growing conviction not only that overexcited feelings could contribute to madness but that they might be, so to speak, the disease itself. Yet, in order to develop moral insanity as a nosological category he had to embed it in his medical theorizing. And this was achieved through a reappreciation of humoralism and the crucial concept of the instincts.

Thomas Hancock and Human Instincts

Up to and including the eighteenth century, instincts had been regarded by many as the base animal counterpart of divine human rationality. At the beginning of the nineteenth century, however, their status was remodelled. For Prichard, the work of the physician Thomas Hancock (1783-1849) was of decisive importance. The two men had studied together at Edinburgh, had remained friends ever since, and expressed praise for each other's writings.[25] Hancock was a Quaker, born in Ireland. Once his studies were completed he moved to London where he worked as physician to the City of London and Finsbury Dispensaries. He participated in the medico-philosophical debates of the London medical establishment, writing articles on medical and other subjects which gained him a reputation as a judicious thinker.[26] In his *Essay on Instinct and Its Physical and Moral Relations* – published in 1824, two years after Prichard's first book on insanity – he rescued the instincts from their low status in brutish nature. Working within the framework of Thomas Reid's and Dugald Stewart's philosophy, Hancock asserted that instincts were characteristic of man as well as animals.[27] It was wrong to see them as the equivalent in the animal kingdom for human rationality;[28] they belonged to that part of the constitution of which the living creature, human as well as animal, was not consciously aware.[29] Both a cause and a corollary of Hancock's views was his conviction that Locke's philosophy of the human mind bore dangerous resemblances to Hume's dubious scepticism.[30] Hancock, therefore, rejected Locke's idea that the mind started off as a tabula rasa. At the same time, however, he admitted that it was unrealistic to assume that the mental faculties of man, and in particular the moral sense, were fully developed from the beginning of each individual life. It had been the mistake of Stewart and Reid to stipulate just that, and for this reason their common-sense philosophy encountered many criticisms. Hancock regarded it as his job to apply necessary corrections. For this purpose he introduced a metaphor through which he hoped to delimit the notion of inbred faculties: it was the image of the "seed".

Seeds were, so to speak, archetypical objects of the Romantic era. A philosophical outlook which laid more emphasis on "becoming" than on "being" was liable to consider the notion of the seed as highly significant.[31] In his *Essay on Instinct* Hancock wrote: "it can hardly be doubted that the enlargement of the intellect and the development of the mental capacities bear some analogy to the evolution, growth and expansion of the several parts of the ovum and of a seed or germ".[32] He held that it was wrong to deny the existence of innate faculties. They were there from the beginning, albeit in an undeveloped form:

> as the growth of a plant proceeds from one degree to another by its inherent powers, without human assistance ...; so in the development of the mind, the internal seeds, faculties, or talents, may be gradually unfolded.[33]

Reid and Stewart were right in supposing the existence of inbred faculties, but, like a seed, in each individual they had to ripen over time. Hancock put forward a philosophy of the moral sense which first dissociated morality from reason, and then went on to show that the seed of the moral sense was implanted in every human being. Whether or not it developed to perfection depended on external influences. "Art may ripen, but it does not implant the seed" which was sown "by the Creator, in every mind." If man preferred virtue to vice it was not thanks to the inscription through education on Locke's "cold and insensible marble tablet" but as "the effect of sacred immutable obligation, or rather of warm original impulse in the mind". Obviously, those faculties he had in mind were God-given gifts. For Hancock, "Conscience", the "Moral Sense", "Light of the

World", "the Divine Principle of Truth" were interchangeable expressions for the "Spirit of God in the Soul". In short, human morality was an inbred seed, implanted into the human fabric as the instincts were ingrained in an animal.[34]

This theory of natural instincts which ran parallel to, and explained, the Quaker doctrine of the "inner light", helped Prichard to elucidate his own ideas on the human mind. "Reason", Hancock wrote, "does not enable man to fulfil the ends of his creation." God had implanted a moral standard or "spiritual principle" in the human constitution; it formed part of man's instinctive fabric.[35] But although they were innate, instincts were modifiable. While Hancock contemplated the loss of instincts that domestication brought about in animals,[36] Prichard reflected on the role instincts played in the human mind, coming to the conclusion that the human species had an inbred propensity to madness. Referring to Hancock, he declared: "it may be said in one sense that a preparation is made for this species of derangement [madness] in the constitution of the human mind".[37] The human instinct that was liable to disorder was the innate moral sense.

Prichard accepted the widespread notion that with the increasing refinement of society, madness was also increasing.[38] Hancock helped him account for that phenomenon in a manner which would not call into question the perfection of Creation. A propensity to madness was nothing less than a necessary corollary of the human ability to survive. While in animals the sense of self-preservation operated unconsciously or instinctively, human nature was endowed with the faculty of foresight: "hope and fear, anxiety respecting the future", wrote Prichard, "are the principles in human nature by which the care of self-preservation is insured".[39] Hope, fear, and anxiety were deeply ingrained in the human psyche, being inherent in men's nature and hence beyond the control of rationality. The theory did not only inscribe insanity into the human condition, it also had a desirable side-effect: Etienne de Condillac and his followers thought that animal instincts were reducible to habit and experience. Thus, bolstering the role of the instincts as part of the body's constitution as a whole amounted to a refutation of sensationalism and its derivative schools.

Thanks to Hancock, Prichard gradually learnt to appreciate theories which emphasized the significance of madness as a phenomenon of the body's essential make-up. To be sure, that was a slow process: although he wanted to refute phrenological tenets he could not easily bring himself to believe that the brain might play only a secondary role in the onset of madness. Mental operations were performed by the brain, so that was where madness had to be centrally located. At the same time, however, Prichard was on the lookout for other theories that might, as it were, deflect attention from the brain, thus curbing the triumphalism of phrenologists and other materialists who used anatomical evidence testifying to the correlation between visible cerebral lesions and impaired mental faculties: "doubts interpose themselves", he wrote, "whether the phenomena of insanity are really the results of changes discovered in the brain. May it not be supposed that these changes are the effects of mental disorders rather than their cause?"[40]

It was with great interest that Prichard learned of those doctors who located the causes of insanity in bodily parts other than the head. Quoting Pinel, he contemplated in 1822 whether some forms of madness such as epilepsy were – "in some unknown way" – ultimately referable to an "irritated portion of the stomach or intestines" or "disease in the liver, and other abdominal viscera" – and therefore not primarily to some lesion of the cerebral structure.[41] Elsewhere he reflected on the seat of the passions, though he concluded that "these notions, respecting the locality of the passions, are very vague and undefined". The elements of the theory that was later to crystallize as the concept of moral insanity were present in 1822, though not endorsed as such. "I am at present acquainted with no fact, either in physiology or pathology, which furnishes any ground for presuming that those mental phaenomena, which are termed *passions*, take place through the instrumentality of any corporeal processes whatever", Prichard wrote, "*it seems to me probable that they are affections of the soul, or immaterial principle*, and that primarily, and without the cooperation of any part of the corporeal structure."[42] Speculations about a type of insanity involving only the "active powers" and not the intellect, Prichard said, would require a "very different theory".[43] While, in this context, he mentioned Pinel, there were other alienists who advanced similar notions. These were those German somatists, already mentioned, whom Prichard later called "the school of Nasse".[44] They included Christian Friedrich Nasse, Maximilian Jacobi, Franz Francke and others.

The School of Nasse and Diseases of the Passions

The doctrines of this group were derived from the Idealist philosophy of mind. Unlike Pinel's theory of "mania without delusion", that of the Nasse school addressed a wider range of emotional disorders which comprised not only states of "exalted mania", but all possible sorts of emotional aberration, ranged on a scale from excess to depression. In the 1820s, in the course of contemplating the nature of madness and the make-up of the mental faculties, Prichard grew familiar with these tenets. They spelled out many of his own implicit assumptions about the cultural meaning of madness and arguably helped him to come to terms with the notion that mental faculties could be diseased like any other part of the body. Their theory of somatic pathology did not – like that of Gall – regard the functions of the soul as reducible to the structure of the brain. Prichard, of course, recognized the importance of the brain as the seat of madness,[45] but resisting reductionist theories, he stressed that the whole phenomenon must be viewed within a wider context that might involve lesions of the viscera, in particular those of the abdomen and the thorax.

The Nasse school had as its mouthpiece a periodical edited by Nasse, initially called *Zeitschrift für psychische Ärzte*, and from 1823 *Zeitschrift für die Anthropologie*.[46] Published in Leipzig from 1818, it was reckoned the first high-quality periodical on insanity to be set up in Germany.[47] In 1824, the journal included an excerpt from Prichard's book on nervous disorders.[48] The footnotes in the *Treatise on Insanity* reveal that Prichard paid a lot of attention to the *Zeitschrift* and the articles of one of its most eminent editors, Maximilian Jacobi.[49] Deeply involved in Romantic philosophizing, the *Zeitschrift's* contributors tried to support what they perceived as real and inner human values against superficial French rationality. Practising in Halle and Bonn, Nasse (1778-1851) was a pupil of Johann Christian Reill.[50] Jacobi (1755-1858) was the son of the philosopher who had been a companion of Goethe.[51] Their politics of the body bolstered the notion of a holistic interplay between all parts of the body and the soul, while at the same time, they believed in a distinct hierarchy in which the soul was constantly at odds with the flesh. According to the Nasse school, at the onset of most cases of madness there existed a derangement of the emotions, brought about by a disease in parts of the organism. This could – but need not necessarily – lead to a deranged understanding. While the latter illness was indeed seated in the brain, dislocated emotions signified a disease of the visceral organs, be it the heart, the liver, the stomach or a part of the intestines.[52]

In pitting derangements of the passions against those of the intellect, the Germans relied heavily on humoralism.[53] As a faculty whose functioning was clearly dependent on the brain, the understanding was open to anatomical investigations. Not so the passions: their expression was a matter of the body's physical constitution. Humoralist doctrines were used to theorize and classify them. In Jacobi's words, the task was to investigate "the temperaments as somatic basis of the affective powers and the passions". He contended that "the impact which the brain exerts on the psyche [was] far less well established" than that of the temperaments: the particular humoral constitution of the body determined his moral conformation.[54] It governed, in other words, what Thomas Hancock called moral instinct. Although Prichard was very reluctant to acknowledge his indebtedness to German somatists, his praise of Hancock arguably went together with a kind of increasing adaptation to German theorizing on his part. Besides, he was not the only physician to be influenced by German theories of madness. Philippe Pinel, too, was manifestly impressed by German doctrines, and he too had developed a notion of emotional disorders.[55]

If there was a specifically German approach to notions of the human mind as well as of madness this was to some extent a question of language. The German word "Gemüt" has no exact equivalent in English; sometimes it may mean "mind", Prichard, by contrast, translated it as "sentiment", but "Gemüt" is more than that. It refers to the emotional disposition or the moral framework of man and relates to the understanding, as heart relates to brain. Hence German semantics suggested a classification of madness which naturally included the notion of diseased emotions.[56] In the theories of Jacobi and the Nasse school, physiological tenets joined with the repertoire of Romantic criticism. To regard madness primarily as a disease of the viscera was a corollary of the fact that Romanticism considered the understanding as the inferior, merely instrumental part of the human character. Accordingly, the brain as the instrument of the understanding was of lower transcendental value than those organs which were symbiotic with the emotions. As Jacobi put it, "the holiest powers of man which constitute his actual value, his humanity, reside in his sentiment [Gemüth]".[57] For the German somatists, the visceral organization of the body had more to do with the transcendental nature of man than had the brain, and this was the idea behind Jacobi's remark that "there are certain morbid changes in the organisation" which ultimately lead to an impairment "of moral freedom".[58]

Thus, the Nasse school provided what may be seen as the moral undergirdings to the theory of moral insanity. If it had not been for their somatist theories that medically reduced lunacy to visceral complaints, Prichard might have acknowledged their merit a lot earlier than he actually did. If he instead explicitly associated moral insanity with Pinel and Esquirol this may have been for reasons that were not strictly professional: Esquirol was not only one of the most influential alienists of his time, he also held conservative social outlooks that agreed more with Prichard's own opinions than the liberal progressivism of the German somatists. In fact, regarding the politics of medical doctrines it was rather undesirable for Prichard to be associated with the Nasse school whose representatives were widely derided for their physicalism (or somatism) which was viewed as denying the existence of the soul. Their adversaries, the mentalists (or psychicists), headed by the alienist Johann Christian August Heinroth (1773-1843), tended to place the aetiology of mental illnesses in the soul. It was a difference mirrored in their politics: their liberalism placed the somatists opposite the rather conservative outlook of Heinroth and his followers which led them to view mental disorder as a product of immorality.[59] Significantly, they all spoke as one when it came to fighting "the one-sided, physically-oriented, 'mind-less' medicine of the *Aufklärungs* era".[60] This explains why the writings of both schools, that of Nasse as well as that of Heinroth, appealed to Prichard. He could not subscribe wholeheartedly to a theory which so much emphasized the role of the bodily constitution in insanity as did that of the Nasse school. It was necessary to fight the phrenologists, but not at the expense of letting in materialism through the back door in the guise of somatism: once the forces of the body were unleashed, they appeared to threaten his dualist world-view. The other possibility, however – that of supporting Heinroth's understanding of madness as sin – was too far off the course of the scientific objectivity Prichard professed to follow. In this respect he was torn between personal taste and professionalism: although Heinroth's notions were "rather theoretical or speculative than the result of actual observation", and although they were "singular and absurd" in some of their "most fundamental principles", Prichard quoted his *Lehrbuch der Störungen des Seelenlebens* (1818) frequently and held it "worthy of consideration".[61] Like most eclectics, Prichard was not the man to grant unconditional allegiance to any one theory, rather he would waver between various standpoints, and fashion his own opinions from single elements of diverse doctrines. Despite this practice, and his reticence towards somatism, he finally endorsed the similarities between moral insanity and related theories of the Nasse school.

Reconciliation with Jacobi's Theory

It was in the years around 1840 that Prichard made up his mind and yielded to the theories of the Nasse school, accepting moral insanity as a disease of the viscera. This was instanced in his contribution to

Alexander Tweedie's *Library of Medicine* (1840-42), where he remarked that "disorders of the different viscera and of the functions of physical life are in a very curious manner connected with states of the mind".[62] In 1844 he published a brief article reporting a typical case of moral insanity and revising his former position. Now he praised Jacobi wholeheartedly "for the practical sense as for the deep philosophical investigation" of his works:

> Jacobi has not expressed his opinion precisely in this manner; but it would appear ... that he looks upon effects produced upon the sensorium and the mind, through the medium of the stomach, or any of the viscera of physical life, as not less immediately brought about by the action of the material organism on the intellectual or sensitive power, than the impressions produced in the mind by a blow on the head, or by any powerful agency exerted immediately on the brain.[63]

If we ask why Prichard finally admitted common ground with the Germans, an explanation may lie in his frustration with the French medical scene. Alienists such as Pinel and Esquirol had been interested in the relation between passions and mental derangement. But this phase lasted for only two decades. After Esquirol's death in 1840 his pupils who, much more than their teacher, employed physicalist theories which were not tempered by religion, led the debate. By the 1830s, French theorizing upon madness was dominated by the anatomical approach and the attempt to depict correlations between cerebral lesions and mental disorder.[64] Prichard did not conceal his exasperation with contemporary trends in anatomy. In 1844, he regretted that "in England and France, the principal, if not the almost undivided attention of anatomists has been directed to the discovery of morbid changes in the brain". The Germans, even though they were generally neither "more practical" nor "sound", had at least taken "a different course": the school of Nasse, in particular, Prichard wrote, found many connections between insanity and physical lesions of the viscera which were discovered at post-mortem dissections. Now he asserted that "the principal and fundamental cause of insanity is, in many instances, to be sought, not in the brain, but in some other region of the body".[65] Prichard's little 1844 article concluded the issues which have been discussed so far, namely his defiance of the phrenologists through the theory of moral insanity, and his increasing conversion to the notion that moral insanity was tied to a disorder in the viscera and thus to the entire constitution of the body. "The phenomena of moral insanity", he wrote,

or of a disordered state of the affections and moral feelings, without
any corresponding lesion of the understanding, or of the reasoning
faculties, furnishes, or appears at least, *prima facie*, to furnish a firm
ground whereon to maintain the negative position in regard to the
participation, or, at least, the primary influence of the brain, in the
development of an extensive series of psychological phenomena.[66]

This statement was very different indeed from Prichard's earlier
insistence on the pivotal role of the brain. The links between the
theory of insanity and his implicit belief systems are revealed by the
following example. In 1844, Prichard presented the pathological
findings in question as if he had only been waiting for anatomical
evidence to prove that moral insanity arose from a disease of the
viscera. He cited the case of "a lady highly accomplished, and of great
mental endowments, pious, affectionate, and sincere" who suddenly
became "low-spirited and hypochondriacal". At the same time she
refused to eat. When her friends and family urged her, she
complained about pains in the abdomen. "Her whole temper and
character became changed. Formerly devoted to her duties, and to
works of benevolence to others, she now thought only of herself, and
her complaints." Finally, she was sent into an asylum where she "was
induced, though not without great difficulty, and a constant threat of
compulsion if she resisted, to take a moderate quantity of the most
nutritious and digestible food". Subsequently she died. The
dissection showed that her intestinal canal was full of ulcers and
tubercles. Now, instead of concluding that this woman was not mad,
but did indeed suffer terrible pain and therefore had reason to reject
food, Prichard took the abdominal evidence as testifying to the truth
of his theory on moral insanity:

> the perpetual complaints made by the patient of pain and suffering
> in the abdomen had an organic cause, and were not unreal, as it
> had been sometimes suspected. As these complaints had been
> uniform, and had continued from the commencement of the
> disease, it may be inferred as highly probable that the organic
> disease in the intestinal canal had been coeval with the mental
> disorder, and the foundation of the whole train of morbid
> symptoms.[67]

It is significant that Prichard described the patient as being self-
obsessed – "she now thought only of herself". Identification of self-
centredness as a feature of insanity was common among the Nasse
school. Thus Jacobi wrote that the "forces of selfishness" strive in

man "against revelation"; only by overcoming the "forces of nature" could man's soul liberate itself. But time and again, nature proved stronger. "Nothing", Jacobi concluded, "can stop man in this temptation, which threatens shattering and extinction, but the firm belief in the truth ... of revelation."[68]

Unlike Esquirol's pupils in France, the somatist branch of German Romantic physiology explicitly and persistently referred to metaphysical convictions; in their understanding, insanity was concomitant, as it were, with a break-up of the ties linking an individual to his transcendental nature.[69] In that sense, Prichard and Jacobi had a common cause. Both of them partook seriously of the anxieties of their age, the uprooting of traditional hierarchies, subsequent social upheavals, a burgeoning acquisitiveness hitherto unknown, scientific materialism – it all was indicative of far-reaching moral depravity. In a speech in 1835, Prichard sighed about "these days, when intellect is deified and worshipped as the sole divinity".[70] The country which seemed to furnish ample reason for misgivings was France. In the wake of the French Revolution, religious observance had reached an all-time low. Selfish passions were no longer held in check. Jacobi implicitly conflated socially egoistic behaviour with the exaggerated self-centredness of the insane. In the end, both were attributed to loss of religion. Prichard saw things similarly. He translated a passage from Jacobi on the moral debasement of the French: "the generality of men have their understanding impaired through the influence of lower passions, and of vices" which Jacobi considered as "so much the more prevalent" now the Christian moral standard was on the decline.[71] As this quotation shows, in spite of his liberal politics, Jacobi was critical enough of modern times to appeal to conservative minds. While Prichard found his misgivings concerning the state of religion mirrored in Jacobi's words, his social apprehensions were – characteristically perhaps – expressed by a Frenchman, namely, the famous Esquirol himself.

Madness: A Post-Revolutionary Disease

Esquirol, in his time the greatest and most influential authority on alienation in France, was politically conservative enough to provide Prichard with rich quotations on the detrimental effects of moral decline. But unlike Jacobi, Nasse, and Prichard, Esquirol showed some sympathy towards French positivism, and his theories did not revolve around notions of redemption and life after death. Hence Esquirol's misgivings as to the contemporary state of morality were tied rather more to the course of civilization than to the individual's readiness to transcend his own self.

By the time Napoleon had been safely despatched to St Helena, it was permissible for conservatives to cite Rousseau. For Esquirol, backed by Rousseau, it was evident that civilized man had so far departed from propriety and decency that madness must be on the rise. Prichard chose Esquirol's texts[72] to express his own misgivings: "during the last thirty years", Prichard stated through the words of Esquirol, "the changes which have taken place in our manners in France, have been productive of more cases of insanity than our political torments". With the demise of religious observance in France, Esquirol stated, "demonomania and superstitious madness have disappeared". But instead of ushering in an epoch which was mentally saner, this change had caused the reverse to happen. The pivotal role of religion in the sustenance of social order was an early nineteenth-century commonplace. Esquirol had established what happened in a country with weak religious foundations: "the influence of religion over the conduct of the people being weakened, in order to keep men in obedience governments have had recourse to police". This had dire consequences: now "it is the police which haunts weak imaginations. Asylums are filled with monomaniacs, who, fearing this authority, have gone mad upon the subject, and believe that they are constantly pursued".[73] Esquirol deplored the substitution of selfishness for virtue:

> A cold egotism has dried up all the sources of sentiment: there no longer exist domestic affections, respect, attachment, authority, or reciprocal dependencies; every one lives for himself; none are anxious to form those wise and salutary provisions which ought to connect the present age with those which are destined to follow it.[74]

The Burkean overtones in this passage are evident. But Burke's target, the Revolution, was history. Esquirol was talking about another kind of social lesion, he called it "perfect selfishness",[75] Jacobi called it "Selbstsucht"[76] – it was the disease of the age of capitalism. Many contemporaries perceived that they were living through a phase of change. The way in which they theorized this is indicative of their political standpoints as well as of their ontology. Some attributed the apparent change of manners to a reorganization of society as a whole, or to a changed mode of production. Others would not follow the turn to sociological analysis which, as they saw it, played down morality, ruling it out as an explanatory category. The notion of alienation was widespread. But some philosophers – most famously, of course, Karl

41

Marx – came to see this as a socio-economic phenomenon, whereas such philosophizing physiologists as Prichard, Jacobi and Esquirol regarded it as a phenomenon staged *within* human consciousness. It expressed itself in terms of a separation between men's social identity and their metaphysically grounded morality.

An awareness of this problem characterizes not just Prichard's medicine, but also his anthropology. He accounted for the different varieties of mankind by linking humoralism and environmentalism. Thus he could reject the notion of distinct human races, while at the same time eschewing the pitfalls of external, "materialistic", determinism. In both anthropology and medicine, he was concerned to combat the growing importance attached to the brain and consequently the construction of hierarchies along the lines of increasing cerebral complexity, the latter amounting, in his eyes, to an erosion of individual moral responsibility.[77]

Prichard's deep piety was tied to the framework of natural theology. He was involved in a scientific theodicy, questioning for instance why it had pleased God to inflict madness upon man. We have seen how he took his views on this matter from Thomas Hancock's *Essay on Instinct*, and how he explained insanity as part of the human constitution and as a necessary corollary to the human ability to entertain fear for the future. It was, however, not just the "anticipation of wants" which was implanted in the human soul, but also the expectation of "a state of existence after death".[78] Human beings were endowed with foresight to enable them to survive during their earthly existence. Equally, awareness of the Fall and of a future Day of Judgement was given to them so that they could govern their behaviour in such a manner as to deserve redemption on the day of atonement. Indeed, Prichard conceived of an inherent and eternal fear which was constitutionally implanted in men's mental fabric: "there is one feature" common to all men, he wrote, "their prevailing character is gloomy ... A persuasion of moral demerit or a consciousness of guilt has been deeply impressed upon the minds of men in all ages".[79]

It was certainly no accident that the word "gloom" also appeared in the context of insanity. In his contribution to Tweedie's *Library of Medicine*, Prichard mentioned melancholy as characteristic of patients suffering from moral insanity: "persons in this state have no relish for the enjoyments of life; they express *no feelings of consolation or happiness in the prospect of a future existence*, they view everything through a medium of gloom".[80] In the 1835 *Treatise*, Prichard specified: "a considerable proportion among the most striking

42

instances of moral insanity are those in which a tendency to gloom or sorrow is the predominant feature".[81] But, for him, the matter also touched on the transcendental. If gloom, then, tormented the sound as well as the unsound, what was the difference between the two states of mind other than a question of degree?

When Prichard suggested that a disposition to madness was part of the human constitution, this might be understood as his way of saying that mankind paid with madness for the Fall. Without anxiety, fear, and gloom, men would not behave as they should in order to ensure their survival as well as redemption after death.[82] But these very qualities were, so to speak, too much for the human constitution. Mental sanity did not prevent the sound-minded from sharing in the gloom of damnation with which the diseased were inflicted. The difference was only that the sane managed to pull themselves together and fulfil their daily duties, while the morally insane "remain ... moping and silent in their beds".[83]

The Social Significance of Moral Insanity – A Concept Put to the Test

It has been shown that moral insanity must be understood as a corollary of Prichard's conservatism in a struggle which was taking place on many levels: reform versus counter-revolution; materialist physiology versus organismic holism of body and soul; purely sociological versus "moral" or psychological explanations; secularization versus metaphysics. For Prichard, moral insanity was a moral perversion in both senses, leading to a dislocation of the moral sentiment and of morality. When talking science Prichard did not want to moralize, yet he could not help finding some truth in Heinroth's theory that insanity rose out of sin: "vices, inordinate passions, and the want of mental discipline", Prichard conceded, tended "to increase the prevalence of insanity".[84] He believed that the causes of moral insanity were, more often than not, of a moral rather than a physical kind.[85] Fully in line with this view that the disposition to madness was part of the human fabric, was his statement that mere eccentricity was already a sign of madness: "if ... we are obliged to discuss the question, whether eccentricity is in general allied to madness, and even a modification of that state or not, there is no doubt that the decision would be in the affirmative".[86] For an alienist who had the duty and the power to confine mad people to an asylum, a definition as broad as this opened the way to boundless activity. But Prichard did not jump to this conclusion: for him, confinement was necessary only when the behaviour of the patient was dangerous.[87]

Prichard recommended the adoption of moral insanity in both penal and civil law. He believed that many individuals convicted for murder actually suffered from "homicidal madness", a variant of moral insanity.[88] They did not deserve to be subjected to the death penalty, but should be locked up and receive treatment. In civil law, by contrast, Prichard advocated confinement only in those cases when the insane's behaviour was too outrageous:

> The question which jurors will have to determine is, not whether the person whose case is under examination is afflicted with insanity according to any abstract definition, or general notion, as to the nature of that disease, but whether his mental state is individually such as to render him unfit to be at large, and to be entrusted with the care of himself and his property.[89]

This brings us to the social implications of moral insanity. What should be done with the morally insane? Discussing the expediency of confinement, Prichard stated: "confinement is unnecessary for such a person, who is in no way dangerous to society. If the management of his property – for such individuals are generally possessed of property – could be so settled as to ensure his having the usual supports of life, this would be sufficient".[90] Buried in this sentence is an interesting aspect of moral insanity. Prichard never spelled it out in detail, but it seems that he regarded moral insanity as a disorder characteristically afflicting the affluent. And it was a disorder which was a lot more respectable than other forms of mental unsoundness. In a way, moral insanity served to create a class of patients who were not liable to be confounded with beastly imbeciles.

The notion of a civil disease for the refined strata of society can be seen as linking up with Prichard's hesitation over recommending confinement: it pandered to the attitudes of an educated class of possible clients. Asylums had in those days a poor reputation, and it was very much in the interest of an alienist (who did not own a madhouse) to play down the importance of confinement.[91] Hence Prichard's claim that in some forms of moral insanity it was sufficient to take the management of his property out of the hands of the disturbed individual. To see moral insanity in this manner as a somewhat polite form of madness, was a concomitant of his assumption that the disorder was characteristic of civilization.[92] The lives of brute men – savages as well as peasant folk – were not refined enough for the "cold egotism" which held sway in modern society and which was to a large extent responsible for the rising numbers of madmen. Moreover, the particular type of anxieties modern men suffered from, loss of fortune or professional ambition, were not to be found in primitive societies. "The apparent increase is everywhere so striking", Prichard commented,

> that it leaves on the mind a strong suspicion ... that cases of insanity are far more numerous than formerly .... It is encouraged by the reflexion that the state of society is, in most countries, such as appears likely to multiply the existing causes of madness. ... Sufficient evidence has arisen to confirm in a great measure the remark made, many years ago by M. Esquirol, that insanity belongs almost exclusively to civilized races of men: it scarcely exists among savages, and is rare in barbarous countries.[93]

What applied to insanity broadly speaking and to different stages of civilization, was true for moral insanity as well. Given that Prichard considered civilized peoples as such to be liable to the disease, he probably assumed that the "more civilized" strata of society were more at risk than the lower classes.[94] The aetiology of moral insanity covered many symptoms which were not dependent on social status. Yet an old tradition had it that the refined classes were more susceptible to feeling than ordinary folk. Moral insanity, defined as a disease of the passions, had therefore the tendency to be prevalent among refined and propertied people. With moral insanity, Prichard devised a model illness which explained in psychiatric terms the deplorable moral corruption of his times and, in particular, of the affluent, who had the means to indulge in "moral debasement" until they were mad. Paradoxically, this very aspect of the disease was apt to make it more palatable to the public. The creation of the concept could appear a cunning selling strategy, except that its formulation was rather a result of Prichard's views on human nature and his despair with the moral depravity of his time.

There is yet another respect in which the consideration of property was pivotal in Prichard's thought. He put forward his pleas for confinement in certain cases, first of all, in the name of social order: "of all these arrangements the maintenance of public order is the principal object, and the second is the preservation of the property belonging to the lunatic and the interest of his family".[95] It is notable that Prichard's concern circled around notions of property and the avoidance of social upheaval.[96] Esquirol, by contrast, had put much greater emphasis on moral propriety. His theory was suitable for post-revolutionary French society where the aristocracy as well as the high bourgeoisie were trying to re-establish distinct social hierarchies. For him, much more than for Prichard, nymphomania and satyriasis were complaints characteristic of civil society.[97] Private property was not one .of the topics which specially preoccupied Esquirol. For Prichard, however, it was not social hierarchy but the preservation of peace and order which was central. Legal action was needed when a mentally disturbed person threatened to harm himself, other people or their property. Society had not only the right, but the duty to interfere with persons who, like Symonds's gentleman patient mentioned at the beginning of this chapter, squandered their possessions and threatened to throw their families into poverty.[98]

Insanity was, for Prichard, a prevalent menace. It was not an exceptional misfortune, but rather a predicament society had to live with. All eccentric behaviour was indicative of a disordered mind. Since many eccentrics did no harm to anybody, their behaviour could be tolerated. But for the sake of social cohesion society had to defend itself when its law and order were attacked. This is why Prichard chose the preservation of social order, of property and personal safety, as the criteria for certification.

Moral insanity arose initially out of his theological interest in sustaining the doctrine of the immaterial soul. As we have seen, the concept was expressive of his views on the precarious morality of modern man rather than of his desire to draw definite dividing lines between the sound and the unsound. For Prichard, man's mental health was ultimately tied to his religion. He was a medical dualist who thought that medicine had not much to do with the mind. Insofar as madness was excited by physical disease, medicine could cure it. That failing, it could aid the law in preserving social order.

Prichard's suggestion was in vain. In English legal practice, moral insanity failed to become an accepted category. His attempt to support the legal enforcement of morality proved fruitless. The M'Naughten Rules of 1843 confirmed the persistence of the orthodox definition of madness which presupposed outright delusion.[99] It was in the theories of many later psychiatrists that moral insanity lived on. But they appropriated it in a manner Prichard would not have countenanced. His zealous endeavour to sustain the doctrine of the soul against contemporary forms of medical materialism inadvertently supported another form of secularization of.the mind. Prichard had referred the mechanisms of psychology to the body in order to preserve the soul's untainted immateriality. In the second half of the nineteenth century alienists would enlarge upon ideas which formed the physicalist part of Prichardian anthropology.[100] The notion of atonement, however, which included the whole of humanity, was lost. While Prichard had fought phrenology, his successors were to integrate it with moral insanity. In the later decades of the nineteenth century, theories about hereditary mental degeneration were spreading. Accordingly, men were doomed by birth, not metaphysically but in terms of their physical heritage. How easily these notions could be combined with moral insanity is exemplified in the articles of John Kitching who, in the 1850s, served as the medical superintendent of the York Retreat. In his contributions to the *British Medical Journal* he applied doctrines of phrenology and hereditary degeneration to the concept of moral insanity. Madness was for him solely a question of "disordered functions of the brain". Moral insanity was the "arrested development in those parts of the brain, which are concerned in the due performance of the moral and instinctive faculties".[101]

While Prichard had managed to uphold a careful balance between the organic sources of the disease and its effects on man's morality on the one hand, and the organic implications of man's metaphysical framework on the other, subsequent generations confined moral insanity entirely to the physical sphere. Moral insanity, Prichard's legacy to medical psychiatry, was employed in conceptualizations of madness which overrode the transcendental nature of man. References to the soul were to become at best the philosophical superstructure in the belief systems of individual alienists. But on the whole, metaphysics was severed from medical theories – a development which, had he lived to witness it, would have confirmed Prichard's worst misgivings.

Notes

1 See Mareta Linden, *Untersuchungen zum Anthropologiebegriff des 18. Jahrhunderts* (Bern: Herbert Lang, 1976).

2 A larger version of this chapter appeared in 1996 in *Medical History*. As will be apparent, in the light of further research and thinking, I have somewhat amended the conclusions.

3 Roy Porter, *Mind-Forg'd Manacles. A History of Madness in England from the Restoration to the Regency* (London: Athlone Press, 1987); Akihito Suzuki, "An Anti-Lockean Enlightenment?: Mind and Body in Early Eighteenth-Century English Medicine". In *Medicine and the Enlightenment*, ed. Roy Porter (Amsterdam: Rodopi, 1994), pp. 226-59.

4 Prichard, "Insanity". In *The Cyclopaedia of Practical Medicine*, ed. J. Forbes, A. Tweedie, J. Conolly, 4 vols (London: Sherwood, Gilbert, Piper, 1833-35), 2: 10-32, 847-75.

5 Prichard, *A Treatise on Insanity, and Other Disorders Affecting the*

Mind (London: Sherwood, 1835). For his visit to Ivry, see his article on "Temperament". In *Cyclopaedia of Practical Medicine*, 4: 159-74, p. 172.

6   Prichard, *A Treatise on Insanity*, pp. 48-50.

7   Prichard, *Treatise on Insanity*, pp. 6, 23-24. See also Prichard, "Insanity". In *The Library of Medicine*, ed. Alexander Tweedie, 8 vols (London: Whittaker and Co., 1840-42), 2: 102-42 – henceforth quoted as "Insanity"

8   Eric T. Carlson, Norman Dain, "The Meaning of Moral Insanity". *Bulletin of the History of Medicine* 36 (1962): 130-40, p. 134; Joel Peter Eigen, *Witnessing Insanity: Madness and Mad-Doctors in the English Court* (New Haven: Yale University Press, 1995), p. 77; Nigel Walker, Sarah McCabe, *Crime and Insanity in England*, 2 vols (Edinburgh: Edinburgh University Press, 1973), 2: 208; and, most recently, German E. Berrios, *The History of Mental Symptoms. Descriptive Psychopathology Since the Nineteenth Century* (Cambridge: Cambridge University Press, 1996), p. 426.

9   Prichard, *Treatise on Insanity*, p. 15.

10   Philippe Pinel, *A Treatise on Insanity*, trans. D. D. Davis (Sheffield: Cadell and Davies, 1806). There were a number of German authors whom Prichard credited with having formulated theories resembling that of moral insanity. These were J. C. A. Heinroth, Johann Christian Reil and Johann Christoph Hoffbauer; the latter two had edited contributions to moral treatment, Hoffbauer was a collaborator of the Nasse school which will feature below. Yet Prichard preferred the theories of these doctors to that of Pinel. All of them, including Esquirol, Prichard wrote, "have not recognized moral insanity under so general a character as we have ascribed to it". See his article "Soundness and Unsoundness of Mind". In *The Cyclopaedia of Practical Medicine*, 4: 39-55, p. 49. Cf. also his *Treatise on Insanity*, pp. 5-6. For Pinel see Dora Weiner, "'Le geste de Pinel': The History of a Psychiatric Myth". In *Discovering the History of Psychiatry*, ed. Mark S. Micale, Roy Porter (Oxford: Oxford University Press, 1994), pp. 232-47; *idem*, "Mind and Body in the Clinic: Philippe Pinel, Alexander Crichton, Dominique Esquirol, and the Birth of Psychiatry". In *The Languages of Psyche. Mind and Body in Enlightenment Thought*, ed. G. S. Rousseau (Berkeley: University of California Press, 1990), pp. 331-402.

11   Jean Etienne Dominique Esquirol, "Monomanie". In *idem, Des maladies mentales considérées sous les rapports médical, hygiénique et médico-légal*, 2 vols (Paris: J.-B. Baillière, 1838), 2: 1-130, p. 5. For Esquirol see Jan Goldstein, *Console and Classify. The French*

Psychiatric Profession in the Nineteenth Century (Cambridge: Cambridge University Press, 1987); G. Swain, *Le sujet de la folie* (Toulouse: Privat, 1977).

12 For the role and influence of phrenology, see Roger Cooter, *The Cultural Meaning of Popular Science. Phrenology and the Organization of Consent in Nineteenth-Century Britain* (Cambridge: Cambridge University Press, 1984).

13 Franz Joseph Gall, Gaspar [sic] Spurzheim, *Anatomie et physiologie du système nerveux en général, et du cerveau en particulier, avec des observations sur la possibilité de reconnoître plusieurs dispositions intellectuelles et morales de l'homme et des animaux, par la configuration de leurs têtes*, 5 vols (Paris: printed by F. Schoell for the Bibliothèque Grècque-Latine-Allemande, 1810-19), 4: 256. Unless otherwise stated all translations are mine.

14 Prichard, *A Treatise on Diseases of the Nervous System, Part the First: Comprising Convulsive and Maniacal Affections* (London: Thomas and George Underwood, 1822), note on p. 35. The second part of the treatise was never published. The debate between Prichard and the phrenologists went on for a considerable time. For attacks against Prichard's anti-phrenological position, see three articles by Andrew Combe, published anonymously in the *Phrenological Journal*, 2 (1824-25): 47-55; 8 (1832-34): 649-57; 11 (1838), 345-58; see also Edmond Sheppard Symes, "Abstract of Address to the London Phrenological Society Containing Strictures Upon Prichard's Article...". *Zoist* 2 (1845): 448-49.

15 *Ibid.*, p. 25.

16 *Ibid.*, p. 119 (Prichard's emphasis). Following common-sense philosophy, which he surely learned in Edinburgh, Prichard divided the mental faculties into judgement and reasoning on the one hand and the passions, appetites, propensities, and volition on the other. At the beginning of his *Treatise* he attempted to prove why these innate mental faculties could be affected by such disorders of the nervous system as madness only in so far as the bodily framework was instrumentally important for the operation of the mind.

17 *Ibid.*, pp. 37-38, 128-32.

18 *Ibid.*, pp. 23-24, 30-31. The same dualist distinction between organic influences and immaterial forces stood at the centre of his discussion of the vital principle whose existence he denied; see his *A Review of the Doctrine of a Vital Principle, as Maintained by Some Writers on Physiology with Observations on the Causes of Physical & Animal Life* (London: John and Arthur Arch, 1829).

19 For the development of neurological anatomy see W. F. Bynum,

"Varieties of Cartesian Experience in Early Nineteenth Century Neurophysiology". In *Philosophical Dimensions of the Neuro-Medical Sciences*, ed. S. F. Spicker, H. T. Engelhardt (Dordrecht: Reidel, 1976), pp. 15-33. See also Edwin Clarke, L. S. Jacyna, *Nineteenth-Century Origins of Neuroscientific Concepts* (Berkeley: University of California Press, 1987). Excellent for the French context is Goldstein, *Console and Classify*.

20 For general accounts of humoralism in the epoch see Antoinette Emch-Dériaz, "The Non-Naturals Made Easy". In *The Popularization of Medicine 1650-1850*, ed. Roy Porter (London: Routledge, 1992), pp. 134-59; William A. Lishman, *Organic Psychiatry* (Oxford: Blackwell, 1990); Owsei Temkin, *Galenism: Rise and Decline of a Medical Philosophy* (Ithaca: Cornell University Press, 1973), pp. 180ff. Nasse, too, professed his adherence to humoralism. See Nasse, "Ueber die Benennung und die vorläufige Eintheilung des psychischen Krankseyns". *Zeitschrift für psychische Ärzte* 1 (1818): 1-48, pp. 39-40.

21 Prichard, "Insanity". In *The Cyclopaedia of Practical Medicine*, 2: 847. The descent into madness proper was the result of accidental circumstances which Prichard in line with medical doctrines of his time conjoined to a "constitutional disposition, whether hereditary or originating with the individual". Among those accidental circumstances "moral causes" held a prominent position. He believed that causes such as stifled hopes or great losses were more apt to incite madness than most other influences that did not only act through the physique but were a mere matter of physicality (see his *Treatise on Insanity*, pp. 157, 174).

22 Prichard, *Treatise on Insanity*, p. 3.

23 See note 18 above and Prichard, *Diseases of the Nervous System*, p. 41.

24 Prichard, *Treatise on Insanity*, pp. 6, 11. He talked of "disordered" or "disturbed" faculties.

25 Symonds, *Some Account*, p. 7. For Prichard's esteem of Hancock's theories, see his *A Review of the Doctrine of a Vital Principle*, p. 63. Cf. also Prichard, *Researches*, 3rd ed., 1: 175; *idem, Treatise on Insanity*, p. 189. For Hancock see Thomas Hancock, *Essay on Instinct and Its Physical and Moral Relations* (London: William Phillips, George Yard *et al.*; Edinburgh: W. & C. Tait, 1824), note on p. 420.

26 See his obituary in *London Medical Gazette* 8 (1849): 790.

27 Hancock, *Essay on Instinct*, pp. 52-101.

28 That view had been asserted, e.g., by William Smellie, in his translation of Buffon's *Natural History*, published in 1785.

29 Hancock, "The Ascending Scale of Instinctive or Unconscious

Motions". In *Essay on Instinct*, ch. 6.

30　See his obituary in *London Medical Gazette* 8 (1849): 790.

31　It would be worthwhile to study the metaphorical usage of the term "seed" systematically. Thomas Arnold, for instance, was "looking anxiously round the world for any new races which may receive the seed (so to speak) of our present history into a kindly yet a vigorous soil...". See his *Introductory Lectures on Modern History* (Oxford: John Henry Parker, 1842), p. 28.

32　Hancock, *Essay on Instinct*, p. 230.

33　*Ibid.*, pp. 263-64.

34　*Ibid.*, pp. 334, 228, 293, 406.

35　*Ibid.*, pp. 173, 315, ch. 9 ("Of the Divine Spirit in the Soul") and part 2 ("Of the Moral Relations of Instinct").

36　*Ibid.*, p. 109.

37　Prichard, *Treatise on Insanity*, p. 189.

38　*Ibid.*, pp. 174-75.

39　*Ibid.*, pp. 350, 189.

40　*Ibid.*, p. 234.

41　*Ibid.*, pp. 242, 323.

42　Prichard, *Diseases of the Nervous System*, p. 30 (original emphases).

43　*Ibid.*, p. 135.

44　Prichard, "Observations on the Connexions of Insanity with Diseases in the Organs of Physical Life". *Provincial Medical and Surgical Journal* 7 (1844): 323-24, p. 323.

45　Prichard, *Treatise on Insanity*, pp. 247-49.

46　The new title highlights the eminent role the concept of anthropology held in Germany.

47　The American alienist Pliny Earle saw it as the first German journal on insanity of any standing. See his *Institutions for the Insane in Prussia, Austria and Germany* (New York: Wood, 1854), pp. 19-26, 28-29. Cited in Richard Hunter, Ida Macalpine, *Three Hundred Years of Psychiatry*, 1963 (Hartsdale: Carlisle Publ., 1982), p. 1015.

48　Prichard, "Beobachtungen über die Beziehung des Gedächtnisses zum Gehirn". *Zeitschrift für die Anthropologie* 7 (1824): 243-50.

49　Prichard, *Treatise on Insanity*, pp. 32, 116-17, 138, 169, 178, 184, 194-98, 237-42, 248.

50　For biographical details of Nasse see Werner von Noorden, *Der Kliniker Christian Friedrich Nasse 1778-1851* (Jena: G. Fischer, 1929).

51　For Jacobi's theory see Klaus Dörner, *Bürger und Irre*, 2nd rev. ed. (Frankfurt: Syndikat/EVA, 1984), pp. 270ff; Gerlof Verwey, *Psychiatry in an Anthropological and Biomedical Context. Philosophical*

Presuppositions and Implications of German Psychiatry, 1820-1870
(Dordrecht: Reidel, 1984), pp. 27-30. Biographical data can be
found in the otherwise – i.e. politically – totally unacceptable
Johannes Herting, *Carl Wigand Maximilian Jacobi, ein deutscher Arzt
(1755-1858): Ein Lebensbild nach Briefen und anderen Quellen*
(Görlitz: Starke, 1930).

52   Carl Wigand Maximilian Jacobi, *Sammlungen für die Heilkunde der
Gemüthskrankheiten* (Elberfeld: Schönian'sche Buchhandlung, 1830),
part 1, pp. 43, 58, 34. Jacobi's *Sammlungen* comprise three texts: his
translation of Samuel Tuke's description of the York Retreat to which
he wrote a programmatic introduction (1822); *Ueber die physischen
Erscheinungen und ihre Beziehungen zum Organismus im gesunden
und kranken Zustande* (1825); *Beobachtungen über die Pathologie und
Therapie der mit Irreseyn verbundenen Krankheiten* (1830). As Dörner
notes, the cornerstones of Jacobi's theory were already developed in
1822; see Dörner, *Bürger und Irre*, p. 277.

53   Even though Jacobi asserted that the second volume of the
Sammlungen dealt mainly with the temperaments (*ibid.*, part 2, p.
vii), this side of his theory has hardly yet been given any
consideration. An exception is Edward Hare, "The History of
'Nervous Disorders' from 1600 to 1840, and a Comparison with
Modern Views". *British Journal of Psychiatry* 159 (1991): 37-45, pp.
41-42.

54   Jacobi, *Sammlungen*, part 1, p. 70; *ibid.*, part 2, p. 137.

55   Weiner mentions that Crichton too was an avid student of German
texts. But much as he emphasized the role of the passions for the rise
of insanity, he did not hold that the passions themselves might be
diseased. See Dora Weiner, "Mind and Body in the Clinic", pp. 334-
36, and Alexander Crichton, *An Inquiry into the Nature and Origin
of Mental Derangement, Comprehending a Concise System of the
Physiology and Pathology of the Human Mind and a History of the
Passions and their Effects*, 2 vols (London: T. Cadell Jr and W. Davies,
1798), 2: 95ff.

56   Traditional British nosology was based on the differentiation
between the "active" and the "intellectual" powers of mind. Cf.
Roger Smith, *Trial by Medicine. Insanity and Responsibility in
Victorian Trials* (Edinburgh: Edinburgh University Press, 1981), p.
38. But as Prichard's *Treatise* of 1822 illustrates, this division
introduced no genuine differentiation in the analytical treatment of
the two. Spurzheim was one of the first to assign two different seats
– both of them, of course, situated in the brain – to the emotive and
the intellectual faculties respectively; cf. Sigrid Oehler-Klein, *Die*

Schädellehre Franz Joseph Galls in Literatur und Kritik des 19. Jahrhunderts, Soemmerring Forschungen 8 (Stuttgart: Gustav Fischer Verlag, 1990), p. 330.

57 Jacobi, *Sammlungen*, part 1, p. 43. "Gemüth" is the old spelling of "Gemüt".

58 *Ibid.*, p. 34.

59 Dörner has emphasized the liberal politics of the "somatic school" among German alienists, some of whom indeed came to sit in the first democratically elected parliament of the Frankfurt Paulskirche that was established as a result of the revolution in 1848. He does not, however, give their religious ethics its due; see his *Bürger und Irre*, pp. 273-79.

60 Verwey, *Psychiatry*, p. 8. L. S. Jacyna, too, has pointed out that the juxtaposition of "moral" theories of insanity and a physicalist aetiology is "over-simple". See his "Somatic Theories of Mind and the Interests of Medicine in Britain, 1850-1879". *Medical History* 26 (1982): 233-58, p. 233.

61 Prichard, *Treatise on Insanity*, p. 8.

62 *Idem*, "Insanity", p. 137.

63 *Idem*, "Connexions of Insanity". *Provincial Medical and Surgical Journal* 7 (1844): 323-24, p. 323.

64 Weiner, "Mind and Body", p. 388.

65 Prichard, "Connexions of Insanity", pp. 323-24.

66 *Ibid.*

67 *Ibid.*

68 Jacobi, *Sammlungen*, part 2, p. 316.

69 For the political and social implications of French medicine see Charles Coulston Gillispie, *Science and Polity in France at the End of the Old Regime* (Princeton: Princeton University Press, 1980); Martin L. Gross, "The Lessened Focus of Feeling: A Transformation in French Physiology in the Early Nineteenth Century". *Journal of the History of Biology* 12 (1979): 231-71.

70 Prichard, "An Address Delivered at the Third Anniversary Meeting", p. 39.

71 Jacobi, *Sammlungen*, part 1, pp. 24-25. Cited in Prichard, *Treatise on Insanity*, p. 196 (Prichard's translation overstates the role of vices).

72 Especially when religious issues were touched upon, Prichard often expressed his views by quoting others.

73 Prichard, "Insanity", p. 115. Translated from Esquirol, "De la lypémanie ou mélancholie". In *idem, Des maladies mentales*, 1: 398-481, p. 401.

74 See Prichard, *Treatise on Insanity*, p. 192. Translated from Esquirol,

"Monomanie", p. 49.

75 It was one of the ten salient characteristics of moral insanity; see
    Prichard, "Insanity", p. 113.

76 Jacobi, *Sammlungen*, 2: 214.

77 This was an important factor in his attitude to racial theories: see
    Chapter 6.

78 Prichard, *Treatise on Insanity*, p. 189, see also his *Researches*, 3rd ed.,
    1: 175-76.

79 *Idem, Treatise on Insanity*, p. 190. The same idea was expressed in
    idem, Diseases of the Nervous System, p. 375.

80 *Idem*, "Insanity", p. 113 (my emphasis).

81 *Idem, Treatise on Insanity*, pp. 18-19.

82 Cf. Hilton, *The Age of Atonement*.

83 Prichard, "Insanity", p. 113.

84 *Idem, Treatise on Insanity*, p. 238.

85 *Ibid.*, p. 174.

86 *Idem*, "Insanity", p. 112.

87 A few years previously, the young alienist John Connolly condemned
    the indiscriminate confinement of people who were merely eccentric
    or depraved: *An Inquiry Concerning the Indications of Insanity* (1830).
    Prichard referred his readers to Connolly's book: *Treatise on Insanity*,
    p. 383.

88 *Idem, Treatise on Insanity*, p. 384ff.

89 *Idem, On the Different Forms of Insanity, in Relation to Jurisprudence.
    Designed for the Use of Persons Concerned in Legal Questions Regarding
    Unsoundness of Mind* (London: H. Baillière, 1842), p. 65. This
    pragmatic advice originated with John Haslam, *Medical Jurisprudence
    as it Relates to Insanity, According to the Law of England* (London: C.
    Hunter, 1817), p. 63.

90 *Idem, Treatise on Insanity*, p. 402.

91 Two parliamentary enquiries and the subsequent popularizations of
    their findings could not fail to make the public wary of malpractice
    in the asylums. See, e.g., Andrew Scull, *The Most Solitary of
    Afflictions. Madness and Society in Britain, 1700-1900* (New Haven:
    Yale University Press, 1993), pp. 115-46.

92 This conclusion follows from Prichard's writings, although he
    himself did not go to the length of developing it.

93 Prichard, *Treatise on Insanity*, p. 350, see also p. 175 where he
    discusses the truth of this hypothesis. Esquirol early on suggested
    that madness was a typical disease of civilization, see his *Des Passions,
    considérées comme causes, symptômes et moyens curatifs de l'aliénation
    mentale* (Paris: Didot Jeune, AN XIV [1805]), p. 15. For the

historiographical context see Mark D. Altschule, "The Concept of Civilization as a Social Evil in the Writings of Mid-Nineteenth Century Psychiatrists". In *idem, Essays in the History of Psychiatry*, 2nd rev. ed. (New York, London: Grune & Stratton, 1965), pp. 119-39; Jean-Christophe Coffin, "Is Modern Civilization Sick? The Response of Alienists in Mid-Nineteenth Century France". In *Proceedings of the 1st European Congress on the History of Psychiatry and Mental Health Care*, ed. Leonie de Goei, Joost Vijselaar (Rotterdam: Erasmus, 1993), pp. 267-75; Andrew Scull, "Was Insanity Increasing?" In *idem, Social Order/Mental Disorder. Anglo-American Psychiatry in Historical Perspective* (London: Routledge, 1989), pp. 239-49.

94 He did not enlarge on this notion, however, and, on the contrary, enumerated many cases of morally insane patients of the lower classes.

95 Prichard, "Insanity", p. 135.

96 In this he fell in line with contemporary feelings. See Ursula R. Q. Henriques, *Before the Welfare State: Social Administration in Early Industrial Britain* (London: Longmans, 1979).

97 In his doctoral thesis Esquirol explained in physiological terms why the sexual passions were so particularly delicate, see Esquirol, *Des Passions*, p. 12.

98 Cf. Prichard, *On the Different Forms of Insanity*, p. 2; *idem*, "Insanity", p. 112.

99 Eigen has shown that the attempts of consulting alienists to introduce the concept of moral insanity in the courtroom were on the whole unsuccessful. Eigen, *Witnessing Insanity*, pp. 149-52. See also Smith, *Trial by Medicine*, p. 123.

100 Cf. Michael Clark, "'Morbid Introspection', Unsoundness of Mind, and British Psychological Medicine, c. 1830-1900". In *The Anatomy of Madness*, ed. W. F. Bynum, Roy Porter, Michael Shepherd, 3 vols (London, vol. 1 and 2: Tavistock, vol. 3: Routledge, 1985-88), 3: 71-101.

101 John Kitching, "Lecture on Moral Insanity". *British Medical Journal* 1 (1857): 334-36, 389-91, 453-56. For notions of degeneracy in British psychiatry see, e.g., Janet Saunders, "Quarantining the Weak-Minded: Psychiatric Definitions of Degeneracy and the Late-Victorian Asylum". In *The Anatomy of Madness*, ed. W. F. Bynum *et al.*, 3: 273-96.

3

Physical Anthropology:
Natural Similarity

The older Prichard grew, the more he insisted that the mind could not be explained through reference to rationality and utilitarian expediency alone. Nor was it sufficient to blame "passion" – that eighteenth-century goblin-like bastard brother of prudent rationality – for deviations in behaviour and thought. His theory of madness, as we have seen, testifies to the fact that he regarded "gloom" and darkness as intrinsic to consciousness. Whatever his adversaries claimed, he was convinced that it was precisely this side of the human character which proved beyond doubt the unity of mankind: a "persuasion of moral demerit or a consciousness of guilt", and the search for atonement, were engraved onto the mind of all human beings. His ensuing ideas of the psyche he himself considered as the foundation stone of a new science: psychology. Before we can examine this issue more closely, however, we must make ourselves familiar with the wider framework of Prichard's natural history of mankind. This chapter will delineate the background of, and the foundations upon which he based, his belief in the unity of the human species.

The third edition of the *Researches into the Physical History of Mankind* (1836-47) was the mature form in which the results of decades of learning coalesced. Whilst Prichard's theories manifest a high degree of consistency (allowing us in many instances to talk about his opinions *tout court*, in the understanding that they did not change), he had to adjust his ideas to developments in his own outlooks and within the sciences. In the following we shall see in which respects his views evolved between 1808, when his M. D. dissertation was published, and 1847 when the third edition of the *Researches* was completed.

Prichard was a man of convictions, and hence of opponents. The latter were mainly of two different types: materialists, and all those who supported the rising theory of race. From Prichard's viewpoint, both sorts tended to pull at the same end of the rope, for they denied the greater part of mankind their birthright as Adam and Eve's children. The terms used to describe the dispute he was involved in date from a later period: monogenists and polygenists were, respectively, the two conflicting factions who supported or denied the common descent of mankind.

The Monogenist–Polygenist Controversy

Given the abundance of eighteenth-century monogenists, it has been suggested that "the idea of the unity of mankind was hardly contested during the eighteenth century".[1] True as this might be, there were eighteenth-century authors who nonetheless espoused polygenesis. Three trains of thought paved the way for this development. Carl Linné had distinguished between (a) the human species created in the image of God, (b) anthropoid Troglodytes, and other creatures located between the ape-type and (c) mankind as created in the image of God.[2] The assumption of a hierarchy, compatible with the Chain of Being, descending from man through anthropoid creatures to apes, was easily reconcilable with the notion that non-European peoples, those of black skin colour in particular, constituted a specific branch of the human family ranged somewhere between white humans and apes. Linnaeus's approach to nature was imbued by his version of protestantism, comprising the assumption that animals too had souls, while rejecting the notions of original sin and atonement. For Linnaeus who liked to think of himself as "the second Adam", the Troglodytes could assume the role of "lesser" humans – likewise, for many nineteenth-century polygenists, a majority of all non-European "races" held that position.[3]

The other train of thought which led to polygenism was famously supported by the Scottish philosophizing lawyer Henry Home, Lord Kames (1696-1782). A polygenist doctrine was Kames's solution to the problem debated in Scotland in the second half of the eighteenth century: the dispersion of human and animal populations. Instead of holding that mankind had spread across the globe thanks to the agency of Providence, Kames maintained that there were several distinct human races.[4]

Yet another source of polygenist thinking arose in the early 1800s in Gall and Spurzheim's phrenology: if individual faculties were innate and heritable, the same must hold for racial character as well.[5] By assigning "human understanding" to the realm of natural history, the phrenologists underscored the process of levelling the special status in natural history which mankind had traditionally been accorded.[6] By deducing individual psychological conformations from the shape of the cranium, phrenology provided a useful tool for the polygenists. It is surely no accident that France, with its great number of anatomists who sympathized with phrenology, contributed heavily to the rise of racial theory between the 1820s and the 1840s.[7]

Among British religious writers it was commonly assumed that the assault on the unity of species was a typical product of French Enlightenment materialism. Voltaire's outright polygenism and his contempt for religion were regarded as two sides of the same coin.[8] In 1836 the future Cardinal Nicholas Wiseman remarked that Prichard's polygenist opponents were "to be found chiefly among French naturalists, who unfortunately are yet, in part at least, unreclaimed from the sceptical theories of the last century".[9] By the early 1840s, Prichard himself believed that he had been driven into a corner: the influence of French materialism had made itself felt in Britain and, as he saw it, only Germany had not yet been besieged by anti-religious tendencies and egotistical utilitarianism.

In the 1830s the cast of Prichard's theoretical enemies comprised eight principal figures, four of them French.[10] Among the latter were the traveller Jean-Baptiste-George-Marie Bory de Saint Vincent (1780-1846)[11] and the doctor Julien-Joseph Virey (1775-1846), who advanced the idea that mankind was originally divided into the white and the black "species".[12] Add to them Louis-Antoine Desmoulins (1794-1828) who started his physiological career as a protégé of Cuvier at the Muséum d'Histoire Naturelle. In the early 1820s, however, he fell out with his mentor. Vexed and of a stubborn disposition, he sealed his fate by publishing his *Histoire naturelle des races humaines* (1826) in which he asserted the existence of no fewer than sixteen originally different human species. Not only was the number exceptional: Desmoulins detected racial distinctions in the history of civilized Europe itself.[13] That a disciple of Cuvier should have published these ideas did not appear at all curious to Prichard: Cuvier himself, "the pope of bones",[14] was after all on his list of polygenists, for in 1812 he had suggested that Europeans, Asiatics and "Negroes" had survived the Flood on different mountain tops.[15] Although Cuvier was no polygenist, properly speaking, Prichard included him among the culprits.

Those, non-French thinkers whom Prichard scorned for their polygenism included the travelling surgeon Johann Baptist von Spix (1781-1826) and Carl Friedrich Philip von Martius (1794-1868), a naturalist who was to become Professor of Botany at Munich University. On the orders of the Bavarian king, Spix and Martius had accompanied an Austrian expedition to Brazil from 1817 to 1820. In "a very strong" and, as it appeared to Prichard, "an exaggerated" manner they had described the "inhumanising" (his translation of "Entmenschung") of the Brazilians.[16] As his erstwhile esteem for Spix and Martius's exploits waned, Prichard came to doubt even the monogenist mind-set of another South America-traveller: Alexander von Humboldt who was perhaps less of a self-conscious philanthropist than Prichard, but certainly at least as much of a humanist. In his growing exasperation Prichard wrongly counted Humboldt among the proponents of racial differentiations.[17]

Monogenism was obviously a crucial doctrine within Christianity. Most historians have taken this for granted, so much so that accounts of early anthropology pay little regard to exact theological context. That was to be elucidated most clearly by a man who departed from orthodox belief: in his reminiscences of his personal religious strife, Francis Newman (1805-97), brother of the Catholic convert John Henry Newman, explained the pernicious religious implications of polygenism. It contradicted the theory of one original couple, Adam and Eve, and it ran counter to crucial Biblical tenets, including the Noachian as well as the Abrahamitic covenant, the doctrine of original sin, and the universal moral submission of mankind under the Christian dispensation. Yet, after a phase of religious qualms, Newman emerged as a polygenist whose creed had become much more liberal than that of the Anglican church. In *Phases of Faith* (1850) he described how Thomas Arnold, the historian and illustrious headmaster of Rugby school who had occasionally clashed with orthodox Anglicans, sowed the seeds of doubt in his heart:

> I had become aware of the difficulties encountered by physiologists in believing the whole human race to have proceeded in about 6000 years from a single Adam and Eve; and that the longevity (not miraculous, but ordinary) attributed to the patriarchs was another stumbling-block. The geological difficulties of the Mosaic cosmogony were also at that time exciting much attention. To my surprise, Dr. Arnold treated all these questions as matters of indifference to religion; and did not hesitate to say, that the account of Noah's deluge was evidently mythical, and the history of Joseph 'a beautiful poem'. I was staggered at this. If all were not descended from Adam, what became of St. Paul's parallel between the first and second Adam [i.e. Christ], and the doctrine of Headship and Atonement founded on it?[18]

Newman – he was a friend of Prichard, teaching Mathematics at

Bristol College[19] – drew the conclusion that it was impossible to hold orthodox Christian beliefs and be, at the same time, conscientious in scientific enquiry. Yet Arnold's example showed him that he need not see himself as a religious renegade.

Newman's was a liberty Prichard never assumed. To demonstrate the validity of monogenesis, the Quaker's son grappled with problems from all the natural and human sciences: anatomy, physiology, biology, ethnology, palaeontology, archaeology, mythology, and philology. Referring humanity to a common lineage, he was obliged to formulate a hereditary theory which guaranteed the unity of the human species while yet accounting for its diversities.

An Anatomy of the *Researches*

The *Researches into the Physical History of Man* was first published in 1813. In two subsequent editions (1826 and 1836-47) Prichard changed "Man" into "Mankind", thereby stressing that it was man as a biological species he was dealing with.[20] In these two editions, each more than twice as voluminous as the preceding, he added to, and amended, his findings in the light of the latest scientific discoveries and the increasing body of travel literature. The third edition was divided into one volume dealing with theory (1836), and four further volumes dealing with the "ethnography" of mankind: in Africa (1837), Europe (1841), Asia (1844), Oceania and America (1847), all of them profusely footnoted. From the second edition, all his ethnological works were embellished with engravings; some of these he had acquired on the recommendation of Blumenbach (including favourites of early ethnography such as the portrait of the native Aethiopian clergyman Abbas Gregorius), others he had ordered himself from the workshop of the Englishman Alexander Day (1773-1841) and from the Belgian painter and lithographer Louis Haghe (1802-85).[21] His friend Hodgkin introduced him to the works of the American painter George Catlin, whose portraits of American Indians were exhibited in London. Hodgkin even helped to arrange for the reproduction of Catlin's pictures in *The Natural History of Man*.[22]

All the illustrations were highly praised, one reviewer of *The Natural History of Man* remarking that the high price of half a crown per instalment of 48 pages was justified (the price for the entire book was £1 10s., equalling two weeks' wages for a labourer).[23] The idea that illustrations were vital for ethnographical descriptions had already been emphasized by Blumenbach. In the late eighteenth century human varieties were characterized not so much by their

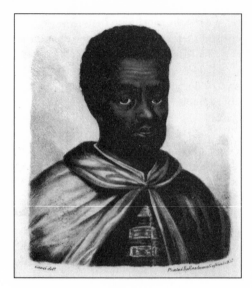

Figure 1
Abbas Gregorius

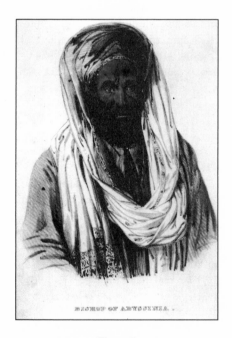

Figure 2
The Bishop of Abyssinia

62

Figure 1
Prichard obtained this portrait of the black clergyman Abbas Gregorius
thanks to Blumenbach who himself had not used it in his own
publications. Aiming to underline the scientificity of his endeavours,
Prichard no longer used anthropological sceneries as Blumenbach had done
around the turn of the nineteenth century. The portrait was inserted in the
second edition of the *Researches of the Physical History of Mankind* (London:
John and Arthur Arch, 1826). The caption informed the spectator that
Abbas Gregorius possessed "frizzy hair, like other Ethiopians".

Figure 2
In the third edition of the *Researches* (London: Sherwood, Gilbert, Piper,
1836-47) Prichard replaced the portrait of Abbas Gregorius by that of a
"Bishop of Abyssinia". He had it produced by the lithographers Alexander
Day (1773-1841) and Louis Haghe (1802-85). While Abbas Gregorius
displayed stereotypical "Negro" features, the Bishop of Abyssinia, though
his skin was black, confirmed Prichard's assertion that many black people
had a rather "European" countenance.

---

specific physiognomy, but by their surroundings.[24] Eighteenth-
century illustrations of "savage" peoples put them into settings akin
to the imaginary landscape of the Garden of Eden,[25] provision for
ethnological and geographical specificities was made by the addition
of characteristic items of clothing, "primitive" dwellings, and plants
allegedly typical of the region. By the 1820s the style of ethnological
iconography had changed: in those illustrations used by Prichard, the
individuals were removed from their picturesque backgrounds, most
of them being depicted only from head to waist. When the third
(posthumous) edition of Cuvier's *Règne animal* came out in 1836-49,
everything from the neck down had disappeared.[26] While many
pictures were included simply because they were available, others
clearly reflect Prichard's intentions and ideas. Thus it was a rather
spectacular choice to use the portrait of a black Indian, Rajah
Ramohun Roy, as a frontispiece to the third volume of the third
edition of the *Researches* that deals with "European" ethnology.[27]

The knowledge Prichard had amassed was staggering. Indeed, it
is easier to enumerate the gaps, rather than the sources, of his
learning. Among the notable omissions in his material is Charles
Darwin's Beagle *Journal* (1839). And whereas Darwin, for his part,
began to study embryology in the late 1830s, Prichard did not take
Karl Ernst von Baer's embryology into account, with rather negative

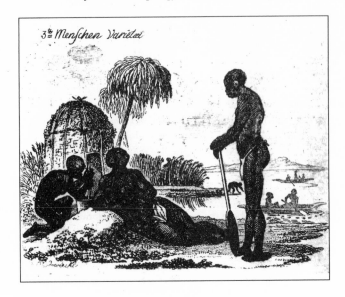

Figure 3
Blumenbach's Ethiopian Variety

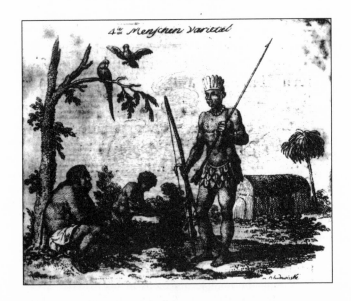

Figure 4
Blumenbach's American Variety

Figures 3 and 4
The third and fourth human varieties of Blumenbach's classification: the
"Ethiopians" and the "Americans". The draughtsman took care to show
entire families, and they are depicted within what at the time was perceived
as their natural habitats. The scenery also shows details of life-style and
acquired arts, such as bow-hunting and boat building. The feathers of the
West Indian head-dress duplicate the equally colourful plumage of parrots.
(From: Johann Friedrich Blumenbach, *Beyträge zur Naturgeschichte*, 2 vols,
Göttingen: J. C. Dieterich, 1790-1811.)

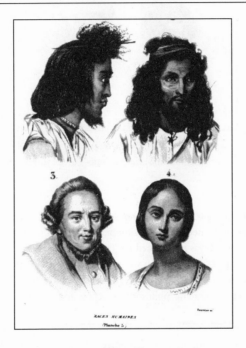

Figure 5
Cuvier's Caucasian Variety – Semitic branch

Figure 5
In Georges Cuvier's multi-volume natural history *Le règne animal* – the third
edition was completed by Cuvier's disciples after the master's death in 1832 –
each human variety, as well as sub-varieties, was depicted in various degrees
of civilization. Thus, the Semitic branch of the Caucasian variety was
represented by the German philosopher Moses Mendelssohn and by barbaric
tribesmen (Jean Victor Audouin *et al.*, *Le règne animal distribué d'après son
organisation*, 3rd ed., 22 vols, Paris: Fortin, Masson, 1836-49, vol. 1).

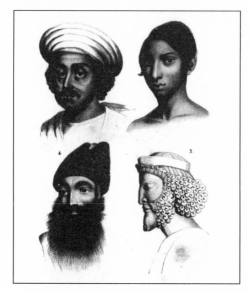

Figure 6
Cuvier's Caucasian Variety – Indo-European branch

Figure 6
The tables in *Le règne animal* were not just synchronically, but also diachronically organised: the Indo-European branch of the Caucasian variety of mankind was represented by (clockwise from the top left) an Indian Brahmin, a "young Indian woman", a statue from Persepolis, and a modern Persian. In 1817 Cuvier wrote that this branch of the "Caucasian race" had excelled more in "philosophy, sciences and arts" than any other human race.

consequences for his ideas of heredity.[28] One of his translators, the German scholar August Wilhelm Schlegel, believed that he was "paradoxical, but erudite", and his knowledge not always up to date.[29] Prichard never ceased quoting from the canon of classical literature. He valued the sagacity of pagan Roman authors and their temporal closeness to the antiquity of mankind. Naturally, he followed travel literature and held accounts of missionaries in especially high regard, for "through long residence ... and by a thorough acquaintance with the language and habits of the inhabitants" missionaries were "well qualified" to write on foreign peoples.[30] Other fields in which he was well read were comparative anatomy and natural history, including the writings of Geoffroy St Hilaire and Cuvier. He rarely explicitly referred to transmutationist doctrines and those of French materialists, of which he was aware and to which he was thoroughly opposed (as will be explained in Chapter 4). Equally, he was familiar with, though not a great admirer of, German physiological writings in the vein of *Naturphilosophie* and transcendental taxonomy. Thus, he never stressed organicism in the manner of the *Naturphilosophen*.[31] If he likened the growth of nations to that of the individual, it was in line with Enlightenment thought, rather in view of education than the biological development of a nation's rise to maturity. From German thinking Prichard expressly adopted only those tenets that passed the test of scientificity. Unlike the more imaginative Carlyle or Coleridge, he never annoyed his countrymen by referring them to the complexities of German philosophy, which in Britain were widely perceived as metaphysical jabbering.

In Prichard's England the inductive method was extolled as the correct approach in the natural sciences.[32] Professing adherence to induction signalled the readiness of the scientist to be guided not by preconceived principles but by evidence and experiment. Prichard favoured proper inductive studies over "the lucubrations of Herder and other diffuse writers", which

> abound in generalisations, often in the speculative flights of a discursive fancy, and afford little or no aid for the close induction from facts, which is the aim of the present work.[33]

To Prichard the "anti-rationalistic"[34] concept of "Volk" appeared dubious in context of anthropological matters. Herder spoke, albeit with reverence, of the Bible as an "old lore ... a national tale".[35] Prichard considered the Bible a sacred document testifying to historical, revealed faith. It was no wonder that Herder's theories appeared to the British doctor vague and speculative.

Nonetheless, the influence of German literature on Prichard's works is striking, Johann Friedrich Blumenbach (1752-1840) being his role model of an anthropological scholar. Later, Christian Carl Josias Bunsen, the philosophical philologist, and the geographer Carl Ritter (1779-1859) also counted among those authors whose writings he would carry around in the roomy side-pockets of his overcoat. In addition he engaged in extensive correspondence with scholars throughout Europe and North America to complete his stock of information.

From his M.D. dissertation, all his enquiries "into the physical history of mankind" were built around the same theoretical core which it is useful first to summarize before discussing its particulars.

Prichard divided the monogenist hypothesis into two necessary propositions which he tried to prove one after the other: first, that, on physiological grounds, all mankind belonged to one species, and second, that they were referable to one single place of origin.[36] He then proceeded to delineate his "methods of inquiry", basing the doctrine of the unity of mankind on four arguments:

(a) Mankind was one because all functions of the human organism took place according to the same "principal Laws of the Animal Economy", including the duration of life, the period of uterogestation, the number of progeny, etc.[37]

(b) All mankind was prone to the same diseases.

(c) Buffon's criterion of hybridity to account for species unity applied to mankind. According to that idea only animals of one and the same species could procreate with each other, so as to engender fertile offspring. Since mixed marriages between individuals of all human varieties fulfilled this prerequisite, all mankind was one species.

(d) The "analogical method" was extremely useful: the laws of the natural history of animals were, *ceteris paribus*, true for mankind as well. Since differences within one animal species were often far greater than those to be found among human varieties, mankind, by inference, was clearly a single species.[38]

Having explained his arguments in favour of the specific unity of mankind, Prichard set out to prove that all humans originated in one quarter of the globe. It is clear that he had the old Biblical terrain in mind. To demonstrate the truth of monogenesis he relied on three methods of investigation:

(a) He discussed the distribution of organized beings, showing that each individual species came from one specific centre of creation.

(b) He ventured into philology to show that all human languages were related and thence referable to one root.

(c) He showed that the myths of all human cultures were so similar that they all must share the same primeval history.[39]

All three editions of the *Researches* follow this outline. In *The Natural History of Man*, however, Prichard departed in certain aspects from this pattern. Published in 1843, the book was intended as a summary of the *Researches*, more easily accessible than the five-volume opus into which the work had grown. It was published in instalments, in the expectation that it would attract a large, and not necessarily very affluent, audience. The calculation proved right: the year 1855 saw the publication of the fourth edition.[40] In *The Natural History of Man* the emphasis of the argument lay on biology. Whereas the second and third editions of the *Researches* start off with a delineation of the distribution of plants and animals, *The Natural History of Man* begins with a detailed discussion of the causes of variation in animals and mankind. Hence, for instance, the issue of changes in instinct is given a more prominent place than in the *Researches*. For Prichard, the rise of racial theory was made possible through materialist philosophy. If it was kept alive by so many physiologists and natural historians, one of the reasons for this was linguistic confusion. From the second edition Prichard was very much aware of the terminological deficiencies and he carefully explained what he understood by the words he used.

"Genus" and "Species", "Race" and "Variety"

The most complex term – disputed to this day – is the concept of "race". The English term is derived from the French. Originally it designated the royal families who governed France from the middle ages. By the eighteenth century the term was often employed as one of several more or less synonymous translations of the Latin "gens" and "genus". Other translations included the terms "stock" and "tribe", "family" and "nation". During the Enlightenment the word "race" was unproblematic because the Latin texts, which determined its meaning, distinguished mainly between nations as political entities and tribes or families as natural entities. The ambiguity of the nineteenth-century understanding of the term "people", with its cultural, genealogical and political connotations, was not at issue in the Latin texts which lay at the basis of pre-modern learning.[41]

The problem with "race", as Prichard saw it, was that the term had no particular meaning. Indeed, natural historians of the eighteenth century had done without clear-cut definitions of crucial terms such as "genus", "species", "variety", and "race". As Goodfield and Toulmin have stressed, in the eighteenth century "species was an intellectual fiction, not a reality".[42] Prichard rightly perceived the desirability of clear definitions:

> The meaning attached to the term *species* in natural history includes only the following conditions, namely, separate origin and distinctness of race, evinced by the constant transmission of some characteristic peculiarity of organization. A race of animals or of plants marked by any peculiar character which has always been constant and undeviating, constitutes a species; and two races are considered as specifically different, if they are distinguished from

each other by some characteristic which the one cannot be supposed to have acquired, or the other to have lost through any known operation of physical causes.[43]

While "species" were explained according to the criterion of lineage, the denomination of "genus" was rather a question of resemblance: "a genus is to be considered as an assortment of tribes, on a principle merely of resemblance, and it may, therefore, include more or fewer species, according to the particular views of the naturalist".[44] How one delineated a genus hinged upon the taxonomic system one followed. Species, by contrast, were, as it were, natural facts. The same applied to varieties:

> Varieties, in natural history, are such diversities in individuals and their progeny as are observed to take place within the limits of species. Varieties are modifications produced in races of animals and of plants by the agency of external causes; they are ... hereditary, or transmitted to offspring with greater or less degrees of constancy.[45]

The last crucial element of Prichard's terminological set-up refers to the notion of "permanent varieties". By this term he understood a specific form of hereditary trait: "permanent varieties are these which having once taken place, continue to be propagated in the breed in perpetuity. The fact of their origination must be known by observation or inference."[46] The man who is likely to have inspired this concept was the Paris physiologist William Frédéric Edwards (1776-1842).[47] As we shall see in Chapter 6, Edwards came up with the notion of permanent racial traits in order to support French liberals who opposed the *ancien régime* aristocracy. To serve his political convictions he introduced racial theorizing into historical inquiry.[48] Later, his doctrines were eagerly taken up by supporters of racial theory. Failing to perceive Edwards's hidden agenda, Prichard credited him for being one of the very few authors who endeavoured to investigate "the physical and moral characters of nations in connection with the races from which they are descended, and the nature of the countries which they inhabit".[49]

Prichard was all the more pleased about this endeavour as he had always, albeit implicitly, assumed the existence of permanent varieties.[50] Otherwise he could hardly have accepted – and then amended – Blumenbach's delineation of five human varieties. To make his viewpoint abundantly clear Prichard explained why he thought that "race" was a category not to be employed by the natural historian of mankind:

The instances are so many in which it is doubtful whether a particular tribe is to be considered as a distinct species, or only as a variety of some other tribe, that it has been found by naturalists convenient to have a designation applicable in either case. Hence the late introduction of the term race in this indefinite sense. Races are properly successions of individuals propagated from any given stock; and the term should be used without any involved meaning that such a progeny or stock has always possessed a particular character. The real import of the term has often been overlooked, and the word race has been used as if it implied a distinction in the physical character of the whole series of individuals. By writers on anthropology, who adopt this term, it is often tacitly assumed that such distinctions were primordial, and that their successive transmission has been unbroken. If such were the fact, a race so characterised would be a species in the strict meaning of the word, and it ought to be so termed.[51]

A few years later, "race" was commonly understood in just this manner. Against the backdrop of contemporary biological knowledge, however, these lines were a powerful refutation of racial theorizing.

Prichard's ideas about which aspect of the human constitution was least liable to variation changed over time. In the first edition of the *Researches*, he believed that skin colour was the most distinctive trait distinguishing the varieties of mankind. By the second edition, he had come to consider the "animal economy" as the most stable part. In the third edition he added human psychology. The important point is that fixity of species, for him, allowed the existence of a certain range of variation. And "permanent varieties" were merely the crystallization of some of these. Time and again he emphasized that the whole range of bodily conformations could spring up in all varieties. This chapter, however, is concerned with the arguments he put forward in order to demonstrate the unity of the human species, and we shall next examine the theoretical strategies he deployed for this purpose and which he himself, of course, considered as the instruments for an analysis of the natural history of mankind.

Prichard advanced several different criteria of species unity which did not all carry equal weight for him. Since the hybridity argument had been attacked by many naturalists, he gave greater emphasis to analogical reasoning. This was important to the way he tackled the problem of man's place in nature. Having adopted it from Johann

Friedrich Blumenbach, he was its foremost proponent in Britain. The significance of the laws of the animal economy had also been ascertained by Blumenbach: in view of species characterization, the dead carcass of an animal was less helpful than the general "habitus" of the living specimen.[52] The notion was in line with the late eighteenth-century conviction that it was not anatomy alone which gave insights into animal physiology, but the physiological mechanisms of the living organisms themselves. Prichard's indebtedness to Blumenbach can hardly be exaggerated.[53] Under his influence he discarded the emphasis which he had earlier placed on physiognomical particulars. From the 1820s his analysis aimed at both "structure and habitudes" of living beings.[54]

Like Blumenbach, Prichard claimed that the similarity of the functions pertaining to the animal economy was a sure indicator of the unity of mankind. What applied to the functions of the animal economy was, as a matter of course, true for its malfunctions as well. In 1813, he had merely speculated on the usefulness of disease patterns as a criterion of conspecificity.[55] By 1826 he had firm opinions on the subject, citing Blumenbach, Thomas Winterbottom (a colonial doctor in Sierra Leone), the Edinburgh-trained Philadelphia physician Benjamin Rush, and the traveller William Keating, in order to establish that, within a certain geographical latitude, all mankind was prone to the same ailments: "if we inquire into the history of the diseases which infect the different races of men, we find nothing which seems to indicate a specific distinction in these races, but on the contrary, a number of facts which render the unity of species the more probable conclusion".[56]

From early on Prichard had a perception of the genuine distinctions between collective characteristics and behaviour on the one hand (including family resemblances and national or typological characteristics), and individual traits on the other. "It appears", he wrote in 1813, "that the principle in the animal oeconomy on which the production of varieties in the race depends, is entirely distinct from that which regards the changes produced by external causes on the individual."[57] Following Blumenbach as well as Buffon, he believed that the individual need not conform in all peculiarities to the definition of its type. In 1813 he evoked Blumenbach's description of the original Egyptian physiognomy in terms of an "if I may so call it, ideal archetype". He also referred to the Indian "prototype".[58]

In his *Beyträge zur Naturgeschichte* Blumenbach had delimited the cognitive bridge between natural fact and the interpretation of the naturalist: "for all the accounts on that point which one adopts, even with the most critical judgment possible, from others, are in reality, for the truth-seeking investigator of nature, nothing more and nothing further than a kind of symbolical writing, which he can only so far subscribe to with a good conscience, as they actually coincide with the open book of nature".[59] Even more than Blumenbach's, Prichard's writings are marked by the assumption that the typical characteristics of any human variety were merely a kind of guide-line for the anthropologist: in reality individuals might deviate in all aspects from the characterization of their particular ethnicity.[60] Empirical descriptions of individual traits, he believed, made it difficult to define the range of typical forms; the variability of nature precluded this. His frequent references to notions of "type" account for his need to create a space where empirical observation and his quest for order could meet. For Blumenbach and Prichard alike, the notion of "type" was a loose category. It offered the possibility of classifying without obliging the naturalist to subsume the totality of any observed population under any typological heading.[61]

Classification, however, was one thing. It was natural connection Prichard was after: the genealogical relationships of human varieties. As we have seen above, his criteria for species unity were tied to a theory of hybridity and a theory of the laws of the animal economy. These provided the natural "laws" at the basis of Prichard's monogenist theorizing. Its other aspects, including the historical proofs he adduced and the mechanisms that allowed for the development of variation within the human species, will be dealt with in other chapters. Here we are concerned with the question of how Prichard turned to analogical reasoning as well as the hybridity argument, and how he applied those concepts to his particular cause. Since there were some authors who asserted that one and the same species could have originated from various geographical areas, he also set out to prove that this was wrong, and that every species came from a single centre of creation. This discussion, which was couched in contemporary biogeography, will also be considered in detail here.

The "Analogical Method" and the Argument from Hybridity

In the Linnaean tradition, theories of hybridity were neatly intertwined with deliberations as to the natural origin of species.[62] On the assumption that the world was originally peopled only by "genera", Linnaeus was compelled to believe that all species were engendered by way of hybridization.[63] Crossbreeding animals of different genera produced new species, these in turn were the propagators of yet further species.

As Linnaeus subsumed humans and apes under the common category of quadrumana it was arguable that both kinds had common generic roots. In the eighteenth century this idea did not have many followers. Only figures as eccentric as Lord Monboddo and Jean-Jacques Rousseau would "bend the stubborn neck of man down to the earth" and toy with the idea that mankind had sprung from apes.[64] In order to disprove their allegations Blumenbach resorted to exempting the human species from the genus of quadrumana, assigning to them the denomination of "bimanus" – two-handed.[65] Other naturalists corrected the Linnaean natural philosophy by means of re-interpreting the theory of hybrids.

Far from accepting hybridization as the source of species evolution, Buffon (1707-88), John Hunter (1728-93), the Italian physiologist Lazzaro Spallanzani (1729-99), as well as Eberhardt August Wilhelm Zimmermann (1743-1815) and Immanuel Kant (1724-1804) adopted cross-fertility as a species criterion.[66] Those animal groups belonged to one species, their argument ran, which could procreate with each other and engender fertile offspring. Soon after this theory was put forward it was denied by the British naturalist Thomas Pennant (1726-98) and the German Peter Simon Pallas (1741-1811).[67] The difficulty of properly classifying closely related animals, such as dogs, wolves and jackals, or the horse, mule and ass, gave rise to manifold speculations concerning the conspecificity of dogs and the fertility of mules. Dubious reports about fertile hybrids were circulating. Buffon himself admitted that there were some animals, such as the horse and ass, whose breeding habits seemed to contradict the theory.[68] Blumenbach, for his part, doubted that all dogs belonged to one species. Consequently, he provided the monogenist doctrine with yet another leg to stand on: the "argument from analogy" came into play.[69] As this chapter deals with the grounds on which Prichard established the unity of mankind, only those aspects of analogical reasoning will be explained here that furthered the argument. In the next chapter we shall explore the limits he set on analogies between humans and lesser animals.

Conventionally, the term "analogy" was used to denote the relationships between the known and the unknown. In 1736 Joseph Butler (1692-1752) published his *Analogy of Religion, Natural and Revealed, to the Constitution and Course of Nature.* Nature itself was a visible analogue for the inscrutable wisdom of God. Another much-used analogy compared the mechanisms of the animal economy to those of national economies. Naturalists working in the Linnaean mould founded taxonomies on the criterion of resemblance. After the turn of the century, however, the discovery of morphological or functional analogies came increasingly into fashion.[70] Departing from Newton's method of setting out "axioms", reasoning from analogy was deemed congenial to nature, narrowing the gap between the human mind and natural creation. With the rise of comparative anatomy, the value of the "analogical method" was proved, comparative anatomy being, as it were, a specific branch of it.

The analogical idea was conceptually attractive for two reasons: it presented the world as a harmonious network of interrelated phenomena, and it seemed to provide a method for an understanding of the book of nature. Prichard's friend Thomas Hodgkin praised "the doctrine of analogies, and of an unity of plan pervading the whole animal kingdom".[71] Applied to the question of monogenesis the analogical method worked in the following manner: if any characteristic differences between human varieties could be found to exist within one single animal species, it was inadmissible to evoke it as a proof of polygenism.[72] Therefore, Prichard delved into animal physiology, convinced that he could understand human nature only through the pathology as well as the physiology of animals: whether all humans belonged to the same species could be answered only through knowledge of the animal realm. There were two questions: what were the criteria for species unity in the animal realm? And did the result apply to mankind?

Taking up Buffon's theory of hybridity, Prichard noted that there was, indeed, a growing number of examples of seemingly fertile hybrids. He discounted, however, their importance. Yet he was well aware that Buffon himself had found reason to doubt his own theory. Prichard remarked that doubts were also raised by the Swedish botanist Anders Sparrman (1747-1820), the Frenchmen Cuvier and Geoffroy Saint-Hilaire, and the Germans Gottfried Reinhold Treviranus (1776-1837), who coined the term "biology", and Carl Asmund Rudolphi (1771-1832).[73] The latter produced a long list instancing all the fertile hybrids known to natural history.[74]

When still at the height of his research activity Prichard avoided tackling "instances" that were "quite sufficient to shake our confidence" in Buffon's doctrine. Instead of seriously engaging with the problems inherent to the hybridity argument he contemplated the beauty of creation: if different species could interbreed, the world might present "a scene of confusion". Since that was apparently not the case there must be some natural principle that "maintains the order and variety of the animal creation".[75]

Other writers asserted that there was a natural repugnance

prohibiting mutual attraction between members of different human families.[76] Prichard, by contrast, insisted that all human populations were devoid of that sort of repulsion. In fact, certain cultures preferred spouses from foreign ethnic groups: "it is said, indeed, that the Turks and other people of the East, choose Negro women for their harems, and it is well known that black men often prefer white women". The latter could be perceived even in England: "indeed, most of the black men who come to England from the West Indies as domestic servants, and continue to reside here, contrive to get English wives" – at this point a polygenist might have interrupted, suggesting that it was no wonder if blacks had a taste for superior species. Nipping the objection in the bud, Prichard continued that the penchant of black men for white women "is a proof, not only of their own good taste in this respect, but also that our countrywomen, the lower orders of them at least, have no invincible repugnance to the Negro race".[77]

The subject of natural repulsion against other human "races" is crucial because, for a while, it held a central place in the arguments of racial theoreticians. From the middle of the nineteenth century it formed part of the idea that it was detrimental to racial development if this supposedly natural barrier between the races was breached. Nineteenth-century racialists were obsessed with purity of race. Arthur de Gobineau (1816-82), the eccentric writer on history who styled himself a count, believed that the infusion of alien blood had been the reason for both the development of European culture but also the subsequent degeneration of European races.[78] The Scottish anatomist Robert Knox (1791-1862) was less equivocal, considering racial mongrels as a "monstrosity of nature" destined for extinction.[79] Contrast these notions with Prichard's insistence that intermixture among human varieties was good, and that, in no small measure, the Europeans owed their favourable physical and mental endowments to it.

In the third edition of the *Researches* and in the *Natural History of Man* Prichard devoted an entire section to the topic of "mixed human races" (denying the scientific significance of the term "race", he would use it interchangeably with "tribe", "nation", or "people").[80] Intermixture between human populations was not only possible: it was desirable. Experimenting animal breeders had discovered that crossbreeding was necessary to keep up the quality of a horse breed. The idea had been put forward by Peter Simon Pallas (1741-1811), the German geologist and natural historian, who held, as a reviewer put it, "all our domestic animals to be strictly mongrels, combining the good points of numerous independent wild species".[81] A similar remark was made by the Spanish naturalist Felix de Azara (1742-1821), whom Prichard frequently cited in the second and third edition of the *Researches* to illustrate his assertion that "the intermixture of varieties is well known occasionally to improve the breed in both the vegetable and animal kingdoms".[82]

From the 1830s Prichard laid increasing weight on the discussion of human intermixture. Quoting Azara's insights into horsebreeding, he emphasized that intermarriages were wholesome for the stock: "in Paraguay, the mixed breed constitutes, according to Azara, a great majority of the people termed Spaniards or white men; and they are said to be a people superior in physical qualities to either of the races from which they have sprung, and much more prolific than the aborigines."[83] The same was true nearer home: the intermixture between Celtic, Slavonic, and "German or Teuton" tribes "has produced breeds physically superior to the majority of either ancestral race".[84]

While it was fine to claim the positive results of interbreeding, Prichard also had to demonstrate that interbreeding was, as it were, all the more natural for mankind as it had started out as one single family, in one geographical spot.

Biogeography: The Single Origin of Mankind

After having established on bio-medical grounds the unity of mankind, Prichard went on to show that all human varieties had been engendered in one geographical location. He did not doubt that mankind had survived in an ark and that it had subsequently dispersed across the globe during many centuries of migratory movements.[85] With respect to animals, however, this belief was already heavily contested during the eighteenth century: there were so many populations whose habitats lay much too far away from the region where Noah supposedly had built the vessel – how could they have entered the ark? How was it possible that, after their release, they did not immediately fall prey to each other? Eberhardt August Wilhelm Zimmermann (1743-1815), Professor of Physics at the Brunswick Caroline College, had claimed, in 1777, that the story of the ark could hardly be true.[86] Pallas also rejected it, assuming instead that all living beings came from different centres of creation.[87] Multiple creation, as the doctrine was called, found an increasing number of adherents.[88] The point was reiterated by Azara and by Cuvier's follower, the polygenist Julien-Joseph Virey, who maintained that there were six originally distinct human races, each of which came from a different centre.[89] Christoph Meiners (1747-1810), Professor of Philosophy at Göttingen University, evoked the analogical method to support polygenism: if it was granted that plants and animals were created in different sites the same was certainly true for men.[90] Having committed himself to analogizing Prichard was obliged to show that mankind and the larger land animals were descended from one particular location.

In the first edition of the *Researches* (1813) Prichard's account of animal dispersion encompassed only land animals. He concluded that Buffon was right in maintaining that animal species "have particular local relations, and were placed by the Creator in certain regions for which they are in their nature peculiarly adapted". No "one animal", he stated, "was originally common to the warm parts of the Old and New World". (With respect to the cold tracts of northern Asia and America Prichard conceded that one and the same species was found on both continents, suggesting that "the opposite points of Asia and America were formerly joined".[91])

By the second edition Prichard had extended his investigations into the distribution of animals to include all organized beings and not just, as in 1813, the mammals. "No writer, as far as I know", he maintained somewhat boldly, "has yet brought together the various facts which are likely to illustrate the distribution of organized beings."[92] By the 1820s, biogeography had not yet gained much ground in Britain.[93] On the Continent, however, there were many naturalists who probed the correlations between geography, physical appearance and physiology, aiming to unravel the laws governing the distribution of organisms.

In the second edition of the *Researches* (1826) Prichard, too, put great effort into collecting biogeographical information, ploughing through accounts of the distributions of plants, insects, birds, marine animals, quadrupeds and reptiles.[94] He followed Linnaeus' and Buffon's example, believing that there was a close link between the form of an animal and its physical abode. Echoing the theories and observations of Buffon and Zimmermann, as well as those of younger, mostly French naturalists such as Cuvier, the entomologist André Latreille, the naval explorer François Péron, and Charles Alexandre Lesueur, he argued that each genus of plants and animals had been created for a particular geographical habitat.

By the 1820s Prichard had developed a great admiration for Alexander von Humboldt (1769-1859) whose theoretical network of correlations between climate, topographical station and animal physiology had done much to build up a modern *systema naturae*. At the beginning of the century Humboldt explored the subject of meteorology, explaining vegetable distribution resulting from an interplay between climatic influence and plant physiology. He won lasting fame with his account of his travels to South America, where his reckless ardour had induced him to climb Chimborazo without so much as a hat on his head. His writings, executed in a more sober spirit, demonstrate "the emergence of natural science out of natural philosophy".[95] Although Prichard felt ambivalent about Humboldt's alleged polygenism, he was greatly impressed by the correlations the German drew between altitude and specific organisms. The other authors on the subject whom Prichard rightly considered as most important were Augustin-Pyramus de Candolle (1778-1841) as well as the Briton Robert Brown (1773-1853), both of whom inquired into the original station of plant families by means of counting the number of genera flourishing at any given location.[96] In fact, what Humboldt, Candolle and Brown did for the vegetable realm, Prichard aimed to do for man. He took a plunge into biogeographical literature, investigating the distribution of plants and animals, correlating their habitats to environmental circumstances, and drawing inferences as to their likely places of origin. Finally, he came up with three conclusions:

(a) Linnaeus was wrong in assuming that all animated beings had been created in one spot. There were several centres of creation spread across the globe.

(b) There was a marked correlation between the bio-climatic conditions of these centres and the physical conformation of the organized beings dwelling in the area.

(c) Each species, mankind including, had only one original habitation.[97]

There remains one issue which has not yet been addressed and which for Prichard himself lay beyond the problem of distribution *per se*. Where precisely, he enquired, did each individual species originate? With respect to plants and to the "lesser" animals as well as to migratory fish and birds, the question could be disregarded: Prichard simply assumed that the wind and the waters had carried them across the globe.[98] Problems arose only in view of larger land animals and mankind – those creatures, in other words, which supposedly had survived the Deluge in Noah's ark. Hence Prichard's frequently expressed adherence to the theory of Buffon and others who maintained that "the more perfect tribes of animals belong chiefly to the old world".[99]

The Geographical Origin of Mankind
and the Caucasian Mystery

Prichard located the original station of mankind on "the banks of the Euphrates". In Biblical times at the mouth of the Euphrates there lay the city of Ur in the land of Chaldaea, Abraham's birthplace. Genesis indicated that the Garden of Eden was crossed by four rivers, one of which was identified as the Euphrates. Avoiding the embarrassment of displaying outright Biblicism, Prichard did not mention the Garden of Eden, though he endorsed the tenet, summarized by Saint Augustine, that mankind "sprang from the family created on the banks of the Euphrates, which was preserved in an ark, and survived upon the mountains of Armenia".[100] To his dismay, however, this was not universally agreed upon: many scholars thought that they knew better than the Bible. By the beginning of the nineteenth century the origin of mankind was located in various geographical areas other than Mount Ararat.[101]

Mixing up different Biblical stories, Linnaeus had maintained that all species had been created in single pairs on a mountain-top; the remaining territory of the world, he believed, lay under water. It was, as Brooke has said, "a conflation of the creation and flood narratives ... It was a flood without Noah".[102] For Linnaeus that mountain had been Ararat. Later, other mountains were suggested. On the basis of Buffon's *Les Epoques de la nature* (1776), many authors concluded that mankind must have begun to flourish in Asia, thus returning to tenets of the early Middle Ages which located Paradise somewhere to the east. Another theory which referred the origin of mankind to Asiatic mountains was founded on the story of the Deluge: when the waters of the Flood subsided, it was this region where terrestrial life started to develop first, the Himalayas being the highest mountains on Earth. The French astronomer Jean Sylvain Bailly (1736-93) proposed yet another idea. In 1775 he maintained that human civilization originated in the Delta of the Ganges with "the old dynasty of the Brahmins".[103]

Some of these theories were so fanciful that they did not survive the turn of the nineteenth century. Only a few of them remained in circulation. One was what Thomas Huxley later called the "Caucasian mystery".[104] The idea that European humans had originated on Mount Caucasus was embraced by many writers of variously powerful religious conviction. Some were monogenists, others believed that in addition to Mount Caucasus there had been other peaks on which non-Europeans had survived the flood.

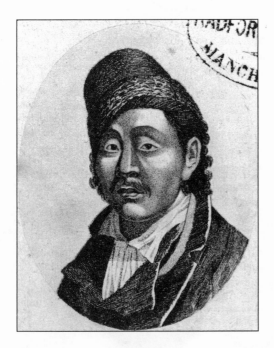

Figure 7
A Caucasian

Figure 7
An engraving of a Turk, representing Blumenbach's Caucasian variety of mankind (see Blumenbach's *De generis humani varietate nativa*, 3rd ed., Göttingen: Vandenhoeck and Ruprecht, 1795). In later decades, the features of the man would have easily passed as characteristically "Mongolian". That was no accident: to choose a Turk as a representative of the Caucasian, i.e. European, variety of mankind fell in line with notions put forward by writers such as the Comte de Buffon and the geologist Peter Simon Pallas who believed that the cradle of the human race was to be found in Asia. In 1819, the surgeon and anthropological writer William Lawrence included Blumenbach's portrait of the Turk in his own *Lectures on Physiology, Zoology, and the Natural History of Man* (the portrait is reproduced from the 3rd edition of that book, London: printed for James Smith, 1823).

Being opposed to all anti-Biblical theorizing Prichard had to take issue with the Caucasian hypothesis. One version of it appeared especially pernicious to him because it seemed to support polygenism:

Georges Cuvier stipulated that there was not one original centre of mankind but three. Geologists had shown that there were sea-shells to be found in high mountaneous regions. Cuvier fell in with the majority of contemporary naturalists who regarded this a proof of a universal inundation. Immersing himself in studies of the fossil record, he came to the conclusion that there might have occurred many catastrophes of that kind, culminating finally in the Deluge to which the Sacred records as well as many mythological narratives bore testimony. Despite his strong Protestant faith Cuvier believed that there were three resting-places for human beings who had managed to rescue

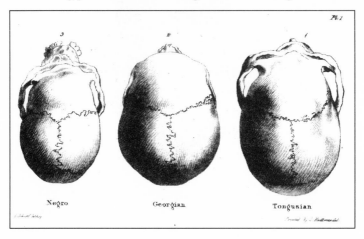

Negro   Georgian   Tongusian

Figure 8
The main cranial types, according to Blumenbach

Figure 8
Although Prichard did not endorse racial classifications that denied the variability of human varieties, he believed that there were anatomical peculiarities characteristic of a majority of any given population. One such was the formation of skulls. Initially, he followed Blumenbach in examining the "breadth of the horizontal section of the vertex" – that is, he measured skulls as seen from above. This illustration shows Blumenbach's three main human varieties: the "Negro", "Georgian", and "Tongusian" (or Mongolian), as reproduced in the 2nd edition of Prichard's *Researches* (1826). Although the same illustration was also included in the third edition, Prichard had, by then, dropped Blumenbach's top-view perspective. Instead he endorsed the approach of the anatomist Richard Owen, considering "the view of the basis of the skull" as decisive.

themselves from the latest Flood. They were to be found in the mountain chains of Caucasus (between the Black and the Caspian Seas), Atlas (in north-west Africa), and Altai (the natural border between Russia and Mongolia). Cuvier suggested that the Mongol races came from the Altai, "Negroes" from the Atlas, and white nations from the Caucasus.[105]

This idea can be traced back to Johann Friedrich Blumenbach. In his attempt to classify human varieties Blumenbach chose the formation of the skull for the most undeviating and most reliable criterion. His specimen collection was much admired. Unlike the anatomist Petrus Camper,[106] Blumenbach did not measure the facial angle, but the "breadth of the horizontal section of the vertex", that is, he measured skulls as seen from above. On the outcome he founded his system of three main varieties – Caucasian, Mongolian, and Ethiopian – as well as two intermediate varieties, the American and the Malay. What he called the "Caucasian" skull he deemed the most beautiful type, thus legitimating the very usage of the word Caucasian that referred to the populations of Europe and Lesser Asia, including the Semitic nations.[107]

It would be wrong to accuse Blumenbach of having deliberately sparked off the vast array of speculations on the Caucasian origin of mankind. In eighteenth-century Europe the Caucasus ballooned on the map of imaginary geography. As Blumenbach's proto-typical skull came from the region, it accordingly gave its name to the human variety. Besides, the choice was backed by one of the greatest living naturalists: for Buffon "the most handsome and most beautiful people in the world" flourished "between the 40th and 50th degree of latitude". This notion in itself coincided with eighteenth-century appreciations of benevolent climates. But Buffon's list of countries that fell under this description in the first volume of his *Natural History* (published in 1748) was remarkable: "Georgia, Circassia, the Ukraine, Turkey in Europe, Hungary, the south of Germany, Italy, Switzerland, France, and the northern part of Spain".[108] Hence Blumenbach would have been familiar with the idea of regarding Georgia as the first country mentioned in connection with the European type of mankind. It was not his desire that his theory should be read as a deviation from the Scripture report (1. Genesis, 8:3) that the ark rested on Ararat. He was far from replacing Mount Ararat with Mount Caucasus.[109] This was a twist of the argument which Cuvier imposed on Blumenbach's theologically inoffensive terminology.

Cuvier's theory greatly annoyed Prichard's sense of historical truth. He rightly perceived that the Caucasian hypothesis was a mongrel of ill-understood philological and anatomical tenets, "a mixture of somewhat vague notions, partly connected with physical theories, and in part derived from history, or rather from mythology".[110] Not only did Prichard disagree with the assumption of three centres of human civilization; he also believed that Cuvier's choice of the Caucasus meant betraying the Bible: "I cannot remember any tradition among the fabulists or historians of Greece, which admits of a construction answering to the hypothesis of M. Cuvier or deducing the human race from Mount Caucasus", he wrote in an essay contributed to the first volume of the *Reports* published in 1833 by the British Association.[111]

In 1844, in the fourth volume of the *Researches*, Prichard concluded his criticism of Cuvier with the statement: "the authentic narrative of the Hebrews lead [sic] us certainly to Mount Ararat, in Armenia, for the resting-place of the ark; but that is far from Caucasus".[112] The entire region to the east of the Caspian Sea is very mountainous. In picking the name of the Caucasus chain Blumenbach and Cuvier had chosen the highest and most prominent of mountain ranges in the area. In context of the story of the Deluge this made sense. The quarrels between traditionalists and the supporters of the Caucasian hypothesis were, indeed, not so much about geography, but about concepts of cultural predominance.

Prichard did all he could to deflate the Caucasian hypothesis. Discussing the "Asiatic nations", he asserted that the Georgians were not related to the civilized races of Europe and India, being "an ever barbarous and unintellectual race".[113] Thus he attempted to dissociate Blumenbach's Georgian proto-type of the Caucasian variety from the Europeans. But his criticism received no support. When the third edition of the *Researches* appeared, Cuvier's suggestion had already been taken up by many French physiologists dabbling in anthropology. Bernard de Lacépède (1756-1825), a specialist on fish and reptiles, as well as the polygenists Jean-Julien Virey and Louis-Antoine Desmoulins, were well-known supporters of the idea that the Europeans came from Mount Caucasus. In Britain, quite a few of Prichard's peers adopted the idea, including the physician and anthropological writer William Lawrence (1783-1867), whom Prichard otherwise considered as his ally against the polygenists.[114] Like the hybridity argument, the Caucasian hypothesis was yet another instance in which Prichard failed to establish his views.

In arguing the case of monogenism Prichard relied on proofs derived from the eighteenth century. But thanks to his untiring quest for new information, he was able to furnish numerous examples corroborating Buffon's and Blumenbach's teachings on the animal economy and the production of hybrids. Biogeography developed only in the nineteenth century. Yet it fitted perfectly within the framework of Prichard's views on the interdependency of culture and physiology: geographical station was the animal equivalent of the climatic and cultural conditions which stood at the centre of the proto-sociology practised by Montesquieu and Scottish Enlightenment philosophers.

Thus, Prichard's argument concerning the proof of monogenesis derived from the natural history of mankind was complete. Reasoning from analogy, he had shown that all mankind was subject to the same biological laws, suffered from the same diseases, and originated from the same spot which Prichard located in the region around Mount Ararat. But that, for him was not enough: he also ventured to show that an examination of the course of history, as it was reflected in the development of languages and mythological belief systems, underscored the cultural unity of mankind. And finally he aimed to show that mankind was one not just in its bodily manifestations, but also in its mental framework, sharing the same hopes and sorrows and the eternal quest for the redemption of those feelings which told every single one that they were but poor guests of this world and of little merit. At the beginning of this chapter stood the announcement that Prichard endeavoured to introduce psychology as a sub-discipline to the natural history of mankind. Now it is time to explain what he understood by psychology and in what respect it ties in with his approach towards the natural history of man.

The Discovery of Psychology

"Psychology is", Prichard wrote, "with respect to mankind, the history of the mental faculties."[115] A comparison of human populations from a physiological point of view, he suggested, ought to be complemented by a similar comparison from a psychological perspective: "the comparative physiology and psychology of different races of men had never been made expressly the subject of inquiry, until the publication of my work", he claimed in the introduction to the third edition of the *Researches*.[116] It was an ambitious task which, in Victorian appreciation, secured him his role as father of British ethnology. But, to pre-empt the conclusion, as far as psychology was concerned he did not fulfil the promise.[117] Instead he used psychology merely to emphasize the unity of mankind, because in his treatment of the subject it more or less boiled down to the question whether all human populations possessed the same propensity for

85

religious feelings. In this, Prichard was a trendsetter: numerous British ethnologists after him posed the question whether "savages" were able to receive the word of Christianity – it was to be the core question of Tylorian ethnology.[118] For Prichard, the answer was easy. Always engaged in highlighting the transcendental potential of human nature, he embedded his notion of the human psyche within a religious framework. On the following pages we shall see how he came to develop his particular concept of psychological unity.

In Chapter 2 it was explained why Prichard believed that moral insanity resided in the distortion of the innate emotional framework. It was a lesion in that part of the mind which he referred to, in his anthropological writings, as man's "psychical character".[119] If his medical theories of madness changed under the influence of both the Nasse school and Thomas Hancock, it appears quite likely that his psychological ideas ripened together with his theories of madness. Prichard never referred to such contemporary philosophers of psychology as Maine de Biran, Victor Cousin, Thomas Brown or Sir William Hamilton. His understanding of psychology was, indeed, not derived from philosophy but from theorizing about instinct. In 1829 he was already aware that a psychical principle existed in man and animals alike. But he had no word for it.[120] Not until 1836 did he find the term he was looking for.

As Prichard realized with dismay, the omnipresent spectre of phrenology was already encamped on the field. A zealot, where craniology was concerned, he took up the fight, in an Appendix to his 1835 *Treatise on Insanity*, published a year before the first volume of the third edition of the *Researches* came out. Grudgingly he recognized the attractiveness of Gall and Spurzheim's treatment of human sentiments: their system combined the attempt to explain the degree of intellectual capacity through the cranium, with an endeavour to locate the entire emotive and instinctive system in the brain, thus connecting the science of mind to anthropology.[121] Prichard admitted that Gall had founded nothing more and nothing less than "comparative psychology": the human psyche was explained on the grounds of analogical comparisons to the animal realm. It was, by and large, the same sort of analogical reasoning which had been put forward by the supporters of the analogical method, Buffon, Blumenbach and Prichard himself. "The point of view in which Dr. Gall and the phrenologists have contemplated the mental faculties may be termed that of *comparative psychology*", he summarized,

it discovers analogies in psychical phenomena between the brute tribes, and traces in them the rudiments of those properties which in the highest degree of development and taken collectively form the human character, and which in lower degrees and various relations constitute the distinctive nature of each of the inferior kinds. This is a new view of the mind and its powers, founded on a principle analogous to that which comparative anatomy applies to the structure of the body.[122]

So far, Prichard had no quarrel with Gall. The trouble with phrenology was its simplistic reductionism. The eighteenth century took it for granted that moral habits followed physical surroundings. The Romantic age related moral habits to particular physical conformations of the body. The interplay between human physiology and the natural surroundings afforded a certain latitude of development: the same environmental stimuli had different effects on different constitutions.[123] Within humoralist patterns of medicine, the interplay between body and psyche was regarded as an intricate network of physico-psychological dependencies. As we have seen in the previous chapter, the phrenological system seemed to provide a shortcut, ruling out the influence of the bodily organs and concentrating on craniological conformation for explaining the prevalence of particular sentiments, passions, and talents.[124] Phrenology lent itself to establishing hierarchies: "white people", an anonymous contributor wrote in the *Phrenological Journal,* "have distinguished themselves in all climates, every where preserving their superiority".[125] And why was this so? The phrenologists knew the answer: "if the brain be large, healthy, and of good quality, the mind will display itself vigorously in every part of the world".[126] Phrenology was a doctrine that, in W. F. Bynum's words, "made polygenism an obvious conclusion".[127]

The ontological implications of the phrenological system, Prichard thought, were appalling and proof enough for the hideousness of the entire approach. It seemed so ludicrous to him, that he was moved to one of his rare outbursts of irony:

> Shall we say, after tracing the operations of a constructive instinct so wonderfully displayed by the beaver, or in the cells in which the bee lays up its honey, that an impulse to action precisely similar gave origin to the pyramids of Egypt or to the building of Constantinople? Shall we venture to affirm that the tunnel under the Thames owes its existence to a burrowing propensity resembling that of the rabbit or the mole? Shall we conclude that Parry and Franklin sought the regions of the north impelled by the instinct of the

migratory rat, and that Magellan and De Gama traversed the southern oceans directed by an influence analogous to that which moves the flight of swallows?[128]

It was as ridiculous as the opposite idea that animals were endowed with reason. The Bristolian admirer of Magellan concluded that it was wrong to see human and animal actions such as travelling or building houses as analogous to each other. The mental faculties of mankind and animals were comparable, although not in view of particular abilities and designs, but in respect of the general make-up of the mind, the changes it underwent and the connection it bore to the rest of the animal economy.

Any analogizing between animals and humans must necessarily bridge the ontological gap between the two. Prichard summarized the philosophical problem thus: "we must, then, either elevate the brutes or lower the superiority of mankind". Lambasting the phrenologists for the latter he himself chose to see it the other way round: instead of referring mankind to the animal realm he contended that animals, too, had souls, insisting "that a psychical principle, or a principle in its nature distinct from organized body, exists in all sentient beings".[129] Consequently, he introduced the concept of animal psychology.

While Enlightenment philosophers such as Erasmus Darwin (1731-1802) set out to prove that animals were endowed with rationality, Prichard followed Thomas Hancock in playing down the importance of rationality. In accordance with this conviction he compared the mental faculties of animal and mankind not in view of reason but regarding "psychical endowments" by which he understood "the whole of the sensitive and perceptive faculties of animals, their intellect, or what in them approaches most nearly to the nature of intellect, as well as their instincts, feelings, propensities, and habitudes of action; all that corresponds in the lower orders of the creation, to the powers and attributes of the mind in man".[130] Rational behaviour, by contrast, was not even one of Prichard's ethnological categories. It is, indeed, striking how little emphasis he placed on the artifices of civilization: when he came to ask in what respects precisely human psychology was unified, he did not emphasize intelligence, but relied more on the universality of men's moral sense.

"Savage" peoples were sometimes denied the ability to rise to Christianity, on the grounds of their supposed intellectual deficiency.[131] Against this assumption Prichard asserted that, on the contrary, all peoples were capable of receiving Christian instruction and gaining an understanding of the Christian dispensation. Although he allowed for diversities in the degree to which intelligence was distributed among human populations, he considered these variations rather as a result of environmental circumstances.[132] And in any case, in his opinion, their significance was overridden by the impressive uniformity of religious sentiments.

The Anthropology of Atonement

Whilst other authors were keen to range all humans into an ascending scale of intellectuality, Prichard stipulated that the capacity of pagans to understand the niceties of Christian theology was proof enough of common intellectual potential.[133] To establish this point Prichard evoked accounts of physiognomically very diverse primitive populations: if they all showed themselves open to the Christian message, this, he argued, was a strong proof for the unity of mankind. Prichard chose three groups: African Hottentots, Greenland Eskimos, and African "Negroes". On the basis of reports mainly by missionaries, he described the spread of Christianity among these heathen nations. High-minded as he was, he insinuated that culture came after Christianity. The way he expressed himself it appeared as a necessary consequence of the refinement of mind brought about by the introduction of Christian doctrines. This is exemplified in a passage on "the Introduction of Christianity among the Hottentots". Prichard reported:

> So rapid has been the spread of civilization around the settlements of the United Brethren ... as to have given rise to a general notion that the missionaries of that church direct their endeavours in the first place to the diffusion of industry and social arts, and make religion a secondary object of attention. This, however, they uniformly deny.[134]

If cultural refinement came with conversion to Christianity, other monotheistic creeds such as Islam had the same effect. Indeed, Prichard believed that all those "Negro nations who have embraced Islam, are in a very different state of society" from those who were "still idolators" and "completely savages".[135] After having related a number of conversion stories among the Eskimos and Negroes, he concluded "that races so nearly allied and even identified in all the principal traits of their psychical character, as are the several races of mankind, must be considered as belonging to one species".[136]

The inbred sense of morality was a safe argument in favour of monogenesis. Unfortunately, it was accompanied by a sense of gloom, that melancholy disposition featuring so prominently in

Prichard's philosophy of psychology and mental illness. It is striking to observe how deeply Prichard was convinced that this sorry trait in mankind furnished the most powerful argument to reconcile the natural history of the species with the theory of monogenesis as laid down in Genesis. "It would be very interesting to inquire, what is the origin of this prevailing apprehension of evils in contemplating the imagined scenes of future existence?" he wrote, "there seems to be no obvious cause for it in the nature of circumstances." Why was it that the fear of punishment was so central to the representations of the ancient mythologists? "The solution of this problem appears to be, that the superstitions of mankind have not been merely the creations of the fancy, but principally of the conscience"[137] – a conscience implanted by nature or, as we may translate it, the Creator.

In the context of discussing psychological endowments Prichard came very near to spelling out his views on the links between human sentiments, innate morality, universal psychology, and its foundation in a natural order that was pre-ordained. It is a very important passage that bears being cited in full:

> If we could divest ourselves of all previous impressions respecting our nature and social state, and look at mankind and human actions with the eyes of a natural historian or as a zoologist observes the life and manners of beavers or of termites, we should remark nothing more striking in the habitudes of mankind, and in their manner of existence in various parts of the world, than a *reference* which is everywhere more or less distinctly perceptible *to a state of existence after death*, and to the influence believed both by barbarous and civilized nations to be exercised over their present condition and future destiny by invisible agents, differing in attributes according to the sentiments of different nations, but universally believed to exist. *The rites every where performed for the dead*, the various ceremonies of cremation, sepulture, embalming, mummifying, funeral processions, and pomps following the deceased, during thousands of successive years in every region of the earth ... the prayers and litanies set up in behalf of the dead as well as of the living, in *the churches of Christendom, in the mosques and pagodas of the East, as heretofore in pagan temples* – the power of sacerdotal or consecrated orders, who have caused themselves to be looked upon as the interpreters of destiny, and as mediators between the gods and men – sacred wars, desolating empires, through zeal for some metaphysical dogma – *toilsome pilgrimages performed every year, by thousands of white and of black men*, through various regions of the earth, *seeking atonement for*

guilt at the tombs of prophets and holy persons – all these and a
number of similar phenomena in the history of nations, barbarous
and civilized, would lead us to suppose that all mankind sympathize
in deeply impressed feelings and sentiments, which are as mysterious
in their nature as in their origin. These are among the *most striking
and remarkable of the psychical phenomena*, if we may so apply the
expression, which are peculiar to man, and if they are to be traced
among races of men which differ physically from each other, it will
follow that *all mankind partake of a common moral nature, and are
therefore*, if we take into the account the law of diversity in psychical
properties allotted to particular species, proved, by an extensive
observation of analogies in nature, to constitute *a single tribe*.[138]

This statement is impressive: theologically anything but narrow-
minded, Prichard granted true religious feelings to peoples usually
decried for their idolatry and desultory paganism. This appreciation
of pagan religions is reminiscent of eighteenth-century Deism;
Prichard had supplemented the Quaker doctrine of "inner light"
with a further doctrine, that, so to speak, of inner gloom. He insisted
that humans were psychologically unified by virtue of their common
belief in an after-life, in supreme forces watching over their existence
before and after death, and in the idea that in some manner they were
answerable to these forces. Yet, the argument bears being turned
around: by arguing for the unity of mankind Prichard also bolstered
the foundations of religion. Evidences of God and the case of
monogenesis were mutually supportive.

So pleased was Prichard with his psychological theory that we
find him stating that the "peculiar psychical qualities ... are even
more distinct, and therefore more characteristic of particular species,
than peculiarities of bodily structure".[139] Mankind's common
"psychical qualities" became one of the cornerstones of his
anthropology. The same kind of religious sentiments were so
prevalent in all societies because "they are the result of principles
deeply laid in the constitution of human nature".[140] Even Voltaire had
summoned a Capuchin priest when on his death-bed.[141] This view
did not only determine his scientific approach but it influenced his
very conclusions, irrespective of the fact that he proposed to treat the
history of mankind "as if the testimony of the Sacred Scripture were
altogether indifferent" to it.[142] Prichard was aware that he was – to use
a locution of the seventeenth-century Justice of the King's Bench,
Matthew Hale – "discoursing in the outward court of the Gentiles".
But he regularly mentioned the Bible in the *Researches*. In all three

editions he pointed out in which instances Scriptural tenets were either refuted or supported by other sources. In so far as his religious views remained the same his anthropology would also be constant.

Yet such simple formulations to bolster monogenesis were bound to be in vain unless their author contrived to show how varieties had come about among human kind. This implied a discussion of the mechanisms of heredity and the possible influences of the environment. It was a formidable task which Prichard attacked bravely, if ultimately inconclusively.

Notes

1   Urs Bitterli, "Auch Amerikaner sind Menschen. Das Erscheinungsbild des Indianers in Reiseberichten und kulturhistorischen Darstellungen vom 16. bis 18. Jahrhundert". In *Die Natur des Menschen. Probleme der physischen Anthropologie und Rassenkunde (1750-1850)*, ed. Gunter Mann, Jost Benedum, Werner F. Kümmel (Stuttgart: Gustav Fischer, 1990), pp. 15-29, quotation from p. 25.

2   For Linnaeus's anthropology see Gunnar Broberg, "Homo Sapiens: Linnaeus's Classification of Man". In *Linnaeus: The Man and his Work*, ed. T. Frängsmyr (Berkeley: University of California Press, 1983), pp. 156-94; James L. Larson, *Reason and Experience. The Representation of Natural Order in the Work of Carl von Linné* (Berkeley: University of California Press, 1971).

3   See Lisbet Koerner, "Purposes of Linnaean Travel: A Preliminary Research Report". In *Visions of Empire*, ed. David Philip Miller *et al.*, pp. 117-52, see pp. 122, 124.

4   Henry Home, Lord Kames, "Preliminary Discourse". In *idem, Sketches of the History of Man*, 2nd ed., 4 vols (Edinburgh: printed for W. Creech, 1788), vol. 1, preface.

5   Cf., e.g., Steven Shapin, "Homo Phrenologicus: Anthropological Perspectives on an Historical Problem". In *Natural Order. Historic Studies of Scientific Culture*, ed. Barry Barnes, Steven Shapin (Beverly Hills: Sage, 1979), pp. 41-72.

6   See Edwin Clarke, L. S. Jacyna, *Nineteenth-Century Origins of Neuroscientific Concepts*, p. 278. The subject is discussed in depth at the end of this chapter.

7   For the wider ramifications of French physiology see the excellent account in Elisabeth A. Williams, *The Physical and the Moral, Anthropology, Physiology, and Philosophical Medicine in France, 1750-1850* (Cambridge: Cambridge University Press, 1995).

8   Michèle Duchet, *Anthropologie et histoire au siècle des lumières.*

Buffon, Voltaire, Rousseau, Helvétius, Diderot (Paris: F. Maspéro, 1971), p. 288.

9   Nicholas Wiseman, *Twelve Lectures on the Connexion Between Science and Revealed Religion*, 2 vols (London: Joseph Booker, 1836), 1: 181.

10 Prichard, *Researches*, 3rd ed., 1: viif.

11 The dates of his birth and death vary, according to other sources he lived from 1778 to 1840. Bory de Saint Vincent was an influential contributor to the science of man in early nineteenth-century France. His career having taken off during Napoleon's reign, he was later criticized for his imperial leanings

12 For Virey see C. Benichou, Claude Blanckaert, eds, *Julien-Joseph Virey: naturaliste et anthropologue* (Paris: Vrin, 1988).

13 Louis-Antoine Desmoulins, *Histoire naturelle des races humaines ... d'après des recherches spéciales d'antiquités, de physiologie, d'anatomie et de zoologie* (Paris: Treuttel, 1826). The text was ill-received among the members of the Musée as well as in Britain. See "Natural History of the Human Race". *Monthly Review* n.s., 3 (1826): 505-15.

14 Quoted in Glyn Daniel, *The Idea of Prehistory*, p. 34.

15 Georges Cuvier, *Recherches sur les ossemens fossiles de quadrupèdes où l'on rétablit des caractères de plusieurs espèces d'animaux que les révolutions du globe paroissent avoir détruites*, 4 vols (Paris: Deterville, 1812), 1: 106.

16 Prichard, *Natural History of Man*, pp. 494-96.

17 Prichard was delighted when he discovered that his misgivings had been unfounded. Henceforth he admired Humboldt, whose *Kosmos* was translated by Prichard's son, and contained a few references about the judiciousness of Prichard's system. Alexander von Humboldt, *ΚΟΣΜΟΣ. A General Survey of the Physical Phenomena of the Universe*, trans. Augustin Prichard, 2 vols (London: Baillière, 1845), 1: 386-87. Humboldt was very dissatisfied with the botched translation. See Alexander von Humboldt, *Briefe an Christian Carl Josias Freiherr von Bunsen* (Leipzig: Brockhaus, 1869), pp. 68-70.

18 Francis William Newman, *Phases of Faith; or, Passages from the History of my Creed* (London: John Chapman, 1850), pp. 110-11. · For Newman see W. F. Bynum, "The Cardinal's Brother: Francis Newman, Victorian Bourgeois". In *Enlightenment, Passion and Modernity: Essays in Honor of Peter Gay*, ed. M. Micale, R. Dietle (Palo Alto: Stanford University Press, 1999).

19 Cf. Francis Newman, *Lectures on Logic, or on the Science of Evidence Generally Embracing Both Demonstrative and Probable Reasonings, With the Doctrine of Causation. Delivered at Bristol College in the Year 1836* (Oxford: J. H. Parker, London: J. G. and F. Rivington, 1838).

To the fourth volume of the third edition of the *Researches* Prichard appended an essay by Newman: "On the Hebraeo-African Languages".

20   Prichard, *Researches into the Physical History of Mankind*, 2nd ed., 2 vols (London: John and Arthur Arch, 1826); the third edition appeared under the same title: 5 vols (London: Sherwood, Gilbert, Piper; John and Arthur Arch, 1836-47).

21   In the first three volumes of the third edition of the *Researches*, most pictures are signed by Day and Haghe. Yet their contributions to the *Researches* ceased after Day had died in 1841. It is, therefore, rather likely that he, and not Haghe, did the engravings. For Day see Samuel Redgrave, *A Dictionary of Artists of the English School* (London: Longmans, Green and Co., 1874). For Haghe see E. Bénézit, ed., *Dictionnaire des peintres, sculpteurs, dessinateurs et graveurs*, 10 vols (Paris: Gründ, 1976), vol. 5.

22   See two letters Prichard wrote to Hodgkin on 4 and 25 November 1841 quoted in Amalie M. Kass, Edward H. Kass, *Perfecting the World*, p. 390.

23   "Dr. Prichard's *Natural History of Man*". *British and Foreign Medical Review* 13 (1842): 522; "Prichard *on the Natural History of Man*". *British and Foreign Medical Review* 15 (1843): 180-83, p. 183.

24   Cf. the illustrations in Johann Friedrich Blumenbach, *Beyträge zur Naturgeschichte*, 2 vols (Göttingen: J. C. Dieterich, 1790-1811).

25   In that respect, early natural history paintings and ethnological illustrations followed the same patterns, see Martin Rudwick, *Scenes from Deep time. Early Pictorial Representations of the Prehistoric World* (Chicago: University of Chicago Press, 1992).

26   Jean Victor Audouin *et al.*, *Le règne animal distribué d'après son organisation*, 3rd ed., 22 vols (Paris: Fortin, Masson, 1836-49).

27   For a discussion of that aspect of Prichard's ethnology see Chapter 5.

28   While there may not have been any particular reason why Prichard should have taken note of Darwin, von Baer was already a highly acclaimed scientist in the 1830s. The evolutionary thrust of his theorizing in *Über die Entwickelungsgeschichte der Thiere* (1828 and 1837), however, was very alien to the English type of natural historical enquiry. See Ernst Mayr, *The Growth of Biological Thought. Diversity, Evolution, and Inheritance* (Cambridge, Mass.: The Belknap Press of Harvard University Press, 1982), pp. 388, 473.

29   Wilhelm von Humboldt, August Wilhelm Schlegel, *Briefwechsel*, ed. Albert Leitzmann, introd. B. Delbrück (Halle: Max Niemeyer, 1908), p. 155 (Schlegel's letter to Humboldt dated 19 May 1823).

30   Prichard, *Researches*, 3rd ed., 5: 283.

31 For that particular Romantic kind of German anthropology see Karl J. Fink, "Storm and Stress Anthropology". *History of the Human Sciences* 6 (1993): 51-71.

32 Cf., e.g., Richard Yeo, "William Whewell, Natural Theology and the Philosophy of Science in Mid Nineteenth Century Britain". *Annals of Science* 36 (1979): 493-512.

33 Prichard, *Researches*, 3rd ed., 3: iv.

34 Frank E. Manuel, *The Eighteenth Century Confronts the Gods* (Cambridge, Mass.: Harvard University Press, 1959), pp. 291-92.

35 Johann Gottfried Herder, *Ideen zur Geschichte der Menschheit*, 3 parts, ed. Julian Schmidt, 1784-91 (Leipzig: Brockhaus, 1869), part 2, p. 164.

36 Prichard, *Researches*, 2nd ed., 1: 10; *ibid.*, 3rd ed., 1: 9.

37 Prichard, *Researches*, 3rd ed., 1: 114-37. See also *ibid.*, 1st ed., p. 85; 2nd ed., 1: 93-94 (where Prichard referred his opinion to Buffon and John Hunter); *idem, Natural History of Man*, p. 65.

38 Prichard, *Researches*, 2nd ed., 1: 100; 3rd ed., 1: 105-9.

39 These topics are discussed in subsequent chapters.

40 Prichard, *The Natural History of Man* (London: H. Baillière, 1843). A second edition appeared in 1845; a third in 1848; a fourth in 1855.

41 For the construction of meaning of the term "race" see H. F. Augstein, "Introduction". In *eadem*, ed., *Race. The Origins of an Idea, 1760-1850* (Bristol: Thoemmes Press, 1996), pp. ix-xxxiii; Michael Banton, *Racial Theories* (Cambridge: Cambridge University Press, 1987); Immanuel Geiss, *Geschichte des Rassismus* (Frankfurt am Main: Suhrkamp Verlag, 1988); Nicholas Hudson, "From 'Nation' to 'Race': The Origin of Racial Classification in Eighteenth-Century Thought". *Eighteenth-Century Studies* 29 (1996): 247-64; Robert Miles, *Racism* (London: Routledge, 1989), ch. 3; Nancy Stepan, *The Idea of Race in Science: Great Britain 1800-1960* (London: Macmillan, 1982), pp. 137-46. The literature on the subject is obviously vast.

42 Stephen Toulmin, June Goodfield, *The Discovery of Time* (Chicago: University of Chicago Press, 1965), p. 171. Other works on the species concept include Peter Bowler, "Bonnet and Buffon: Theories on Generation and the Problem of Species". *Journal of the History of Biology* 6 (1973): 259-81; Paul L. Farber, "Buffon and the Concept of Species". *Journal of the History of Biology* 5 (1982): 259-84; Phillip R. Sloan, "Buffon, German Biology, and the Historical Interpretation of Biological Species". *The British Journal for the History of Science* 12 (1979): 109-53; *idem*, "From Logical Universals to Historical Individuals: Buffon's Concept of Biological Species". In

Histoire du concept d'espèce dans les sciences de la vie, ed. J. L. Fischer, J. Roger (Paris: Fond. Singer-Polignac, 1986), pp. 101-40.

43 Prichard, *Researches*, 3rd ed., 1: 105. See also *ibid.*, 2nd ed., 1: 90-91. Prichard used the term "race" synonymously with "tribe", "nation", or "people".

44 Prichard, *Researches*, 2nd ed., 1: 92.

45 *Ibid.*, 3rd ed., 1: 108.

46 *Ibid.*, p. 109.

47 See W. F. Edwards, *Des caractères physiologiques des races humaines considérés dans leurs rapports avec l'histoire: Lettre à Amédée Thierry* (Paris: Compère jeune, 1829), pp. 4, 15. Edwards, a half-brother of the naturalist Henri Milne-Edwards, was born in Jamaica. When the shock-waves of the French revolution reached the region, giving rise to slave mutinies, the family quit the colonies, settling in Belgium which was at the time under French rule. Edwards studied medicine in Paris, acquired French nationality and became a respected member of the Paris medical faculty. In 1839 he founded the Société Ethnologique de Paris.

48 For an assessment of Edwards's racial theory see Claude Blanckaert, "On the Origins of French Ethnology. William Edwards and the Doctrine of Race". In *Bones, Bodies, Behavior. Essays on Biological Anthropology, History of Anthropology* 5, ed. George W. Stocking (Madison: The University of Wisconsin Press, 1988), pp. 20-55.

49 Prichard, *Researches*, 3rd ed., 3: iv. Someone else who shared Prichard's positive views of Edwards was his friend Thomas Hodgkin: as early as 1832 he co-translated Edwards's *De l'influence des agents physiques sur la vie* (1824): *On the Influence of Physical Agents on Life*, trans. T. Hodgkin, W. Fisher (London: printed for S. Highley, 1832). Moreover, it might have been Edwards who introduced Prichard to the idea that skin colour was not as permanent a human characteristic as most naturalists had heretofore thought. Cf. Edwards, *Des caractères physiologique*, p. 45. Prichard was not alone in overlooking the fact that his own version of "permanent varieties" was developed on a philosophical basis that was very different from the racial concepts of Edwards. At least one historian of our time has referred to Prichard's "permanent varieties" to depict him as a man who yielded to the increasing tide of racialism. The reader of this book will understand why the allegation does not hold. See Reginald Horsman, "Origins of Racial Anglo-Saxonism in Great Britain Before 1850". *Journal of the History of Ideas* 37 (1976): 387-410, p. 397.

50 Prichard's earliest concept of "variety" appears to have been modelled

on Buffon's understanding of "race". For Buffon, races were those "varieties of the species" whose characters had become hereditary. Cf. Duchet, *Anthropologie et histoire*, p. 273.

51 Prichard, *Researches*, 3rd ed., 1: 109.

52 Mayr, *The Growth of Biological Thought*, p. 262. Dougherty has shown that the notion of the habitus was already fully established in Buffon. Frank W. P. Dougherty, "Buffons Bedeutung für die Entwicklung des anthropologischen Denkens im Deutschland der zweiten Hälfte des 18. Jahrhunderts". In *Die Natur des Menschen*, ed. Gunter Mann *et al.*, pp. 221-79.

53 The title of his M.D. dissertation already indicated how much he was influenced by the German Professor of Anatomy: *Disputatio inauguralis de generis humani varietate*, with its allusion to Blumenbach's treatise *De generis humani varietate nativa*.

54 Prichard, *Researches.*, 2nd ed., 1: 17; 2: 570.

55 *Ibid.*, 1st ed., note on pp. 14-15.

56 *Ibid.*, 2nd ed., 1: 119; cf. *ibid.*, 3rd ed., 1: 114, 150-60. For the same idea in Blumenbach see his *De generis humani varietate nativa*. In *The Anthropological Treatises of Blumenbach and Hunter*, 1795, ed. Thomas Bendyshe (London: Green, Longman, Roberts, and Green, 1865), pp. 67-276, see p. 276. This opinion was by no means shared by all naturalists of the time. Prichard, therefore, conceded that "the predisposition to any given disease is different in different races, as it is known to be", he added cunningly, "in the several families of the same race or nation". See his *Researches*, 3rd ed., 1: 153.

57 Prichard, *Researches*, 1st ed., p. 194.

58 *Ibid.*, pp. 386, 395. Buffon had used the word "proto-type". See Mayr, *The Growth of Biological Thought*, p. 261.

59 Blumenbach, *Contributions to Natural History* (1790-1811). In Thomas Bendyshe, ed., *The Anthropological Treatises of Blumenbach and Hunter*, pp. 277-340, see p. 298.

60 Prichard considered Blumenbach's classification of skulls a tentative endeavour: "with a view of affording merely a general idea" of the character of organization of different tribes of men. Prichard, *Researches*, 2nd ed., 1: 172.

61 This tendency fell in line with a revival of Platonism. For Aristotelianism versus Platonism in the nineteenth century see David Newsome, *Two Classes of Men. Platonism & English Romantic Thought* (London: John Murray, 1974). For Platonism in Blumenbach see Timothy Lenoir, "Generational Factors in the Origin of *Romantische Naturphilosophie*". *Journal of the History of Biology* 11 (1978): 57-100. As the nineteenth century progressed

"type" was to gain an altogether different meaning, turning into a tool of racial systematization. For the confusion surrounding the usage of the term see Janet Browne, *The Secular Ark. Studies in the Historiography of Biogeography* (New Haven: Yale University Press, 1983), p. 160.

62 For the topic of hybridity and crossbreeding see Dougherty, "Buffons Bedeutung"; Nicholas Russell, *Like Engend'ring Like: Heredity and Animal Breeding in Early Modern England* (Cambridge: Cambridge University Press, 1986); Sloan, "From Logical Universals to Historical Individuals".

63 See: John Hedley Brooke, *Science and Religion*, pp. 231-34; Mayr, *The Growth of Biological Thought*, pp. 259-64.

64 "Zimmerman's [sic] *Geographical History of Man*". *Monthly Review* 80 (1789): 678-90, p. 686.

65 Johann Friedrich Blumenbach, *Handbuch der Naturgeschichte*, 4th enl. ed. (Göttingen: J. C. Dieterich, 1791), pp. 49ff.

66 See Mayr, *The Growth of Biological Thought*, p. 262. See also John Hunter, "Observations Tending to Show That the Wolf, Jackal, and Dog, are all of the Same Species" (1787-1789). In *The Works of John Hunter*, ed. James F. Palmer, annotated by Richard Owen, 4 vols (London: Longman, Rees, Orme, Brown, Green, and Longman, 1837), 4: 319-30. For Kant see Hans Querner, "Christoph Girtanner und die Anwendung des Kantischen Prinzips in der Bestimmung des Menschen". In *Die Natur des Menschen*, ed. Gunter Mann *et al.*, pp. 123-36, quotation from p. 127.

67 For Pallas see Dougherty, "Buffons Bedeutung", p. 232. For Pennant see James Sydney Slotkin, ed., *Readings in Early Anthropology* (London: Methuen, 1965), p. 186.

68 Peter J. Bowler, *The Fontana History of the Environmental Sciences* (London: Fontana Press, 1992), p. 183.

69 Blumenbach, *Contributions to Natural History*, p. 292.

70 Cf. Michel Foucault, *The Order of Things. An Archaeology of the Human Sciences* (London: Tavistock, 1970 (1966)).

71 Quoted in Louis Rosenfeld, *Thomas Hodgkin. Morbid Anatomist and Social Activist* (Lanham, Md.: Madison Books, 1992), p. 199.

72 Prichard, *Researches*, 1st ed., p. 14.

73 Prichard, *Researches*, 3rd ed., 1: 139-42.

74 Carl Asmund Rudolphi, *Beyträge zur Anthropologie und allgemeinen Naturgeschichte* (Berlin: Königliche Akademie der Wissenschaften, 1842) p. 160. In 1847 the American doctor George Morton (1799-1851), put particular effort into undermining Prichard's monogenism. He asserted the existence of genuinely different human

races by means of refuting the argument of hybridity. Although
Prichard knew some of Morton's publications, there is no evidence
that he read this article which appeared a year before his death.
Samuel George Morton, "Hybridity in Animals and Plants,
Considered in Reference to the Question of the Unity of Species".
Edinburgh New Philosophical Journal 43 (1847): 262-87.

75   Prichard, *Researches*, 2nd ed., 1: 97; *ibid.*, 3rd ed., 1: 142.

76   Cf. Morton, "Hybridity in Animals and Plants", p. 287.

77   Prichard, *Researches*, 2d ed., 1: 128-29.

78   Michael D. Biddiss, *Father of Racist Ideology. The Social and Political
Thought of Count Gobineau* (London: Weidenfeld and Nicolson,
1970), p. 116.

79   Robert Knox, *The Races of Men*, 2nd ed. (London: Henry Renshaw,
1862 (1850)), p. 88. Other proponents of that notion include the
German Gustav Klemm, the French Victor Courtet de l'Isle, and the
Americans J. C. Nott and George Gliddon. For Klemm see Biddiss,
Father of Racist Ideology, pp. 110-11. For Courtet de l'Isle see
Banton, *Racial Theories*, p. 46. For Nott and Gliddon see their *Types
of Mankind: Or, Ethnological Researches, Based Upon the Ancient
Monuments, Paintings, Sculptures, and Crania of Races...* (London:
Trübner; Philadelphia: Lippincott, Gambo, 1854).

80   Prichard, *Researches*, 3rd ed., 1: 147-50; *idem, Natural History of
Man*, pp. 18-26.

81   "Prichard's *Physical History of Mankind*". *New Quarterly Review* 8
(1846): 95-134, quotation from p. 126.

82   Prichard, *Researches*, 2nd ed., 1: 128. In the first edition the idea was
not yet present: Prichard had obviously derived it from Azara whom
he had not read by 1813. Of Spanish origin, Azara had moved to
Paris during Napoleon's consulate. Since he had already made
himself a name with a natural history of the Paraguayan quadrupeds
– *Voyages dans l'Amérique Méridionale* (1809) – he was welcomed
among the French naturalists. Prichard, too, was greatly impressed
by Azara's work and incorporated the results into the third edition of
the *Researches*. Later Prichard often spelt the name "Azzara". Cf.
Francisco Guerra, "Felix de Azara". In *Dictionary of Scientific
Biography*, 1: 351-52.

83   Prichard, *Researches*, 3rd ed., 1: 147-48.

84   *Ibid.*, p. 149.

85   *Ibid.*, 2nd ed., 1: 89; 3rd ed., 1: 259-60. See also Prichard, "Abstract
of a Comparative Review of Philological and Physical Researches, as
Applied to the History of the Human Species". *Edinburgh New
Philosophical Journal* 26 (1838): 308-26, p. 323.

86 Browne, *The Secular Ark*, pp. 1-27. For Zimmermann see F. S. Bodenheimer, "Zimmermann's *Specimen Zoologiae Geographicae Quadrupedum*, a Remarkable Zoogeographical Publication at the End of the Eighteenth Century". *Archives internationales d'histoire des sciences* 8 (1955): 351-57.

87 Cf. Robert J. C. Young, *Colonial Desire. Hybridity in Theory, Culture and Race* (London: Routledge, 1995), p. 11.

88 Browne, *The Secular Ark*, pp. 112-13.

89 J.-J. Virey, *Histoire naturelle du genre humain*, 2nd ed., 3 vols (Paris: Crochard, 1824), 2: 202ff. Félix de Azara, *Voyages dans l'Amérique Méridionale, depuis 1781-1801*, 4 vols (Paris: printed for Dentu, 1809), 1: 371.

90 Christoph Meiners, *Verschiedenheiten der Menschennaturen (die verschiedenen Menschenarten) in Asien und den Südländern, in den Ostindischen und Südseeinseln, nebst einer historischen Vergleichung der vormahligen und gegenwärtigen Bewohner dieser Continente und Eylande*, 3 vols (Tübingen: J. G. Cotta, 1811-15), 1: 11.

91 Prichard, *Researches*, 1st ed., note on p. 101, pp. 133-34.

92 Prichard, *Researches*, 2nd ed., vol. 1, note on p. 42.

93 Philip F. Rehbock, *The Philosophical Naturalists*, p. 125.

94 Prichard, *Researches*, 2nd ed., 1: chs 2 and 3. See also *ibid.*, 3rd ed., 1: 13-97.

95 Michael Detelbach, "Humboldtian Science". In *Cultures of Natural History*, ed. N. Jardine, J. A. Secord, E. C. Spary (Cambridge: Cambridge University Press, 1995), pp. 287-304, quotation from p. 304. Cf. also Susan F. Cannon, "Humboldtian Science". In *eadem, Science in Culture: The Early Victorian Period* (New York: Dawson and Science History Publications, 1978), pp. 73-110; Malcolm Nicolson, "Alexander von Humboldt, Humboldtian Science and the Origins of the Study of Vegetation". *History of Science* 25 (1987): 167-94.

96 Prichard, *Researches*, 3rd ed., 1: 21. For Humboldt and Candolle, see Browne, *The Secular Ark*, pp. 42-64. For Brown see *ibid.*, p. 62.

97 Prichard, *Researches*, 2nd ed., 1: 3 7, 27, 40.

98 See, e.g., Prichard, *Researches*, 3rd ed., 1: 51-52.

99 *Ibid.*, 1st ed., p. 92. Cf. also *ibid.*, 2nd ed., 1: 62; 3rd ed., 1: 77.

100 *Ibid.*, 2nd ed., 1: 89.

101 See the excellent article by Charles W. J. Withers, "Geography, Enlightenment and the Paradise Question". In *Geography and the Enlightenment*, ed. Charles W. J. Withers, David Livingstone (Chicago: University of Chicago Press, 1999, forthcoming). A good overview, though with no new insights, may be found in Norman Cohn, *Noah's Flood. The Genesis Story in Western Thought* (New

Haven: Yale University Press, 1996).

102   John Hedley Brooke, *Science and Religion*, p. 232.

103   Léon Poliakov, *Le mythe Aryen. Essai sur les sources du racisme et des nationalismes*, rev. ed. (Bruxelles: Editions Complexe, 1987 (1971)), pp. 210-11.

104   Huxley's quip is quoted in: Londa Schiebinger, *Nature's Body. Gender in the Making of Modern Science* (Boston: Beacon Press, 1993), p. 130. For the origins of this theory see H. F. Augstein, "Paradise On Mount Caucasus – How Physiologists Envisioned The Origins Of Mankind: A Contribution To The Prehistory Of Racial Theory". In *Race, Science and Medicine: Racial Categories and the Production of Medical Knowledge circa 1700-1960*, ed. Waltraud Ernst, Bernard Harris (London: Routledge, forthcoming). For the subsequent career of the ethnological term "Caucasian" see Matthew Faye Jacobson, *Whiteness of a Different Color. European Immigrants and the Alchemy of Race* (Cambridge, Mass.: Harvard University Press).

105   Georges Cuvier, *Recherches sur les ossemens fossiles*, 1: 106. For this context see Sandra Herbert, "Between Genesis and Geology: Darwin and Some Contemporaries in the 1820s and 1830s". In *Religion and Irreligion in Victorian Society. Essays in honor of R. K. Webb*, ed. R. W. Davis, R. J. Helmstadter (London, New York: Routledge, 1992), pp. 68-84.

106   Camper's "facial angle" referred to the angle between one imaginary line from the forehead to the nose and another from the nose to the chin. Camper claimed that the degree of intelligence grew proportionally with the volume of the forehead. Blumenbach rejected the idea: Camper's system discredited itself by implying that the owl was more intelligent than most human beings. According to Claude Blanckaert, Blumenbach was responsible for Camper's later reputation as an early racialist. As a matter of fact, however, he invented the facial angle, first of all, to teach his anatomy classes how to draw. See Blumenbach, *A Short System of Comparative Anatomy*, trans. William Lawrence (London: Longman, Hurst, Rees, Orme, 1807 (1805)), p. 56; Claude Blanckaert, "'Les vicissitudes de l'angle facial' et les débuts de la craniométrie (1765-1875)". *Révue de synthèse* 108 (1987): 417-53.

107   Blumenbach, *De generis humani varietate nativa*, 268-76.

108   Georges-Louis Leclerc, Comte de Buffon, *Natural History, General and Particular*, trans. William Smellie, 9 vols (Edinburgh: printed for William Creech, 1780 (1749ff.)), 3: 205.

109   For the Biblical origins of Blumenbach's choice of the term "Caucasian" see Dougherty, "Christoph Meiners und Johann

Friedrich Blumenbach im Streit um den Begriff der Menschenrasse". In *Die Natur des Menschen*, ed. Gunter Mann *et al.*, pp. 89-111, quotation from p. 107; cf. also Schiebinger, *Nature's Body*, p. 131.

110 Prichard, *Natural History of Man*, pp. 133-34.

111 Here Prichard stated for the first time that philology was a necessary complement of anthropological studies. Prichard, "Remarks on the Application of Philological and Physical Researches to the History of the Human Species". In *Report of the First and Second Meetings of the British Association for the Advancement of Science; at York in 1831, and at Oxford in 1832* (London: John Murray, 1833), pp. 529-44, see p. 542.

112 *Ibid.*, p. 542. Cf. Prichard, *Researches*, 3rd ed., 1: 260; *ibid.*, 2nd ed., 2: 603-5. The distance between Ararat and the Caucasus chain amounts to 200 miles.

113 Prichard, *Researches*, 3rd ed., vol. 4, note on p. 261; 3: 507.

114 *Ibid.*, 1: vii. According to the nineteenth-century physical anthropologist Joseph Bernard Davis, in later life Lawrence denounced his former monogenism; see George Stocking Jr, *Victorian Anthropology* (New York: Free Press, 1987), p. 66.

115 Prichard, *The Natural History of Man*, p. 386.

116 *Idem, Researches*, 3rd ed., 1: vi.

117 Nonetheless, one of his chapter headings read "The Psychological Comparison of Human Races". See his *Researches*, 3rd ed., 1: 165.

118 The question whether "savages" were able to receive the message of the Gospel was put forward, and already denied, by Locke. His stipulation "Idea of God not innate" cannot have ingratiated him with Prichard. See John Locke, *Philosophical Works*, 2 vols, ed. J. A. St John (London: George Bell and Sons, 1905-8), 1: 183-84.

119 Prichard, *Researches*, 3rd ed., 1: 167.

120 He called it "immaterial principle". See Prichard, *A Review of the Doctrine of a Vital Principle*, p. 62.

121 Prichard, "Temperament". In *Cyclopaedia of Practical Medicine*, 4: 169.

122 Prichard, *Treatise on Insanity*, p. 465 (Prichard's emphasis).

123 Cf., e.g., Blumenbach, *The Institutions of Physiology*, trans. John Elliotson, 2nd ed. (London: printed by Bensley for E. Cox, 1817 (1810, German orig. 1798)), p. 24.

124 Young pointed out that Gall rejected traditional sensationalism, instead trying to replace the "epistemological psychology" of the sensationalist with "a biological one". Robert M. Young, *Mind, Brain and Adaptation in the Nineteenth Century* (Oxford: Clarendon Press, 1970), p. 15. Gall was, as Cooter put it, "the first to treat mental

phenomena as well as the human passions ... as purely organic problems of neuroanatomy and neurophysiology". Roger Cooter, *The Cultural Meaning of Popular Science*, p. 3.

125 "On the Life, Character, Opinions, and Cerebral Development, of Rajah Rammohun Roy". *Phrenological Journal* 8 (1832-34): 577-603, p. 577.

126 *Ibid.*, pp. 578-79.

127 Bynum, "Time's Noblest Offspring", p. 206.

128 Prichard, *Treatise on Insanity*, p. 468. The passage is reminiscent of the phrenological Lecture in Thomas Love Peacock's *Headlong Hall*: "Here is the skull of a beaver, and that of Sir Christopher Wren. You observe, in both these specimens, the prodigious development of the organ of constructiveness". See T. L. Peacock, *The Novels*, ed. David Garnett (London: Rupert Hart-Davis, 1948), p. 68.

129 Prichard, *Treatise on Insanity*, pp. 468, 466. He adopted the notion from the one-time Bishop of Bristol, Joseph Butler. In the early nineteenth century Butler's *Analogy of Religion, Natural and Revealed* (1736) enjoyed a great revival. It served Prichard's anthropological aspirations particularly well since it helped to reconcile the spiritual and the natural sphere, science and religion, nature and culture. Hilton has aptly remarked that Butler's *Analogy* was so successful during the first decades of the nineteenth century "because he managed to combine the Scottish and evangelical doctrine of conscience with the utilitarian doctrine of consequentialism – put *conscience* into the machine, as it were". Hilton, *The Age of Atonement*, pp. 181-82 (original emphasis).

130 Prichard, *Researches*, 3rd ed., 1: 165. A letter to Thomas Hodgkin shows just how far Prichard had assimilated Hancock's critique of Locke: "the Anti-Lockean system of innate principles", he wrote, "seems to have been almost established as matter of fact, by the remarkable analogy, and almost uniformity, which has been traced among nations the most widely separated, in sentiment and in belief and in some of the most recondite and mysterious phenomena of the human mind"; see Prichard, "Letter to Dr Hodgkin". *Extracts from the Papers and Proceedings of the Aborigines Protection Society* 1, no. 2 (1839): 56-58, p. 57.

131 The ethnologist John Lubbock compiled a list of all those ethnographical authors who assumed that certain aboriginal tribes had no religion. Among them were: Joseph Beete Jukes (1811-69), William John Burchell (1782?-1868), and John Ross (1721-90). See John Lubbock, *The Origin of Civilisation and the Primitive Condition of Man*, 5th ed. (London: Longmans, Green and Co., 1889 (1870)),

pp. 213, 215.

132   This issue will be discussed in depth in Chapter 5.

133   Prichard, *Researches*, 3rd ed., 1: 215.

134   *Ibid.*, p. 183.

135   Prichard, "Observations on the Races of People who Inhabit the Northern Regions of Africa". Paper read on 25 May 1825. In "Abstracts of Papers, & c Read Before the Philosophical & Literary Society Annexed to the Bristol Institution. Beginning With the Paper Read at the Evening Meeting on 6th January 1825". Compiled by the Philosophical and Literary Society. MS B 12361, Bristol Central Library.

136   Prichard, *Researches*, 3rd ed., 1: 215. Cf. also: *ibid.*, p. 376; 4: 612; 5: 548.

137   Prichard, *Diseases of the Nervous System*, p. 375. Already in this 1822 *Treatise* Prichard's religion had crept into his science.

138   Prichard, *Researches*, 3rd ed., 1: 175-76 (my emphases).

139   *Ibid.*, p. 375.

140   Prichard, *A Treatise on Diseases of the Nervous System*, 375.

141   *Ibid.* The story is apocryphal, Prichard cited it from Jacob Grimm.

142   Prichard, *Researches*, 3rd ed., 1: 8.

4

Environmentalism and Heredity:
Natural Variety

"There must, indeed, be some principle", wrote Prichard in 1826, "on which the phaenomena of resemblance, as well as those of diversity, may be explained."[1] We have just seen how he established resemblance in the sense of species identity. The phenomena of diversity, by contrast, were at least as complex as the Schleswig-Holstein question of which Lord Palmerston would say that only three people had fully understood it: one was dead, the other was mad, and he was the third, but he had forgotten.

Diversity existed on several levels: the individual deviated from the type of the family, while whole families or populations deviated from the archetype of the species. As the former did not immediately touch upon the problem of monogenesis, Prichard did not give much consideration to it.[2] The latter, however, was of immense importance. Any natural history of man deserving that name had to elucidate the origins of variations. Prichard followed Buffon, John Hunter, Blumenbach and Georges Cuvier in regarding the natural history of mankind as analogous to the natural history of animals and plants, and hence in comparing animal domestication to human civilization. Against this backdrop he modelled his biological views of heredity, the environment and civilization. In this chapter, we shall trace his attitudes towards these issues through the three editions of the *Researches*. At times this will make complicated reading. But there is much gain to be had from the effort: nowadays, Prichard is habitually quoted by writers on nineteenth-century medicine and ethnology who are not intimately familiar with his works. As a result, his thinking has been misunderstood and the editions of his works jumbled together. To overcome these pitfalls this chapter aims to explain in detail what Prichard thought and when. It is nothing more or less than a guide through the evolution of his theorizing in the natural history of mankind. We shall see how he accommodated new information within his system and how this led him at times into contradictory statements. But, then, his principal starting point had a touch of paradox about it: how could one believe in the unity of species given that human beings looked so different from each other?

1813 – The First Edition

Prichard himself said he owed his interest in the varieties of mankind to Dugald Stewart (1753-1828), whose course on moral philosophy he had attended in 1806-7 at Edinburgh.[3] Stewart, a pious Whig, took offence at the notorious polygenist theory of Henry Home, Lord Kames, who suggested that God might have peopled the Earth with various species of man at various locations.[4] Stewart's counter-arguments were formulated along the lines of entrenched Scottish environmentalism. Accordingly he maintained that mankind was one, and that all differences were referable to external influences which, through some obscure physiological process, left their stamp on physical appearance. A corollary of this theory (nowadays known by the term "soft inheritance") was the assumption that acquired characteristics – such as the scorching of the skin by the sun – could be passed on to the progeny.

For Stewart, the young Prichard, and also the great bulk of Enlightenment naturalists, the main variation among human populations was skin colour.[5] One theory ascribed dark skin colour to a superabundance of black bile, traces of which gave a dark tint to the skin. Another explanation considered pigmentation as a function of climatic circumstances and geographic station: whiteness was reckoned the norm, while all dark human varieties had their skin "burned" by the sun. This theory, pre-eminent among Scottish Enlightenment philosophers, prolonged the tradition of Montesquieu's proto-sociological philosophy which found correlations not only between climate and skin colour, but between the entire environment, on the one hand, and customs and habits on the other. In the Victorian age the concept was dubbed the "environmentalist theory"[6] and was extended to sources as various as Hippocrates, the seventeenth-century gentleman philosopher Sir William Temple, Montesquieu and Buffon.[7] Blumenbach adhered to it too, claiming that the sun drew bodily carbon into the skin whence it acquired a dark colour.[8]

Sophisticated thinking on the mechanisms of heredity was not part of Scottish Enlightenment views on the development of societies and the physical characteristics of mankind. According to an age-old tradition, it was taken for granted that all new traits could be inherited, the sole prerequisite being that the impact of the exciting influences would be strong enough to call forth a change in the hereditary fabric. This idea applied not only to bodily peculiarities but also to moral qualities. When Dugald Stewart evoked the time-worn theory of climate to refute Kames, he extended the notion of the inheritability of particular characteristics to the whole of civilized manners.[9]

As early as 1807 Prichard, by contrast, rejected the idea that any characteristics acquired during an individual's lifetime could become part of the hereditary framework.[10] If those traits became hereditary, he argued, then the whole universe of living creatures would be utterly chaotic, for every single alteration in individual features would have given rise to tribes and families which displayed the same peculiarities. Indeed,

> the evils of all past ages would be perpetuated, and the human race would in every succeeding generation, exhibit more abundant examples of accumulated misery. Every species would have become at this day mutilated and defective, and we should see nothing but men and animals, destitute of eyes, arms, legs, &c. The whole creation, which now displays a spectacle of beauty and happiness, would present to our view a picture of universal decrepitude and hideous deformity.[11]

In reality, however, there was some order in creation. While still at university Prichard did not attempt to pinpoint the natural principles governing the "spectacle of beauty and happiness". Initially, his theory of human varieties turned upon a more simple question: why did different human tribes have different skin colours? In his doctoral dissertation this was the salient criterion of human diversity and, by inference, a conspicuously stable characteristic of human varieties.

If in his early writings he was concerned with colour, this was in part because the different colours of mankind were more striking than all other differences. When as a boy Prichard had strolled along the docks of Bristol, the spectacle of dark-skinned people cannot have failed to impress him. Another part of the answer lies in the fact that his medical interest directed him towards theories about the diversity of complexion – most of which struck him very early on as false.

Having dismissed Stewart's notion that acquired characteristics could become congenital, Prichard set out to explain what heredity was indeed about. His ideas were collated from the doctrines of John Hunter, the Edinburgh physician James Gregory (1753-1821),[12] and others who had written on the animal economy. "It appears", he wrote, "that the principle in the animal oeconomy on which the production of varieties in the race depends, is entirely distinct from that which regards the changes produced by external causes on the individual".[13] Of course, there were variations within the human race which were heritable. However, these variations were not externally induced but part of the human constitution. They were, Prichard asserted, "connate", that is, ingrained into the human fabric before birth.[14]

Unlike Buffon and the Scottish Enlightenment philosophers, he did not believe that such developments were due to "the gradual influence of climate, of situation and peculiar customs".[15] Instead, he referred these variations to alterations in the connate fabric of the parents, claiming that "every part of the corporeal structure has a tendency to become hereditary".[16] Accidental varieties rose spontaneously and did not develop over time as the environmentalists believed: "this deviation is not a change gradually produced by the action of the same causes exerting their influence thro' a long series of generations. Such an imperceptible progress is clearly foreign to its nature. It generally becomes fully established in one generation."[17]

In Prichard's cosmos, nature advanced in leaps, giving rise to accidental variations such as polydactylism or the tall stature of the Prussian king's "giant regiment" of which he had read.[18] They came about suddenly, but once they had sprung up they persisted in the offspring.[19] How precisely they were produced Prichard left to others to solve. His theory of heredity was anything but clear. It was precisely by virtue of its vagueness that its author has been counted among the "forerunners" of Darwin.[20] I wish to argue, however, that Prichard's idea, seemingly so modern from an evolutionist viewpoint, was less an act of prophecy than a blow struck against old enemies. Prichard came up with the concept of "connate" traits to defy the transmutationist form of epigenesis, put forward by Jean-Baptiste Lamarck (1744-1829) and Erasmus Darwin (1731-1802). This stipulated that animal species deviated into each other as a result of climatic influences and an internal drive that Darwin termed "appetancy".[21]

Fighting Transmutationism

Erasmus Darwin excited Prichard's scorn. Thus, he rejected the idea retailed in the *Zoonomia* that dogs whose tails had been docked gave birth to dogs with the same characteristic: "the authors who have brought such examples as these in defence of their opinions, would not probably have thought them worth recording, ... if they had not happened to coincide with the systems they were advocating".[22] Who were "the authors"? The example of the tailless dog originally came from Buffon, but Darwin, too, had quoted the remark when discussing the theory of climate, with the aim of showing that acquired characteristics were generally heritable. From this Darwin concluded that the influence of climate not only furthered new varieties but also new species: "many of these enormities of shape are propagated, and continued as a variety at least, if not as a new species of animal".[23] In 1813 Prichard's attack on Darwin discreetly omitted to mention his adversary by name.[24] By 1829 this had changed. In his book on the doctrine of the vital principle, Prichard expressed his opinion on Darwin's theory very clearly: "what can be more absurd than the notion which this scheme presents to us?"[25]

In establishing a system of heredity that denied the theory of climate, Prichard meant to cut off Darwin's transmutationism at its theoretical roots. He therefore ruled out the influence of climate as a formative agent and was inclined to believe that new human variations sprang up suddenly rather than over a long stretch of time (for time was a factor requisite for the transmutation of new species).[26] To uphold monogenesis Prichard was obliged to explain the rise of different varieties, but he had to do it in a manner which precluded the mechanisms underlying Darwin's theory. Therefore, he resorted to regarding the origins of human variation as a mixture of total predetermination plus a limited degree of accidental variation (its potential being ingrained in the individual constitution).

Prichard took it for granted that the range of possible alterations was held in check through natural laws that forbade monstrous aberrations.[27] Moreover, he believed that the course which the physical history of mankind had taken was unilinear, tending towards the production of increasingly beautiful varieties. This entailed his conviction that the course of nature guaranteed the transformation of black ugliness into white beauty. This notion lay at the centre of his theory of human variations, put forward in 1813, which must now be delineated.

The range of variability was determined in accordance with an analogy between human development and natural history at large. John Hunter had laid down two axioms which Prichard made central to his theory. The notable London surgeon had claimed that, first, the tendency to variation in animals led always from darker to lighter varieties, the reverse being virtually impossible since the original colour of most animals was dark rather than light. Second, he suggested that the predisposition to variability was much more greatly developed in domesticated populations than in their wild counterparts.[28] Prichard applied both notions to mankind, concluding that "the process of Nature in the human species is the transmutation of the characters of the Negro into those of the European, or the evolution of white varieties in black races of men".[29] (When he used the term "evolution" he employed it, of course, in its eighteenth-century sense, implying the development of characteristics ingrained in the human fabric.) Even though Prichard conjectured that the original colour of man might have been black, he saw whiteness as a quality which in one way or other was within the compass of mankind's pre-ordained physical destiny.

Drawing analogies between vegetable cultivation, animal domestication and human civilization, he held that the standard of taste prevalent in individual human populations played a role in the development of white varieties. He explained it by reference to the example of domesticated animals. The production of new varieties in livestock was a natural development. But it was given to the farmer to decide which of the accidental varieties were to survive. What applied to plants and animals had to be true for mankind as well. This was the point at which Prichard's famous theory of sexual selection came into play.[30] From the analogy between cultivation, domestication and civilization he concluded that humans exerted their selective tastes on their own kind as well: according to the reigning taste of any given community, some varieties were regarded as more comely.[31] Individuals endowed with these superior features were eagerly selected as marriage partners and hence were sure to pass on their particular characteristics. Paying tribute to the fact that all civilized peoples were white, Prichard asserted that "the general complexion of savages is black or a dark hue", while "wherever we see any progress towards civilization, there we also find deviation towards a lighter colour and a different form, nearly in the same proportion".[32]

Blackness was not accidental either. Prichard argued that "dark [human] races are best adapted by their organization to the condition of rude and uncivilized nations". By this he did not mean to say that their features had developed as the result of an adaptive process which enabled them to survive under harsh environmental conditions.[33] Instead he surmised that blacks had always been blacks: "the primitive stock of men were Negroes".[34] There was one and only one adaptive variation which Prichard in his early writings allowed in the "evolution" of the human species: in the savage state a tribe would not progress, only civilization brought about physical development.

Once the civilizing process had set in, physical evolution followed. Higher creatures knew two materially different stages: rudeness and refinement. Being artificial, the latter removed humanity from the natural economy which governed over it in its ruder state. In so far as it instanced a development, mankind's natural history commenced only with the history of civilization. For "nations of savages, would never be changed materially in complexion by the influence of climate alone".[35]

It is important to bear in mind that, in the first edition of the *Researches*, new varieties were held to be the immediate products of civilization. Having rejected the influence of external agents, Prichard could not possibly discuss the impact of civilization on the same level as contemporary environmentalists. Rather he averred that the civilized state was particularly conducive to the rise of new varieties in the connate fabric, though he did not consider these alterations as adaptations to the natural surroundings, for such an assumption would yet again have played into the hands of the transmutationists. So it was the teleological principle of the "beneficial tendency" of nature to which Prichard ascribed the fact that the new varieties to which civilization gave rise were "more fitted for their new condition".[36] The process of human differentiation was not one of an adaptive nature, but once new varieties were produced they appeared to be wonderfully adapted to their respective abode.

Having established that it was primarily civilization which predisposed mankind to branch out into new varieties, Prichard nevertheless admitted that climate might exert a similar influence. Hedging his bets, he considered it "not improbable that the effect of climate when conjoined with other causes, as in nations advancing towards a state of civilization, would be more considerable", though its influence was held in check because "mankind is defended by so many arts against the influence of the elements".[37] In summary, Prichard's attitude to climate was governed by his desire to refute traditional environmentalism. But as a factor favourable to the production of connate varieties, he did not entirely disclaim its influence. If the argument appears somewhat laboured, undecided to the point of contradiction, it was yet a remarkable achievement for a man in his mid-twenties who had engaged in a devilishly complicated problem.

1826 – The Second Edition

In 1813 Prichard did not explain how the principle of heredity was supposed to work. Which characteristics were connate and which were not was, for him, a question of empirical investigation. His views on heredity were shaped along the lines of an "evolutionist" or preformist theory of generation which entailed the notion that species developed only within very narrow confines. Initially, adaptation was not part of Prichard's explanatory framework. By the second edition of the *Researches*, published in 1826, he had changed his views in certain respects.

The second edition was twice the length of the first. The ethnological material was greatly enlarged; the philological sections included enquiries into the history of living languages. Prichard's biological views also diverged in several respects from those previously held. Now he acknowledged that the populations of mankind might vary in response to environmental conditions. Why this change? Environmentalism had gained legitimacy in his eyes because most of the important biogeographers of his day were employed in finding correlations between climate and structure. Moreover, he had discovered a theory of generation which enabled him to reconcile a concept of adaptation with his claim that acquired characteristics could not become hereditary. A corollary of his new position was the shedding of Hunter's theory that the domesticated state predisposed to the production of new varieties. These alterations notwithstanding, Prichard upheld his general concerns: his argument still aimed to prove monogenesis. And, although he had troubles with the concept, he retained the theory that new varieties sprang up suddenly and not through a gradual process. His opposition to Darwin's and Lamarck's transmutationism was unmitigated.

The two-volume edition of 1826 was dedicated to Johann Friedrich Blumenbach whom Prichard admired for having founded the "natural history of mankind" as an independent discipline.[38] The Göttingen anatomist had a decidedly non-racialist approach to the natural history of man which suited Prichard's monogenist morality.[39] It was, not least of all, thanks to Blumenbach that Prichard had turned to the "analogical method": the application of rules, derived from the natural history of animals, to the natural history of man. As we have seen in Chapter 3, this method enabled both naturalists to establish species relationships without necessarily having recourse to Buffon's criterion of hybridity. The second edition may be summarized thus. Its most interesting feature will be given further scrutiny.

Discussing the problem of human variation in 1826, Prichard harboured doubts concerning one particular of his hereditary theory of 1813, namely, his claim that all new varieties sprang up accidentally and suddenly. In 1826 he deemed it questionable "whether the degeneration or variation of animals is in fact a mere accidental phaenomenon". It is easy to see why he felt uncomfortable with this idea: accidentality smacked of contingency. Now Prichard pondered "whether the varieties in nature" were a result of external influences "modifying the structure and constitution of races, and adapting them to the physical circumstances under which these races may be destined to exist", or whether they were "only the casual effect of degeneration".[40] His 1826 view was that both were true. He explicitly recognized that this solution appeared contradictory. But thanks to a hereditary theory which he derived from Blumenbach and Kant,[41] Prichard managed to square the circle and reconcile both theories.

As a philosopher in the strict sense of the word, Kant was not only brilliant but also humane. His anthropology and biology, by contrast, regurgitated many prejudices. Modifying the preformist theory, Kant suggested that each species had a determinate number of hereditary "germs". The typical traits of each given species, inscribed onto these germs, would develop in any case. But apart from these, there were other characteristics of minor importance whose unfolding depended on external stimuli.[42] Blumenbach gave a summary of the theory, and Prichard adopted it in the second edition of the *Researches*: "we may remark in general", he wrote with respect to the relative fixity of species,

> that each individual being, through the animal and vegetable worlds has certain laws of organization impressed upon its original germ, according to which the future developement of its structure is destined to take place. These inbred or spontaneous tendencies, governing the future evolution of the bodily fabric, cause it to assume certain qualities of form and texture at different periods of growth. From these predispositions are derived the characteristic differences, and the peculiarities of individual beings.[43]

Thus Prichard claimed that "the organization of the offspring is always modelled according to the type of the original structure of the parent".[44] It was the pattern of the parental type which guaranteed the continuation of species; and yet there was room for variation: "this law of hereditary conformation exists with a certain latitude or sphere of variety, but whatever varieties are produced in the race, have their beginning in the original structure of some particular ovum or germ, and not in any qualities superinduced by external causes in the progress of the developement".[45] Falling in with prevalent gender stereotypes, he suggested that it was the hereditary make-up of the father that guaranteed the prolongation of the species,[46] while extraneous impressions on the mind of the mother could influence the form of the individual foetus: "at, or soon after the time of conception, the structure of the foetus is capable of undergoing modification".[47]

Thanks to this theory of generation Prichard managed to retain the accidentality of new variations, but he physically relegated it to the maternal disposition which was susceptible to external influences.[48] The exact mechanism, however, by which processes of adaptation took place, remained obscure to him. "*How, by what influence,* and *in what manner,* the antecedent circumstances affect in any instance the parents, so as to give rise to the production of some new appearance in their offspring, we shall perhaps never be able to ascertain."[49]

One putative answer had been provided by writers on biogeography. Alexander von Humboldt and Robert Brown harboured the conviction that there were some teleological principles permeating nature which accounted for the fact that particular organic structures were especially fitted to specific geographical locations. Prichard followed this line willingly. Adaptation lost its odious smell. If deviations from the original type were by nature limited because their occurrence was dependent on the range of variation implanted within the constitution, then embracing a theory of adaptation no longer amounted to endorsing transmutationism.

Prichard nevertheless continued to insist on his earlier assumption that there was "a general law of the animal economy, according to which, acquired varieties are not transmitted from parents to their offspring, but terminate in the generation in which they have taken their rise".[50] As proof he cited the case of white settlers in the West Indies as well as the progeny of black slaves raised in Europe: all of them kept the original colour of their ancestors.[51] Sometimes, it seems, Prichard adopted new ideas without being quite able to assimilate them. He was aware that it was paradoxical to embrace a theory of environmental adaptation and yet deny the heritability of acquired traits. His only answer to the problem was yet again the evocation of a mysterious law of the animal economy "which gives rise to an alteration in the breed calculated to fit the race for its new abode".[52] Pondering the nature of adaptive processes, he was greatly inspired by the geographer and natural historian Felix de Azara whom we have encountered in the context of Prichard's espousal of interbreeding. Like the German psychiatrists, Azara was hardly known in England. If Prichard's science was eclectic he at least knew how to make surprising use of original sources.

Travelling through Paraguay, Azara had observed that only wild animals were liable to variation, while "domestic breeds undergo no alteration".[53] The sentence struck Prichard: this was the very opposite of John Hunter's assumption that new varieties sprang up mainly under the condition of domestication. Azara's observation, by contrast, supported the theory that new varieties were brought about by environmental influences.[54]

Since Prichard's approach to the natural history of man was based so largely on applying to man what was true for animals, Azara's theory appealed to him. It suggested that it was not civilization which predisposed to human variations but the rude state of mankind. "It may be noticed, in general", he wrote in 1826, "that fewer variations occur in races of white than in those of darker colour".[55] In 1813, by contrast, he had believed that new varieties rose mainly among domesticated animals. The new theory moreover made sense within the framework of Prichard's notion of how civilized physiognomy had come about: if rude populations were liable to connate variations, this explained how white races had developed: it was not so much an effect of the history of manners as a normal process of natural history.[56]

To sum up: in the 1826 edition new discoveries regarding the natural history of animals, environmentalism and Blumenbach's hereditary theory mutually supported each other. Under their combined impact Prichard turned explicitly towards environmentalism. The replacement of civilization by climatic agencies has been viewed as a major shift in Prichard's theory of the formation of human varieties.[57] In fact, however, the rejection of traditional environmentalism had never been his prime concern. It merely resulted from his urgent desire to dissociate himself from transmutationism. The second edition of the *Researches* suffered from the flagrant contradiction between an endorsement of environmentalism and the insistence that acquired characteristics could not become hereditary – the latter being the basis of resistance against the transmutationist assault. It was only in the third edition that this bastion fell as well. Prichard endorsed all sorts of theories as long as he could establish some or other mechanism to account for the development of species that was different from fully-fledged transmutationism and in line with his broad notions of epigenesis.

1836-1847 – The Third Edition

In the fifth volume (published in 1847) of the third edition Prichard summarized his whole endeavour. With respect to the phenomena of hereditary variation he wrote:

> the principal object of these researches has been to furnish the

groundwork of a comparative inquiry into the physical and psychological characters of various races, with a view of determining how far these characters are permanent or subject to change, and whether they are in their nature specific distinctions, or merely accidental or acquired and transmutable varieties.[58]

What had been true for the second edition applied to the third: Prichard drew an analytical distinction between "accidental" surges of new varieties which were completed more or less within the first generation, and the notion that some characteristics were acquired under the impact of climatic and living conditions. In line with the former proposition he maintained

> that the changes alluded to do not so often take place by alteration in the physical character of a whole tribe simultaneously, as by the springing up in it of some new congenital peculiarity, which is afterwards propagated and becomes a character more or less constant in the progeny of the individuals in whom it first appeared, and is perhaps gradually communicated by intermarriages to a whole stock or tribe.[59]

Thus Prichard had preserved not only his notion of sudden accidental varieties but also the idea that these were propagated through marital selection. However, as in the second edition, he deviated in certain respects from his previous theories. Before this issue can be addressed, a short recapitulation of the general framework of the third edition may be helpful.

The structure of the work follows the pattern of the first and second editions. The first volume provides a theoretical presentation of Prichard's arguments concerning the question of monogenesis from a biological point of view. The remaining four volumes contain a host of ethnological information, ranging from physical anthropology to philology. Among the criteria which proved the unity of mankind Prichard included the human psychological make-up, epitomized by the shared belief in a universal Creator, the notion of an after-life and the feeling of guilt.[60] Coterminous with the psychological criterion came his conviction that external features – pigmentation and integuments – were unreliable, because highly mutable, indicators of anthropological typology. As we shall see in the next chapter this change of mind was reinforced by first-hand observations Prichard made when he encountered the Indian Rajah Ramohun Roy whose complexion defied the assumption of a correlation between social standing and external appearance. Besides, the thrust of Prichard's intellectual development went into the direction of discounting the importance of external features in favour of inner characteristics. From the 1830s he concentrated on the inner make-up of mankind, that is, psychology and bone structure:

> It is in the external and less essential parts that varieties principally take place. In the texture and coverings whether hairy or woolly of the skin, the absence or presence and the size of horns and other appendages, the colour or complexion, and in some instances in the number of fingers and toes.[61]

Since these parts were so much liable to change they did not furnish any stable information upon which to found a classification of mankind.[62] Instead, Prichard adopted the perspective assumed by Blumenbach and systematically explored by the German physical geographer Carl Ritter, who had developed a system of geographical conditions which, in varying degrees, were conducive or detrimental to civilization.

In the third edition of the *Researches* Prichard classed mankind according to its geographic stations.[63] His ethnological scheme will be discussed at a later stage where Ritter will figure prominently. In the context of biology, the German professor was important because he reintroduced social theories of a type that Prichard had encountered at Edinburgh. Revealing a pious mind which considered the world from a teleological point of view, Ritter's system explained the prevalence or absence of civilization as a function of more or less favourable geographical confines. Somesuch notions rekindled Prichard's memories of Scottish Enlightenment philosophy.

Renewed reliance on the impact of culture on living conditions, and hence bodily conformation, helped Prichard to revise his views on another front. In the third edition he finally accepted that characteristics acquired *post natum* might become hereditary. The same had been advocated by Cuvier's pupil François Désiré Roulin (1796-1874).[64] In a paper presented to the Paris Académie des Sciences in 1828, the French natural historian, referring to dogs, horses and cattle, had asserted two striking points. First, he showed that some animals passed on to their offspring "instincts" which they had artificially acquired. Habits which had been imparted "with care and art upon their ancestors" were transmitted to their posterity. This was true, for example, for barking: "wild dogs do not bark", noted Prichard, "they only howl". Roulin had shown that barking was an "acquired hereditary instinct".[65]

Secondly, he advanced an idea which proved Ritter's cultural environmentalism from the viewpoint of the naturalist. On a voyage through Venezuela and other parts of the Spanish territory of New Grenada, Roulin had observed that cows, abandoned by the first colonizers more than a century earlier, had lost their ability to provide an abundance of milk, having reverted to the original state. "A restoration of domestic animals to the wild state", Prichard stated, "causes a return towards the original characters of the wild tribe."[66] He considered this as a major insight. Indeed, it helped to overturn his previous views on the variability of wild and domesticated animals.

The Decay of Domestication

In 1813 Prichard had assumed that it was mainly the domesticated or civilized state that gave rise to new variations; by 1826, he had come to believe that domesticated animals and civilized men no longer changed to any great degree. Both hypotheses were reconcilable with his biological interpretation of civilization as a unilinear process. Now, however, the possibility loomed that civilization was – like domestication – a reversible state. In 1829 he claimed: "the facts related by M. Roulin respecting the effect of a change of climate, and the return to a wild state of domesticated races which had been transported to South America, are highly important".[67] Nowadays, Roulin is hardly known, but at the time his findings were warmly praised by Geoffroy Saint-Hilaire.[68] Being also a protégé of Cuvier, Roulin was a scientist not to be ignored. In consequence, Prichard abandoned the idea that acquired characteristics could by no means become hereditary. Obviously, they could. Roulin's observations in South America further diluted Prichard's idea that all variations made their first appearance suddenly, due to an immediate surge in one individual germinated ovum. He did not discard this theory, but he added another one to it, namely, that the environment might act slowly and gradually on all individuals of a given population at once, thus fashioning the latter according to the exigencies of the surroundings.[69]

Since Carl Ritter had given credence to the theory, Prichard admitted that adaptation to climatic circumstances was a beneficial institution of nature, enabling all human populations to bear the particular circumstances of their living conditions. Therefore, the observations of people like Roulin or the British zoologist and horticulturalist Thomas Andrew Knight (1759-1838)[70] had to be reckoned with. The idea that adaptation could, even in human populations, result in the loss of previously improved features was confirmed by "an excellent paper on the population, &c. of Ireland" which Prichard had read in the *Dublin University Magazine.* Its author asserted that native Irish who in the seventeenth century were "driven into the mountains" had, after "two centuries of degradation and hardship", acquired a "physical condition" which reflected their general "deterioration". The skulls of their descendants had approached to the least civilized, the prognathous form, "their advancing cheek-bones and depressed noses bear barbarism on their very front". On the whole they displayed "the worst effects of hunger and ignorance, the two great brutalizers of the human race".[71] Prichard was not anti-Irish – on the contrary, he praised the Irish for their early civilization.[72] His point was rather that civilized human populations, thrown back into wretched living conditions, survived through their physical adaptation to a different environment. (That this had, indeed, an impact on skull formation we shall see in the next chapter.)

Until the late 1820s he had taken it for granted that civilization was a unilinear process. If it were reversible, however, the natural historian had to change his outlooks entirely: the task would no longer be to establish the genealogy of an ascending line towards civilization and refinement, but explaining ethnological features within a framework of deviations. In the second edition Prichard had considered the development of varieties mainly under two aspects: either they were "deviations" from a "common standard", a "common original", a "common character", a "primitive type", a "general character", and a "common type".[73] Or they were deviations "towards a lighter shade", towards "a lighter and different hue".[74] This way of expressing himself mirrored his opinion that "fewer variations occur in races of white than in those of darker colour".[75] By the third edition, the term "deviation" was no longer pointing simply in the direction of increasingly light skin colour. Since Prichard had adopted the notion of "permanent varieties", the variations he described had ceased to refer to the original type of mankind. Instead he employed the word mainly to indicate differences. He spoke of deviations in "structure", or in "form and structure".[76] Organisms deviated in both directions, towards the development of refined features as well as towards a ruder physiognomy.

As with the degeneration of the Irish, the deviation towards the "African" type was regarded by Prichard as a degenerative process towards the worse. But since it was reversible the doctor must not be mistaken for a racial degenerationist (indeed, he tended to use the term "deviation" instead of "degeneration"). He believed that all human varieties possessed a certain potential for development either towards rudeness or towards refinement. External influences, whether climatic or cultural, largely determined to what extent human characteristics and faculties unfolded.

We have seen above that it was a peculiar characteristic of Prichard's anthropology that he came very near to considering civilization as an epi-phenomenon of Christianity, and that he regarded religion on the whole as an element of the instinctive or psychological propensities of mankind. In this respect he differed markedly from mainstream Enlightenment anthropology, which considered civilization primarily as a result of artifice and reason. If his growing exasperation over the un-Christian behaviour of colonials did not influence his biological views, it was yet reflected in the fact that his attitude towards civilization grew increasingly ambiguous: civilized manners did not, after all, go hand in hand with moral behaviour. With cool heads and starched collars civilized men went about exterminating helpless foreign peoples.

Civilized Rudeness

Prichard's moral misgivings will be examined in the next chapter. Suffice to say here that they surfaced even in his discussion of the origins of skin colour. In the third edition of the *Researches* he maintained that a light complexion was an effect of comfortable living conditions – "persons at ease" who were sheltered from the climates, acquired a lighter tint. Being "at ease" was certainly no ethical achievement. He made the point quite obvious when referring to the variations within the Malayans: the lower castes, he said, were dark, being "continually exposed to the agency of the climate". By contrast, "the chieftains and the people of a higher grade in the same islands lead an indolent and luxurious life. They have attained the average stature of Europeans, and in some instances exceed it."[77] Civilized existence, he let his readers know, was accompanied by "an indolent and luxurious life". The explicit comparison between European and Malayan features mirrored what Prichard thought of the Europeans themselves. There were numerous instances in the 1830s when he referred to the abject morality of civilized society.[78]

Civilization had as it were two "appearances", an internal and an external. The former implied a vision of true religion; the latter, by contrast, Prichard identified with "wealth and conveniences",[79] furthering indolence, moral depravity, and selfishness. To him it looked as if this second face, the decadent image of civilization, was outstripping the first. This opinion coloured his theory of madness and, as will be shown in the next chapter, it also imbued the

120

foundations of his ethnology.

Until the third edition of the *Researches* Prichard saw no reason to question his belief, characteristic of the late Enlightenment, that the course of history led from rudeness to refinement, in manners as well as in bodily shape. Once he had acknowledged that the unilinearity of human development was threatened, the potential consequences for civilization were massive: driving Roulin's observations concerning the return to the wild state to their full consequences would have meant that white Europeans could revert to the physical features of the Africans. But this was a conclusion Prichard avoided: "it will not immediately follow that the climates of Africa are capable of transmuting other races of men into Negroes or Hottentots".[80]

Roulin had shown the impermanence of animal tribes. Prichard was not, however, prepared to accept that this might apply to mankind. This meant that the analogical method faltered when it came to the eminently important question of the extent to which the rise of new varieties was possible. In 1836, he posed himself the question: "are the varieties in mankind more permanent than in the lower tribes?"[81] His answer was that there were so many different degrees of species permanency in the animal realm itself, that it was futile to compare animals to mankind in that respect.[82] Thus he got himself off the hook in view of the disconcerting consequences that an application of Roulin's theory to the variations in mankind would have had. In *The Natural History of Man*, when he expressly confronted Roulin's theory,[83] he dismissed its consequences for human development at a stroke: "the influence of the mind must be more extensive and powerful in its operations upon human beings than upon brutes. And this difference transcends all analogy or comparison."[84]

According to his own standards this argument was weak: it was not sustained by any further reflections, and it defied that principle of analogy which Prichard had extended in the third edition of the *Researches* to encompass a comparison between the psychology of mankind and animals. The analogical method, one of the mainstays of his anthropology, was overridden by Prichard's insistence that, in the last event, the mind triumphed over mere physicality. To give him his due, it must be said that he did not, as it were, accidentally stumble upon this way out of a calamity. From the 1830s Prichard's work in the field of natural history placed ever greater emphasis on the immaterial reasoning powers, at the expense of mere physicality.

As he gradually relinquished the hope of proving the unity of mankind through arguments directly derived from physical aspects of natural history, he lost interest in the latest developments in the field of heredity – hence his failure to develop a consistent theory of heredity, capable of negotiating the conceptual gap between environmental stimuli and their influence on the hereditary fabric. How little he was anxious to solve the problem is instanced by his entire neglect of embryology, which was gaining ground from the 1830s. This shift of emphasis is not devoid of irony. For, as Prichard increasingly relied on the cultural aspects of anthropology, his reputation as Britain's foremost ethnologist was established.

His achievements in biological theory lie less in the answers he suggested than in the questions he posed. Being scrupulously aware that the problem of the origin of human variations had more facets than a fish had scales, he found himself stranded on the shore where, some decades later, Charles Darwin's amphibia would scramble onto the land, gradually turn into mammals, then into humans, and then into historians, some of whom would pick up the shells of Prichard's theory and call them anticipations of evolutionary theory. Both his notion of "connate" traits as well as his concept of marital selection reminded them of Darwinism. As we have seen, they had in fact precious little to do with it. The truth is that they flowed from his quest for new mechanisms of variation through which he tried to demonstrate that there was an alternative to the structured rigidity of polygenism.

Notes

1 Prichard, *Researches*, 2nd ed., 1: 91.

2 *Ibid.*, 1st ed., p. 194.

3 *Ibid.*, 1st ed., p. ii.

4 J. Borthwick, "Notes from A Course of Lectures on Moral Philosophy. Delivered by Dugald Stewart Esq. 1806-7", pp. 365-66. MS Gen. 843. Special Collections, Edinburgh University Library.

5 For the problem of skin colour see Renato G. Mazzolini, "Anatomische Untersuchungen über die Haut der Schwarzen (1700-1800)". In *Die Natur des Menschen*, ed. Gunter Mann *et al.*, pp. 169-87; *idem*, "Il colore della pelle e l'origine ell'antropologia fisica". In *L'Epopea delle soperte*, ed. Renzo Zorzi (Florence: Leo S. Olschki, 1994), pp. 227-39.

6 Herbert Spencer has been credited with having coined the term "environmentalism". See Armin Hajman Koller, *The Theory of Environment, an Outline of the History of the Idea of Milieu, and its Present Status* (Menasha: University of Chicago Press, 1918), p. 5.

7 Ronald Meek, *Social Science and the Ignoble Savage* (Cambridge: Cambridge University Press, 1976); Robert Shackleton, "The

Evolution of Montesquieu's Theory of Climate". *Revue internationale de philosophie* 9 (1955): 317-29; Waldemar Zacharasiewicz, *Die Klimatheorie in der Englischen Literatur und Literaturkritik von der Mitte des 16. bis zum frühen 18. Jahrhundert* (Wien: Braumüller, 1978).

8   Blumenbach, *De generis humani varietate nativa*, p. 211.

9   For Kames see William Lehmann, *Henry Home, Lord Kames, and the Scottish Enlightenment: A Study in National Character and in the History of Ideas* (The Hague: M. Nijhoff, 1971).

10 Prichard, "Of the Varieties of the Human Race", p. 133.

11 Prichard, *Researches*, 1st ed., p. 199. Cf. also: *Researches*, 2nd ed., 2: 542.

12 Prichard attended one of his courses at the University. See the Matriculation Indexes. MS Da 35, Edinburgh University Library, Special Collections.

13 Prichard, *Researches*, 1st ed., p. 194.

14 *Ibid.*, p. 25. Cf. also: *idem*, "Of the Varieties of the Human Race", p. 98.

15 Prichard, "Of the Varieties of the Human Race", p. 101.

16 *Ibid.*, p. 103. Cf. also his *Researches*, 1st ed., pp. 25-27.

17 Prichard, "Of the Varieties of the Human Race", p. 97.

18 *Ibid.*, pp. 107, 109.

19 Prichard, *Researches*, 1st ed., p. iii.

20 See E. B. Poulton, "A Remarkable Anticipation of Modern Views on Evolution". In *idem, Essays on Evolution* (Oxford: Clarendon, 1908), pp. 173-92; Annemarie de Waal Malefijt, *Images of Man. A History of Anthropological Thought* (New York: Alfred A. Knopf, 1974), p. 267.

21 In the 1790s ideas about the mutability of species were much flaunted. See R. W. Burckhardt Jr, "Lamarck, Evolution and the Politics of Science". *Journal of the History of Biology* 3 (1970): 275-98; *idem, The Spirit of System: Lamarck and Evolutionary Biology* (Cambridge, Mass.: Harvard University Press, 1977), pp. 202-9.

22 Prichard, *Researches*, 1st ed., p. 198. Jacques Roger explained why and how Buffon placed limits upon organic changes. Peter Bowler has even suggested that Buffon's theory of generation, presupposing a fixed internal mould, was reconcilable with preformationist theories. However true that may be, Prichard considered Buffon's theory of generation as absurd. Janet Browne's characterization of Prichard as "one of Buffon's greatest admirers" seems to be exaggerated. Peter Bowler, "Bonnet and Buffon"; Browne, *The Secular Ark*, p. 156; Jacques Roger, *Buffon* (Ithaca: Cornell University Press, 1997 (1989)).

23 Erasmus Darwin, *Zoonomia or, the Laws of Organic Life*, 2 vols (London: printed for J. Johnson, 1794-96), 1: 501.

24 Wells, therefore, erroneously denied that Prichard might have discussed Lamarckian ideas. See Kentwood D. Wells, "Sir William Lawrence (1783-1867). A Study of Pre-Darwinian Ideas on Heredity and Variation". *Journal of the History of Biology* 4 (1971): 319-61, p. 359.

25 Prichard, *Doctrine of a Vital Principle*, p. 227. His criticism included Lamarck as well.

26 Prichard rejected the theory of the Chain of Being because it brought man and apes into too great proximity. Transmutationism did the same, and was even more dangerous than the Chain of Being because it implied a genetic relationship instead of a mere classificatory one.

27 Cf. Prichard, *Researches*, 1st ed., p. 75.

28 For Hunter see S. J. Cross, "John Hunter, the Animal Oeconomy, and Late Eighteenth Century Physiological Discourse". *Studies in the History of Biology* 5 (1981): 1-110.

29 Prichard, *Researches*, 1st ed., p. 233.

30 Cf. Bynum, "Time's Noblest Offspring", p. 87. Such a theory had already been put forward by the Edinburgh-trained Philadelphia doctor Samuel Stanhope Smith in his *An Essay on the Causes of the Variety of Complexion and Figure in the Human Species* (1787).

31 The observation tallied with the late eighteenth-century tendency to regard sexuality as "social institution". See Alan Bewell, "'On the Banks of the South Sea': Botany and Sexual Controversy in the Late Eighteenth Century". In *Visions of Empire*, pp. 173-93, see p. 173.

32 Prichard, *Researches*, 1st ed., pp. 236-37. Theories about the race-forming capacity of marital selection were prevalent among Scottish Enlightenment philosophers. Prichard's novel approach lay in the combination of this theory with laws of natural history.

33 Prichard, *Researches*, 1st ed., p. 235.

34 *Ibid.*, p. 233. The point is of particular importance for Bynum; see "Time's Noblest Offspring", pp. 101-4; cf. also Stocking, "From Chronology to Ethnology", pp. liv, lxv-lxviii.

35 Prichard, *Researches*, 1st ed., pp. 222-23.

36 *Ibid.*, p. 235.

37 *Ibid.*, pp. 222, 209.

38 Prichard, *Researches*, 2nd ed., 1: vi; *ibid.*, 3rd ed., 1: v.

39 See Frank W. P. Dougherty, "Johann Friedrich Blumenbach und Samuel Thomas Soemmerring: Eine Auseinandersetzung in anthropologischer Hinsicht". In *Samuel Thomas Soemmerring und die*

Gelehrten der Goethezeit, ed. Gunter Mann, Jost Benedum, Werner Kümmel (Stuttgart: Gustav Fischer, 1988), pp. 35-56; *idem*, "Christoph Meiners und Johann Friedrich Blumenbach im Streit um den Begriff der Menschenrasse".

40 Prichard, *Researches*, 2nd ed., 2: 575. For Prichard's usage of the term "degeneration" see below.

41 For the impact of Kant's philosophy on the natural sciences see Frederick Gregory, "Kant's Influence on Natural Scientists in the German Romantic Period". In *New Trends in the History of Science. Proceedings of a Conference held at the University of Utrecht*, ed. Robert Visser *et al.* (Amsterdam: Rodopi, 1989), pp. 53-66. Blumenbach himself said about his theory of generation that it constituted "*the union and intimate coexertion of two distinct principles in the evolution of the nature of organized bodies, – of the PHYSICO-MECHANICAL, with the purely TELEOLOGICAL*". See Blumenbach, *The Institutions of Physiology*, p. 336 (original emphases). For the philosophical background of Blumenbach's natural history see Karl J. Fink, "Storm and Stress Anthropology"; Timothy Lenoir, *The Strategy of Life, Teleology and Mechanics in Nineteenth Century German Biology* (Dordrecht: Reidel, 1982).

42 For the generation theory of Kant and Blumenbach and the points where they did not meet see Phillip R. Sloan, "Buffon, German Biology, and the Historical Interpretation of Biological Species". For Kant in particular see Peter McLaughlin, *Kant's Critique of Teleology in Biological Explanation* (Lewiston: E. Mellen Press, 1991).

43 Prichard, *Researches*, 2nd ed., 2: 536.

44 *Ibid.* Cf. also: *idem, Doctrine of a Vital Principle*, p. 139. Note that Prichard did not expressly name Blumenbach as the source of this theory. That it was gleaned from Blumenbach, however, is extremely likely, not least because Prichard developed it only once he had assimilated Blumenbach's texts. For his previous assumptions see his *Researches*, 1st ed., p. 231.

45 Prichard, *Researches*, 2nd ed., 2: 545.

46 *Ibid.*, p. 551.

47 *Ibid.*, p. 555.

48 It is not particularly fruitful to address Prichard's writings in terms of a gendered analysis. Still, it was obviously in line with contemporary notions of masculinity that it was the male who ensured the constancy of species.

49 Prichard, *Researches*, 2nd ed., 2: 548 (Prichard's emphases).

50 *Ibid.*, p. 532. Prichard explicitly extended this law to "acquired varieties of constitution". See *ibid.*, p. 547. His definition of species was formulated accordingly: "two races are considered as specifically

125

different, if they are distinguished from each other by some peculiarities, which one cannot be supposed to have acquired, or the other to have lost, through any known operation of physical causes". *ibid.*, 1: 90.

51 *Ibid.*, 2: 582.

52 *Ibid.*, pp. 582, 566. Now he admitted that "it does not appear to be very important in respect to the general conclusion to be drawn [that is, monogenism], whether the deviations we observe are found to display themselves at once in strongly marked examples, or take place by slow and imperceptible degrees". This means that he did not deem it necessary that a particular complexion sprang up at once in a tribe. It was conceivable that it was the result of a process comprising several stages; *ibid.*, 1: 102.

53 Prichard, *Researches*, 2nd ed., 2: 551.

54 Azara and Hunter agreed only in respect of the original colour, which they imagined to have been dark rather than light. Cf. Prichard, *Researches*, 2nd ed., 2: 560; cf. also: *ibid.*, 3rd ed., 1: 341.

55 Prichard, *Researches*, 2nd ed., 2: 583.

56 On these grounds Prichard surmised that the well-being of an individual enhanced the colour of his complexion. This was exemplified in the skin of black slaves working on the plantations: the skin of field slaves was of "a dusky hue", while those working in the house were a lot blacker. "The better a Negro is fed and clothed", Prichard wrote, "and the more healthy he is, the darker is the colour of his skin." *Researches*, 2nd ed., 2: 536. The observation fits ill with Prichard's other remarks about skin colour – little as he contradicted himself over time, he yet managed to do it in one and the same publication.

57 Bynum, "Time's Noblest Offspring", p. 107; Stocking, "From Chronology to Ethnology", p. lxxx.

58 Prichard, *Researches*, 3rd ed., 5: 547.

59 *Ibid.*, p. 550.

60 *Ibid.*, p. 548, see also p. 612.

61 *Ibid.*, 1: 113.

62 Prichard would be too reticent to mention it, but we may safely assume that this list also included the length of the penis: it was generally supposed that the genitals of dark-skinned men were particularly sizeable, which in turn fuelled the idea that people of colour possessed more animal spirits, while Europeans and their American cousins were endowed with superior reasoning qualities. Cf. Blumenbach, *De generis humani varietate nativa*, p. 249; Charles White, *An Account of the Regular Gradation in Man and in Different*

Animals and Vegetables... (London: printed for C. Dilly, 1799), p. 61.

63 For the importance of Ritter see Hanno Beck, *Carl Ritter. Genius der Geographie* (Berlin: Dietrich Reimer Verlag, 1979); Karl Lenz, ed., *Carl Ritter – Geltung und Deutung. Beiträge des Symposiums anläßlich der Wiederkehr des 200. Geburtstages von Carl Ritter November 1979 in Berlin (West)* (Berlin: Dietrich Reimer Verlag, 1981). Prichard quoted from the second edition of Ritter's description of Africa, published in 1822, and from the seven-volume enterprise in which Ritter demonstrated the physical geography of Asia: *Die Erdkunde im Verhältniß zur Natur und zur Geschichte des Menschen, oder allgemeine vergleichende Geographie*, 7 vols (Berlin: G. Reimer, 1832-43).

64 Roulin translated Prichard's *Natural History of Man* into French: *Histoire naturelle de l'homme* (Paris: J.-B. Baillière, 1843). Prichard became acquainted with Roulin's article shortly after publication. See his *Doctrine of a Vital Principle*, p. 225.

65 Prichard, *Natural History of Man*, pp. 35-36. Cf. François Désiré Roulin, "Mémoire sur quelques changemens observés dans les animaux domestiques transportés de l'ancien monde dans le nouveau continent, lue à l'Académie Royale des Sciences le 29. Sept. 1828". *Annales des sciences naturelles* 16 (1829): 16-34.

66 Prichard, *Natural History of Man*, pp. 39-40.

67 Prichard, *Doctrine of a Vital Principle*, note on p. 228.

68 Etienne Geoffroy Saint-Hilaire, "Rapport fait à l'Académie des Sciences sur un mémoire de M. Roulin...". *Annales des sciences naturelles* 16 (1829): 34-44. For an excellent exposition of Geoffroy's biology see Toby Appel, *The Cuvier–Geoffroy Debate: French Biology in the Decades before Darwin* (Oxford: Oxford University Press, 1987).

69 Prichard, *Researches*, 3rd ed., 5: 549-50. Unlike the *Researches*, *The Natural History of Man* referred explicitly to the doctrine of "acclimatization". See *Natural History of Man*, p. 39. For the notion of acclimatization see David Livingstone, "Human Acclimatization: Perspectives on a Contested Field of Enquiry in Science, Medicine and Geography". *History of Science* 25 (1987): 359-94.

70 Thomas Andrew Knight, "On the Economy of Bees...". *Philosophical Transactions* 97 (1807): 234-44; *idem*, "On the Hereditary Instinctive Propensities of Animals...". *Philosophical Transactions* 127 (1837): 365-69. For Prichard's reception of Knight's theory see his *Researches*, 3rd ed., 1: 374; *idem, Natural History of Man*, pp. 70-72. Indeed, the idea that domesticated animals might revert in their instincts to the original state was not new for Prichard. See his *Researches*, 1st ed., p. 115. As he acknowledged in

1829, Blumenbach and Azara had made "many parallel remarks". See Prichard, *Doctrine of a Vital Principle*, note on p. 28. What may be called Prichard's teleological view of natural history, however, had hitherto precluded him from considering the question whether domestication and civilization were reversible processes. It was not that he could not *think* the possibility – he simply did not see the need to do so (for the only exception, Noah's immediate posterity, see Chapter 5).

71 Prichard, *Researches*, 3rd ed., vol. 2, note on p. 349.

72 Prichard, "On the Recent Progress of Ethnology" (Anniversary Address for 1848 to the Ethnological Society of London). *Edinburgh New Philosophical Journal* 46 (1848): 53-72, p. 72. The imaginativeness and artistic talent of the Celts was a Victorian topos. See Mary Cowling, *The Artist as Anthropologist. The Representation of Type and Character in Victorian Art* (Cambridge: Cambridge University Press, 1989), p. 136.

73 Prichard, *Researches*, 2nd ed., 1: 111, 234, 241; 2: 37, 558, 570, 587, 590.

74 *Ibid.*, 1: 357; 2: 454.

75 *Ibid.*, 2: 583. As late as 1834 he claimed that "it would be difficult to point out any clearly ascertained fact which proves that the descendants of a white stock have ever become black" while the contrary was very common. See the abstract of Prichard's "Three Lectures on Egyptian Mummies, Egyptian Antiquities, and the Rosetta Stone". Held on 31 March, 2 April, and 4 April 1834 at the Bristol Institution. Richard Smith, "Manuscript Memoirs", p. 650.

76 Prichard, *Researches*, 3rd ed., 1: 242, 246, 110. Deviations occurred in "the character of a parent-stock", in "the original or the prevalent character of each tribe", in "the peculiarities of the stock from which" an individual "sprang". *Ibid.*, 3rd ed., 1: 108, 373; 2: 343.

77 *Ibid.*, 3rd ed., 5: 285.

78 *Ibid.*, vol. 2, note on p. 34. See also: Prichard, "Letter to Dr Hodgkin", p. 57.

79 Prichard, *Manual of Ethnology, Extract from the Admiralty Manual of Scientific Enquiry* (London: W. Clowes and Sons, 1859), p. 13.

80 Prichard, *Researches*, 3rd ed., 2: 340.

81 *Ibid.*, 1: 373.

82 *Ibid.*, 1: 373-74.

83 In part he may have done so to please Roulin, the translator of the book.

84 Prichard, *Natural History of Man*, pp. 75-76.

5

The Third Calling:
Ethnology or The Unity of Mankind in Time and Space

Within the monogenist research programme, ethnology was a historical science. As such, it relied on philology and cultural relics, such as paintings in tombs and on ancient vases. Comparatively speaking, the linguistic history of mankind was thought to be better comprehended than its physical. The oldest languages dating only a few thousand years in the past, this approach was easily reconcilable with the scriptural tenet that Creation had taken place just six thousand years ago.

In the last two chapters Prichard's principles of physiology and natural history have been discussed. In this chapter we shall follow him into the forests of ethnological data. In his case, that means going back time out of mind, pursuing the historical traces left by long-extinct nations: Prichard believed he had got back within a small number of generations from the primeval couple. They were universally imagined as white. But was that also his opinion, given that he had declared that "primitive man" was black? Although in the third edition of the *Researches* he relegated skin colour to a place of secondary importance, classing it with the rapidly changing "integuments", he was still obsessed with pigmentation. The untractable question was further complicated by the sudden appearance of a black Brahmin in Bristol. This chapter will deal with both "black" Adam and Rajah Ramohun Roy. Prichard was never satisfied that he had solved the problem of skin colour. His own classification of human varieties, accordingly, followed geographical rather than purely physiological principles. Finally, this chapter will discuss his attitude to the topic of race, not on theoretical grounds but in the light of existing peoples.

Early Human History

Prichard's investigations led him from the present into the historical darkness of the centuries before the birth of Christ. Tacitus wrote *Germania*, his accounts of the ancient Germans, in the year 98 c.e. Prichard decided that the dialects of those Germans and the Celts

129

must have been formed during "the first millennium before the Christian era", while languages like Sanskrit, Greek, and Latin which had developed from a common original, were of much earlier date – he suggested the second millennium b.c.e.[1] This was when he thought that the great migrations had taken place. However vague these assumptions from the 1830s, the author of the first edition of the *Researches* had not even decided in which millennium language formation and the first great migrations had occurred.

Prichard had a clear idea of what he considered to be historically recorded time. Its pattern was as follows: the Mediterranean and the Nile regions were known back to around 1000 b.c.e. With regard to the centuries before 500 b.c.e., when the Greek and Roman polities began to flourish, he referred to the Biblical chronology which was corroborated by the Egyptian king Ptolomy I (b. 367-66 b.c.e.).[2] Peoples of other continents, Prichard held, had branched off from the Noachic stem before the Indo-European family of nations had broken up into European and Asiatic peoples. This explained why the languages of far-off nations were so different from the Indo-European languages and those which others would call "Semitic" and which Prichard termed the Syro-Arabian family of languages.[3]

Prichard never attempted to indicate when exactly certain peoples had quit their abode to travel into other regions. But he did not doubt that at one time some peoples had left the region of Asia Minor in the direction of India, while others had turned towards Europe. Before that epoch the centre of human civilization was located in the lands between the Ganges and the Nile. The northern limit of this area was the Caspian Sea, and to the south there was the Indian Ocean. In these confines lay "the region in which mankind first advanced to civilization". It was, Prichard conjectured in 1813, "the primitive abode of our species".[4] Following Genesis, he held that at some very early point in history, mankind had branched out into the posterity of Shem, Ham, and Japhet.[5] But, as we will learn, Prichard's own physio-anatomical classification of mankind had nothing to do with these three groups. He merely took these populations as representative of three different cultural developments, their differences being due to their different living conditions. He identified three

> scenes of the most ancient cultivation of the human race… In one of these, the Semitic nations exchanged the simple habits of wandering shepherds for the splendour and luxury of Nineveh and Babylon. In another an Indo-European or Japetic people brought to

its perfection the most elaborate of human dialects, destined to become in later ages under different modifications the mother tongue of the nations of Europe. In a third, the land of Ham, watered by the Nile, were invented hieroglyphic literature and the arts for which Egypt was celebrated in the earliest ages of history.[6]

At yet another stage further back, there were only two original countries: the Biblical realms of Elam and Edom in the era of Abraham, peopled by "the Indo-Persians or Hindus" and the Egyptians, respectively. "As to the quarter whence [mankind] first ramified, the cradle of the stock and perhaps of the human race", he added modestly, "we have no data in history."[7]

Was Adam Black?

Despite the spirit of ignorance hovering above the origins of mankind, Prichard speculated that primitive men were black.[8] Any reader versed in the field knew that the Dutch anatomist Petrus Camper, the geologist Peter Simon Pallas, and John Hunter had suggested the same.[9] In the eighteenth century it was not an uncommon speculation. But since the mid-nineteenth century incredulous commentators have vulgarized the notion, asserting that Prichard took Adam for a black man.[10] That, however, is questionable. He himself never mentioned Adam's name, nor did he speculate about his skin colour. All he said was that "the primitive stock of men were Negroes".[11] Other evidence confirms that Prichard's Adam was not black. Let us consider some of it.

In its discussion of "language", the sixth edition of the *Encyclopaedia Britannica* (1823) referred to the human state before the Fall. Claiming that language was given to man by God, the *Encyclopaedia* explained that the Bible "represents the first human inhabitants of this earth, not only as reasoning and speaking animals, but also as in a state of high perfection and happiness, of which they were deprived for disobedience to their Creator".[12] The Cambridge physician John Elliotson, who translated Blumenbach's *Institutions of Physiology*, was of like mind. In the notes appended to the second edition of the translation (1817), Elliotson commented on the notion of natural perfection. In that context he endorsed Prichard's theory of original blackness, affirming that it was "rendered extremely probable by the analogy of animals, among which Mr. Hunter remarked that the changes of colour were always from the darker to the lighter tints". Then he added: "if we believe that he [man] was created in perfection, we must believe that after the fall his

131

nature experienced the general change; that he became destitute and wretched, and destined to reach perfection by slow degrees".[13] A similar notion was asserted by the Bristol printer, self-styled scholar and active member of the Bristol Literary and Philosophical Society, John Mathew Gutch. In 1827 he gave a paper at the Institution, pointing out that Adam's "faculties would be greatly weakened by the Fall" and that the destruction of the tower of Babel would throw mankind into a "state of barbarism".[14] Despite the impressions of some later interpreters, it seems that, at the time of the first edition of the *Researches*, Britons did not believe that Adam could have been black. It is probable that Prichard shared their views, surmising that "primitive man" was black, whilst Adam was not. As late as 1838 Bunsen understood the author of the *Researches* in exactly this way: "the savage is a degraded man, not man a civilised savage. Pritchard's [sic] work scarcely allows me to sleep."[15]

Prichard did not indicate when the first humans lost their dark skin colour, though as early as the fifth century b.c.e., Herodotus had suggested that the Egyptians had all been black.[16] Prichard held that the trait had been prevalent long before it caught Herodotus's eyes. The great Blumenbach in Göttingen had showed the way to solve the question. In a memoir, published in 1794 in the *Philosophical Transactions* of the Royal Society, Blumenbach had set out that three different physiognomical types were to be perceived in the Egyptian mummies and sepulchral paintings: the Berber, the Ethiopian, and the Indian type.[17] This was grist to Prichard's mill. In 1813 he wrote, quoting Blumenbach, that "the general complexion was black, or at least a very dusky hue", but "a part of the population of Egypt resembled the modern Hindus".[18] This notion tallied with his theory that civilization was a whitening agent: "the Egyptians were a civilized people and we should expect to find examples of a fair complexion among the better orders at least".[19]

What applied to Edom was true for Elam as well: Prichard believed that the ancient Hindus had been just as black as the earliest Egyptians. While the Egyptian evidence had rested on sepulchral remains, in the case of the ancient Indians it was provided by sculptures found in old temples.[20] "There can be no doubt", he wrote in 1813, "that the prototypes from which they were designed, were either Negroes properly so called, or that they were possessed of physical characteristics similar to those of the natives of Africa." Comparison of Indian and Egyptian mythologies, as well as the fact that old Indian pagodas had a significant "pyramidal" shape, seemed to suggest "that the inhabitants of ancient Egypt and of India were separated portions of one kindred stock" and that "both these races possessed originally the characters of the genuine Ethiopians or Negroes".[21]

That the Indians, Ethiopians, and Egyptians were closely allied, was always one of Prichard's pet theories.[22] But, as will be shown in the following section, it was to prove difficult to uphold the notion that their skin colour changed as civilization improved. Moreover, it turned out that Blumenbach had been quite wrong in asserting that the Indian type was to be found among the Egyptians.[23] Criticisms of his analysis were numerous. The sudden abundance of British specialists in the complexion of ancient Egyptians grew in part out of a great exhibition in London in 1821, put together by the traveller Giovanni Battista Belzoni (1778-1823).

Egyptian Antiquities and Skin Colour

What was known as the "Egyptian fever" arose from Napoleon's expedition to Egypt in 1798-99. As a by-product of the Anglo-French wars, both powers settled permanently in Egypt. Pasha Mehemet Ali, the ruling autocrat, shared with Napoleon his year of birth – 1769 – and the ambition of modernizing his country. He invited the French government to help him build up an effective administration. During the 1810s he was also entertaining friendly relations with Britain. By 1822, in the eyes of Europeans, Egypt was very different from the obscure place it had been before the French invasion.[24] An Albanian by birth, Mehemet Ali had no particular reverence for the ancient Egyptian antiquities. If Europeans brought him knowledge, he was happy to reward them with tons of what he considered old rubble.

It was a time when derring-do men could thrive. One such was the Italian athlete and public performer Giovanni Battista Belzoni. Through the agency of Henry Salt, the British consul in Cairo, he had been entrusted to collect as many antique artefacts as he could grab. In 1820 he travelled to Britain to present his finds, sepulchral antiquities from his own excavations near Thebes (Luxor) and from the huge temple sites of Philae and Elephantine in southern Egypt, dating back to the reign of the Ptolomies in the fourth century b.c.e. Nearly two hundred life-size copies of Egyptian monuments as well as 800 copies measuring one to three feet were despatched to London.[25] Belzoni arranged to have his objects exhibited in the fortunately named "Egyptian Hall" erected in 1812 at Piccadilly. The exhibition was inaugurated on 1 May 1821, with the opening of a mummy in front of a select audience of medical men and the press.

Belzoni's greatest achievement was a complete reproduction of a burial chamber, including all the wall paintings and statues. In wax and papier mâché the outer burial chamber of Sethy I (father of Ramesses II – he died ca. 1300 b.c.e.) arose.[26] The exhibition lasted for a year and proved an enormous success.[27]

Thus all London could form its own ideas about the complexion of the ancient Egyptians.[28] It was pointed out that the colour of the figures depicted on the exhibits was dark brown, not black as Prichard had averred. A contributor to *Fraser's Magazine*, for instance, rejected Prichard's theory of the original blackness of man as "not … substantiated" because "on the tomb of an ancient Egyptian king figures of dark-brown complexioned men are drawn, but they have not the *hair* which peculiarly characterises the Negro race of the present age".[29] In his comments, published in a catalogue accompanying the exhibition, Belzoni referred the three different types of skin colour – reddish, dark, and whitish – to Egyptians, Ethiopians, Jews and Persians respectively.[30] Some fifteen years later the librarian and palaeographer Jean-Jacques Champollion-Figeac (1778-1867), brother of the famous Jean-François who deciphered the hieroglyphics, corrected the English interpretation: the bas-relief did not depict the nations conquered by the Pharaohs, but the different "races of men" known at the time.[31] Around the middle of the nineteenth century American racialists relied on that interpretation to support their theory that racial characteristics had been immutable throughout the natural history of man.[32]

In the 1820s anthropology was not so deterministic. Unfortunately we do not know what Prichard would have made out of Belzoni's exhibition; it seems that he did not even visit it. For all Prichard knew about Egyptian tombs by the 1820s, they depicted only two different types: "the tawny Ethiopians" and the "comparatively fair Egyptians".[33] This information was taken from the *Account of Antient and Modern Egypt* (1809) by Lord Elgin's secretary, William Richard Hamilton (1777-1859). He had visited the temples of Philae and Elephantine, and his *Account* attempted to explain the two different types of light and dark coloured "sculptures" he had seen there.[34] Prichard summarized:

> In the temple of Philae, the sculptures frequently depict two persons who equally represent the characters and symbols of Osiris, and two persons equally answering to those of Isis; but in both cases one is invariably much older than the other, and appears to be the superior divinity.[35]

Hamilton – whose book is nowadays deemed "authoritative but extraordinarily dull"[36] – was not interested in ascertaining how the dark and the light varieties of man were related; he merely suggested that they might symbolize the "devolution of sovereignty from father to son, or the communication of religious mysteries from Ethiopia to Egypt".[37] For Prichard, by contrast, the figures had an ethnological meaning: "it is plain", he argued, "that the idea meant to be conveyed can be nothing else than this, that the red Egyptians were connected by kindred, and in fact were the descendants of a black race, probably the Ethiopian".[38]

In 1826 he obviously still believed that light human varieties originated from black ones. Since the history of the Egyptians reached as far back as that of the Hebrews and was, therefore, necessarily almost as old as human history, their development was not just any example but a very strong evidence of the direction human history had taken. When, in the third edition, Prichard came back to this topic, he repeated his central notion.[39] The difference was only that he now called the colour of original men "melanous" instead of "black".[40] (Like many, he thought that terminology made the scientist: dark-skinned varieties were dubbed "melanous", what others called "yellow" skin was "xanthous", and "leucos" referred to white humans.) Yet, as Prichard had grown aware that the case of unilinear physical development was difficult to prove, he would no longer trumpet the idea as he had done in previous years.

That does not mean, however, that he discarded it. It was certainly no accident that he had chosen the illustration of a jet-black man as the frontispiece of the volume on the ethnology of Europe. The choice is highly significant, the illustration meaning to represent European and Asiatic peoples.[41] The man of that picture was the Indian Brahmin Ramohun Roy (ca. 1772-1833[42]).[43] He was an enigmatic figure in the first third of the nineteenth century: an Indian prince who grew up in Bengal, one of the British domains in India.[44] As a teenager he temporarily fell out with his father. His education as well as his acquaintance with the British way of life and Christian religion drove the adolescent into opposition against Indian traditions.[45] He professed his adherence to Unitarianism, translated parts of the Vedas into English and harboured the ambition to equal European scholars. As an envoy of the petty King of Delhi, who had himself called an Emperor, in 1831 Ramohun Roy was sent to Britain to contest "certain encroachments" on the king's rights by the East India Company.[46] In 1832-33 he spent several months in Bristol: and as tends to happen when reality encroaches on

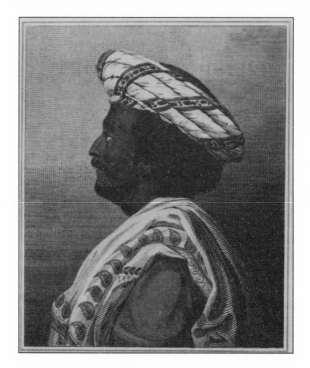

Figure 9
Rajah Ramohun Roy (ca. 1772-1833); he died in Bristol. Defying
contemporary notions of European singularity, Prichard chose the black
prince as a frontispiece to the third volume of the 3rd edition of the *Researches.*

the scholar's mind, Ramohun Roy's presence disturbed the smooth
path of Prichard's theorizing. The interruption, it must be said, was
nonetheless not very great, for an outstanding feature of Prichard's
hypothesizing was a versatility not embarrassed by contradictory
statements. Provided that there were some principles underlying
nature's phenomena and as long as these barred the threat of
contingency, Prichard did not care much which they were. Hence
Ramohun Roy's presence seemed to confirm, rather than to
controvert, his physical history.

When news of the noble Indian convert first reached England, he
was depicted as a gentleman. Part and parcel of the description was
the hint that the Rajah's looks were conformable to the European
standard of taste. As it was summarized in the *Monthly Review,* "he is
particularly handsome, not of a very dark complexion, of a fine

person, and most courtly manners".[47] When the Rajah finally arrived in Bristol, however, he gave a very different impression. Prichard described him thus: "the countenance of a very dark Brahman. Ram-Mohun-Roy was much darker than many Africans."[48] Having set out the idea that civilization (and Christianity) furthered a white complexion, he was certainly somewhat surprised to see that the Rajah in fact was darker than, according to his own scheme, civilized people were.

It had been frequently observed that Indian Brahmins were endowed with a complexion that was lighter than that of lower castes. Eighteenth-century scholars had surmised that they must belong to different populations: contemplating the origins of the caste system, the German historian Arnold Hermann Ludwig Heeren (1760-1842) suggested that the Brahmins were a nation of the north who had, at some stage in history, subdued the darker peoples of the Indian sub-continent. Subsequent racial segregation would have led to the preservation of skin colour in the respective castes.[49]

It characterizes Prichard's disinclination to take up racial theorizing that he did not espouse this idea: as he saw it, Ramohun Roy's features refuted the notion of original racial differences: if the Rajah was as black as any Pariah, why should they belong to different races?[50] In another context Prichard might have evoked social status to account for the Rajah's peculiar skin colour. This, however, was out of the question, as the pious civility of the Rajah, as it were, contradicted his uncouth complexion. Climate, too, provided no answer. Prichard's solution was as simple as it suited his philosophy: he had always been the first to assert that characteristics peculiar to any one population could spring up in any other as well; now, Ramohun Roy came as a living proof of that theory.[51] "The Brahmans", Prichard explained with reference to the Rajah,

> are generally of lighter colour than the low castes, but this is subject to exceptions. The agency of external causes on breeds of animals, and on races of men, is not uniform if we regard individuals. The influence of external conditions is more favourable to the development of one variety than another, and its operation is perceived on a large scale, but not in every individual instance.[52]

Ramohun Roy was an exception to the rule. Of course, exceptions smacked of contingency. But that did not threaten Prichard, for he had elevated his concept of "individual instance" to something akin to a general law. It is only very rarely that we find him raising any doubts as to order in nature. And as it was most manifestly expressed second volume of the *Researches* (1837), Prichard briefly toyed with the question whether the white European variety of mankind might have sprung up accidentally, as a *lusus naturae*, as it were. He reminded his readers of the description of Albino girls in India – they were deemed beautiful by the local people, their white skin might one day dominate the complexion of the region. As a travel writer had suggested: "it is easy to conceive that an accidental variety of this kind might propagate, and that the white race of mankind is sprung from such an accidental variety. The Indians are of this opinion, and there is a tradition or story amongst them in which this origin is assigned to us." Prichard quoted this story not only in the *Researches* but also in *The Natural History of Man*.[53]

It might look to us as though the example of Ramohun Roy threatened Prichard's theories, but in his eyes it was the reverse: on the one hand, he used Ramohun Roy's portrait as a frontispiece to hint at the still looming possibility that the first human populations on the globe had been black. On the other, the Rajah's appearance reassured him that external features were of slight importance when it came to classifying the varieties of mankind. Instead he chose a system that was based on geography and greatly influenced by the teachings of Carl Ritter.

Classifying Mankind:
The Argument of "Geography" and the Argument of "Race"

Prichard's approach to anthropological classification must be seen in the light of his thinking about the environment: he presupposed a number of physical and mental characteristics within which individuality unfolded, and whose scope was held in check by some teleological, and ultimately providential, principle. From the 1830s his analysis of diversity focused on the form of the skull and the pelvis, as well as of the native language. He considered each individual population in view of each of these three criteria. As we shall see, the result was not one single anthropological typology, but two (if not three). They were incongruous, this being exactly what Prichard intended to show: it was impossible to divide mankind into a certain number of different varieties because the main characteristics on which the description of each single variety was founded obliged the researcher to devise different classificatory systems. Since all human varieties were, as Prichard put it, shading into each other it was wrong to assert the existence of distinct human races.

Drawing up his taxonomy Prichard acknowledged that there were seven relatively permanent, distinguishable human varieties which "differ so strikingly from each other, that it would be improper to include any two of them in one section, and there is no other division of the human family that is by physical traits so strongly characterised".[54]

These varieties were:

(1) the "Europeans", including all the nations between the Indian subcontinent and the Atlantic, as well as those nations which Prichard called Syro-Arabians taking in the Semitic nations, Arabs, Egyptians and some African nations[55]

(2) Kalmuks, Mongols, and Chinese

(3) "Native Americans" (excluding the Eskimos)

(4) Hottentots and Bushmen

(5) "Negroes" – comprising all African tribes which were not classified under (1) or (4)

(6) Papuas in Polynesia

(7) Alfourous[56] and Australians[57]

These seven varieties, Prichard argued, mirrored the historical "division of the human family". Much as he endorsed the idea of permanent varieties, he established so many genealogical links among these seven human "divisions" that the notion of permanency was greatly relativized and reconciled to the doctrine of monogenism. We know how bitterly he fought the idea of the Caucasian origin of mankind. Accordingly, he refused to assume a "Caucasian" sub-species. Instead he followed the gentleman linguist Sir William Jones (1746-94) in calling all those peoples included under (1), "Iranians". Iran was Jones's name for the eastern country of Elam, where Prichard located the Indo-Persians. "Iranian" by definition applied to Semitic and Hamite peoples. It designated the core of the old world. Those peoples situated further to the north-east Prichard referred to as "Turanian". This term was derived from the Göttingen-trained geographer Carl Ritter (1779-1859).[58]

In 1817-18 Ritter, whose career began as a history teacher, published two volumes on a discipline which he called "physical geography". It was conceived by analogy to anatomy[59] and delineated a system of geography in which national character was inferred from the climatic surroundings. The publication attracted Alexander von Humboldt's attention, thanks to whom Ritter acquired a chair as Professor of Geography in Berlin. Thus geography was established as a subject taught at university. Like the transcendental anatomists, Ritter aspired to find some "basic forms" in geography,[60] demonstrating why and how particular geographical circumstances shaped human culture.[61] Like Prichard, Ritter started circumstances shaped human culture.[61] Like Prichard, Ritter started off with a modestly short work, but what he termed the "second part" of his endeavour comprised already seven volumes for the geography of Asia alone. His mixture of an environmentalist thrust and an insistence on the human capacity to improve has been termed "possibilism".[62] Firm religious convictions precluded his assuming a determinist position.[63] He has been called one of the last physico-theologians of early nineteenth-century Germany.[64] All these elements endeared him to Prichard. Added to this was Ritter's belief that the geographical circumstances of the old Biblical areas had been especially fortunate: within his physico-geographical philosophy it was no mere accident that the conditions in the ancient homeland of the I sraelites had been ideal for the development of spiritual excellence.[65] Ritter rejected colonization as a method of improving uncivilized African tribes. Instead he advocated missionary activity and the transmission of culture.[66]

In the third edition of the *Researches* Prichard frequently quoted Ritter. His delineations of several geographical regions closely followed Ritter's geographical system. It was most likely under Ritter's influence that he changed from "Iranian" to "Arian", thus aligning himself with a terminology which, innocent at the time, was to gain ominous prominence.[67] Like Ritter, he believed that lack of civilization was to be explained through adverse geographical conditions. More than anywhere else this was true for the African continent, whose "compact and individed form" made extensive travel by water impossible. Quoting Ritter's *Geography* Prichard wrote:

> Africa ... wanting both separating gulfs, and inland seas, could obtain no share in the expansion of that fruitful tree, which, having driven its roots deeply in the heart of Asia, spread its branches and blossoms over the western and southern tracts of the same continent.[68]

Whatever the particular talents of the African nations, their geographical setting was the primordial determinant of their cultural backwardness. With respect to human physiognomy things stood somewhat differently: in part it was a corollary of prevailing living conditions. Prichard held that this applied to the form of the cranium, in particular. Like Blumenbach, he rejected Camper's "facial angle". But he did not adhere to Blumenbach's top-view-perspective either. Instead he endorsed the perspective of the anatomist Richard Owen, considering "the view of the basis of the skull" as decisive.[69] Prichard praised Owen for clearly distinguishing "the quadrumanous type from that of the human skull".[70] Aligning himself with Owen's theory, he delineated three different types of skulls, each of which was, by and large, analogous to one of Blumenbach's three types. Unlike Blumenbach, however, he maintained that the formation of the skull was indicative of a particular stage of civilization. Enlarging on Scottish Enlightenment philosophy, he held that civilization brought about the beautiful oval features of Blumenbach's "Caucasian" variety or of his own "Iranian" one.

The formation of skulls was determined by living conditions. First, there was the "symmetrical or oval form, which is that of the European and western Asiatic nations". The head is "rounder", the forehead "more expanded". Second, Prichard described the "narrow and elongated" shape most unmistakably displayed by "the Negro of the Gold Coast". This type, called prognathous, was the stereotypical picture of the black savage. It was evoked by all those who embraced the idea of a link between black people and apes. Yet, Prichard never intimated such a proximity, insisting that it was not a universal feature distinguishing black populations from other human varieties.[71] There were many blacks, he said, whose features did not conform to the prognathous type with projecting cheek-bones and a "lengthened" upper jaw. His third skull formation was that of the "broad and square-faced" Turanian type, comprising Mongols as well as Eskimos. These skulls were slightly prognathous. Since their base was broader than the forehead, Prichard called them "pyramidal". For him each individual type indicated the relative preponderance of the sentient or the rational faculties. The prognathous as well as the pyramidal formation showed that the intellectual faculties were but moderately well developed. Only civilized peoples, who had full command of their intellectual potential, possessed oval skulls. The next stage down in the scale designated nomadic tribes: they displayed the pyramidal form. The "rudest tribes" represented the prognathous type: altogether uncultivated peoples.[72] Prichard obviously shared in the hierarchized classification that correlated mental faculties in humans with their physical appearance. It is seminal to note, however, that he strongly disclaimed any attempt to classify human varieties along these lines.

Having devised this neat system Prichard had to adjust it to his notions of human history. It was assumed by many, most famously by Georges Cuvier, that the three human variations – Semitic, Hamite, and Japhetic – displayed the three main different features of skulls postulated by Blumenbach. Accordingly, it was commonly believed that the Hamites had prognathous, uncouth features; the Japhetic and Semitic nations were associated with the two other shapes which were distributed according to the pro- or anti-Biblical leanings of the author.[73] Prichard would have none of this, since the admission of original differences among the sons of Noah amounted to acknowledging some sort of polygenist theory. Instead, he claimed that all ancient peoples, including the Ethiopians, Egyptians, Persians, and Hindus, had had oval skulls:

> they were neither nomads nor savages, nor do they display in their crania either of the forms principally belonging to races in those different states of existence. They had all heads of an oval or elliptico-spherical form, which we have observed to prevail chiefly among nations who have their faculties developed by civilisation.[74]

Prichard did not bother to explain why these ancient peoples had "civilized" skulls while their skin colour was not uniformly white (and not, therefore, "civilized"). It was yet another instance in which his various theories were lacking in coherence.[75] We have seen above that he distinguished three seedbeds of culture, associated with the Semites, the Indo-Europeans, and the Hamites. Yet, he did not ground a biological classification on this triad. In 1843 he even warned his readers not to jump to simple conclusions: "we cannot regard these three divisions of the ancient civilised world as representing the three great departments of mankind, as these departments are discriminated by the forms of the skull".[76] He regretted the misleading nature of Blumenbach's distinction between the "Caucasian", "Mongolian", and "Ethiopian", since it implied "that these three varieties of form are characteristic of three distinct human races of mankind".[77]

This was the error which Cuvier had made. As Prichard saw it, Cuvier's classification was singularly confused. "Nothing", he wrote, "can be more vague and conjectural than Baron Cuvier's notices of African ethnography. He not only considers the limitations of races as much more strongly and permanently defined than they really are, but makes the most singular mistakes in grouping and identifying tribes." Cuvier had ignored the fact that not all Africans had "narrow and compressed skulls".[78] Prichard accused him of having advanced a definition of the Negro features which was in line with European ideas of the great ugliness of black Africans. In reality, the doctor held, there were many African Negroes endowed with handsome traits. He was convinced of this idea, exemplifying it throughout the *Researches.* As a scientist, Prichard was a *bricoleur:* as everybody else classified human skulls, so would he. As a moralist, however, he held firm opinions and strongly disapproved of theorists of race. With the melancholy of hindsight we may see his axioms of physical appearance falling in with the racism of his contemporaries. Yet, at the time he was a stout opponent of racial theory. Unaccountably, some historians have the impression that he gradually resigned himself to some form of racialism.[79] It may be helpful to explain why Prichard was, indeed, adamant and unwavering in his rejection of racial classifications.

Theories of Race

Nineteenth-century racial theories were various but contained certain core elements: first, mankind was divisible into a certain number of "races" whose characteristics were fixed, if only in the sense that they defied the modifying influences of external circumstances (as distinct from changes produced by miscegenation). Second, intellectual and moral capacities were unevenly spread among human races. Third, mental endowments were bound up with certain external traits considered to reveal the inward nature of individuals and populations. This basic definition of modern racial theory was often accompanied by the idea that "race" was the be-all and end-all of history.[80]

As we have seen, for Prichard, the only proper use of the word "race" was as a synonym of tribe or nation. For all he had to say about the skull, he insisted that the intelligence of dark-skinned peoples was not naturally inferior to that of Europeans. And he maintained that "specimens of each kind are to be found in different races of men; whence is to be derived the important conclusion, that no particular figure is a permanent characteristic of any one race".[81] Prichard was convinced that there were no abrupt leaps within the gradation of human physiognomy, and that all peoples of the Earth were linked to each other through imperceptibly changing signs of resemblance. The most "savage" and the most "civilized" looking human tribes were connected to each other through the multifarious peoples whose features combined traces of rudeness and refinement, of northern and southern climatic influences, of good and abject living conditions:

> The different races of men are not distinguished from each other by strongly marked, uniform, and permanent distinctions, as are the several species belonging to any given tribe of animals. All the diversities which exist are variable, and pass into each other by insensible gradations.[82]

In accordance with the mentality of his time Prichard had an idea of perfect ugliness personified by a certain sort of physiognomy of blacks (very dark skin, woolly hair, and the so-called protruding jaw). But unlike all those authors, including Cuvier, who identified black peoples *in toto* with that type, Prichard differentiated, striving to show that in reality it was more or less confined to equatorial regions.[83] He ascribed European features to African nations, and he also found features of the "Negro" type in European nations: "it may be observed ... that examples might easily be found in which all the peculiarities of the Negro countenance are discernible in the persons of Europeans".[84] As it were, nature had a certain variety of choice in store, and by virtue of environmental stimuli or accidental creation of mutations, these forms came into being throughout all her realm. Given that Britain was engaged in warfare against some of the tribes whose culture Prichard and other philanthropists were vindicating, his theoretical engagement on behalf of these peoples ran counter to prevalent phantasies of ferocious savages. Among the native tribes he defended were the Kaffir nations of the South African Cape. They fought intermittently between 1817 and 1879 against British soldiers.[85] Prichard, however, praised some Kaffir peoples as exceedingly civilized.[86] He could be sure to find some support for this among the British public; nonetheless somesuch defence of Britain's enemies was out of step with widespread pro-colonial opinions.

When he discussed intelligence as an ethnological characteristic, Prichard underlined, like Blumenbach fifty years earlier, that the existence of one clever person among a tribe of blacks who might otherwise live as thoughtless "savages" was sufficient to prove that his kin were not naturally inferior to whites.[87] In 1837 Prichard demanded that "the Negro ought to occupy a different situation in society from that which has been declared to belong to him by the British government and we may add, by the unanimous acclaim of the British nation".[88]

Besides, Prichard believed that black populations, too, had had their cultural acme. He referred to ancient Egypt. And for those among his readers who discounted the theory that there had been blacks among the ancient Egyptians, he named the African Mandingos[89] who were, in his view, more civilized than many European tribes had been in antiquity: "the civilization of many African nations is much superior to that of the aborigines[90] of Europe during the ages which preceded the conquests of the Goths and Swedes in the north and the Romans in the southern parts".[91]

Prichard's fight against that perception was formed by his

antiquarian habit of collecting ethnological data. He had been a member of the British Association for the Advancement of Science since its inception in 1831, attending the Section "Anatomy and Medicine". But from the late thirties he devoted all his energy to ethnology, pressing for its recognition as an independent subject. This goal he partially achieved in 1842 when ethnology was officially made part of the Section "Zoology and Botany"; not until 1846, however, was the discipline finally admitted as a subsection in its own right.[92] Backed by the BAAS, Prichard took part in drawing up a manual of ethnological questions to be sent out to missionaries, explorers, and governmental employees in the colonies.[93] Neither this nor a successive draft, however, yielded any meaningful results. Her Majesty's subjects were not interested in ethnological fieldwork concerning religious rites or the origins of physical diversity, and they certainly did not make "repeated inquiries, to ascertain, if possible, whether such diversities are merely accidental varieties, or are connected with any distinction of tribe or caste".[94]

Canvassing support for this manual and in order to boost the cause of Hodgkin's newly-founded Aborigines Protection Society (motto: "ab uno sanguine"), dedicated to the defence of native peoples against colonial abuse, Prichard gave a lecture at the 1839 meeting of the BAAS in Birmingham. It was called "On the Extinction of Human Races" and described in gruesome terms the imminent demise of many endangered human varieties.[95] If Europeans condemned these peoples to death and extinction, he argued, the least they could do was preserve a memory of their languages and cultures. George Stocking suggested that Prichard's "scientific impetus outweighed the humanitarian".[96] That seems to be rather a harsh judgment on a man who was truly distressed at the treatment non-European nations suffered at the hands of colonists. In 1839 he wrote a letter to Thomas Hodgkin, apologizing for his absence at the Anniversary Meeting of the Aborigines Protection Society in London. The letter was intended for public reading. It is true that the occasion called for a philanthropic commitment, but Prichard went far beyond polite lip-service, identifying the reckless behaviour of European colonists with the crime of Cain:

> what a stigma will be placed on Christian and civilized nations, when it shall appear, that, by a selfish pursuit of their own advantage, they have destroyed and rooted out so many families and nations of their fellow creatures … . For such a work, when it shall have been accomplished, the only excuse or extenuation will be, just what the

first murderer made for the slaughter of his brother, and we might almost be tempted to suppose, that the narrative was designed to be typical of the time when christianized Europeans shall have left on the earth no living relic of the numerous races who now inhabit distant regions; but who will soon find their allotted doom if we proceed on the method of conduct thus far pursued, from the time of Pizarro and Cortez, to that of our English Colonists of South Africa.[97]

When, in the same year, Prichard addressed the BAAS, his speech exuded the same spirit as his letter to Hodgkin. He enumerated several peoples which had died out during the course of history, or which would do so presently unless Europeans changed their behaviour towards them. In a great historical sweep he bracketed the long-gone Guanches of the Canary Islands with the contemporary Charreas,[98] likewise victims of Spanish conquerors, of whom he had seen "three surviving individuals" when visiting Paris.[99] Outraged, Prichard did not invoke some superior destiny of the white man. He did not explain the extinction of human tribes as a "normal" historical fact. It was, for him, not *history* but *man*, civilized man, that is, who eradicated other peoples. He declared:

> a similar process of extermination has been pursued for ages in South Africa, formerly the abode of numerous pastoral nations of Hottentots, a peaceable and inoffensive race, who wandered about with numerous flocks, in a state of primitive simplicity, and whose descendants are now found in the miserable and destitute Bushmen, condemned to feed upon vermin and reptiles, and rendered savage and cruel by the wretchedness which their Christian conquerors have entailed upon them. Wherever Europeans have settled, their arrival has been the harbinger of extermination to the native tribes. Whenever the simple pastoral tribes come into relations with the more civilized agricultural nations, the allotted time of their destruction is at hand; and this seems to have been the case from the time when the first shepherd fell by the hand of the first tiller of the soil.[114500]

His horror was all the greater since it was Christian nations who committed these crimes. "It is only by *christian* nations", he wrote as early as 1830, "that such a work of total extermination has ever been thoroughly accomplished."[101] Interestingly, there had been no trace of this sentiment in the second edition of the *Researches*. By 1830 Prichard's writings registered that something had changed in his views of civilized men. It was as if he had lost his faith in them. An article of 1830, published in the Bristol Quaker publication *The*

Friends' Monthly Magazine, is the first instance of the ambiguous attitude towards civilization which was characteristic of Prichard's later years. Evidently, the analogy with Cain weighed heavily on him. Unlike Hodgkin or his brother-in-law, the abolitionist agitator John Bishop Estlin, Prichard was no crusader. His way of doing the works which the Bible demanded lay in minute registration of ethnological details. We must not see him, however, as an old-style antiquarian. It was not so much the joy of amassing facts which kept him going, but rather a feeling of duty which characterized the set of evangelicals brought up in the conceptual tradition of guilt, atonement, and redemption.[102] In the moral antithesis of civilization – culture versus luxurious self-indulgence – the balance seemed increasingly to fall down on the side of national self-aggrandisement, utilitarian materialist money-grabbing, and the reckless exploitation of foreign territories. In principle, civilization should enable man to have an understanding of his moral obligations. The reality, however, was quite different. While Prichard felt that Christianity was corrupted by the vagaries of personal interest, he immersed himself in collecting ethnographical details, having in mind that later generations might, perhaps, need to rely on his compilation, in a future age when a great number of the present aboriginal peoples would have perished, "when christianized Europeans shall have left on the earth no living relic of the numerous races who now inhabit distant regions".[103]

Notes

1 Prichard, *Researches*, 3rd ed., 2: 224.

2 As Ptolomy was a contemporary of Alexander the Great, his history of the latter's conquests was generally deemed to be reliable. Even though Ptolomy's text itself is lost, it survived in a later history of Alexander by the Roman poet Arrian.

3 Prichard, *Researches*, 3rd ed., 5: 602-3.

4 *Ibid.*, 1st ed., p. 554.

5 Prichard's use of these terms was not consistent. He wavered between "Shemite" and "Semitic"; and following August Ludwig Schloezer's studies on the Chaldaeans, he spelled the adjective "Japetic".

6 Prichard, *Researches*, 3rd ed., 2: 192.

7 *Ibid.*, 1st ed., pp. 471-72. Cf. *idem, Natural History of Man*, p. 136.

8 Prichard, *Researches*, 1st ed., p. 233.

9 For Camper see Miriam Claude Meijer, *The Anthropology of Petrus Camper* (Ann Arbor: UMI Dissertation Services, 1991), p. 216. For Hunter see Prichard, *Researches*, 1st ed., p. 233. For Pallas see Christoph Meiners, *Untersuchungen über die Verschiedenheiten der*

Menschennaturen, 1: 10-11.

10   For contemporary accounts see [Henry Holland], "Natural History of Man". *Quarterly Review* 86 (1849-50): 1-40, pp. 33-34; John Addington Symonds, *Some Account*, p. 17. For modern authors see Bynum, "Time's Noblest Offspring", pp. 101-4; Odom, "Prichard", pp. 136-38; Stocking, "From Chronology to Ethnology", pp. xliv, lxv.

11   Prichard, *Researches*, 1st ed., p. 233.

12   "Language". In *Encyclopaedia Britannica*, ed. Robert Cox, Thomas Stewart Traill, 6th ed., 20 vols (Edinburgh: A. Constable & Co., 1823), 11: 518.

13   Blumenbach, *The Institutions of Physiology*, trans. John Elliotson, 2nd ed. (London: printed by Bensley for E. Cox, 1817), p. 419.

14   John Mathew Gutch, *Observations or Notes Upon the Writings of the Ancients Upon the Materials which they Used, and Upon the Introduction of the Art of Printing; Being Four Papers Read Before the Philosophical and Literary Society, Annexed to the Bristol Institution, at their Evening Meetings in 1827* (Bristol: J. M. Gutch, 1827), p. 12. As members of the Bristol Institution, Gutch and Prichard met frequently. One may imagine that they agreed in their opinions of the matter.

15   *Memoir of Baron Bunsen*, 1: 482.

16   Cf. Prichard, *Researches*, 2nd ed., 1: 316.

17   John Frederick [sic] Blumenbach, "Observations on Some *Egyptian* Mummies Opened in *London*". *Philosophical Transactions* 84 (1794): 177-95, p. 191.

18   Prichard, *Researches*, 1st ed., p. 388.

19   *Ibid.*, note on pp. 388-89. Cf. also *ibid.*, 3rd ed., 2: 232.

20   *Ibid.*, 1st ed, p. 392.

21   *Ibid.*, pp. 395, 397, 384. Cf. also *ibid.*, 2nd ed., 1: 323.

22   Cf. *ibid.*, 3rd ed., 2: 192-93, 197-98, 207-17.

23   *Ibid.*, 2nd ed., 1: 324.

24   Cf. Jack A. Crabbs, *The Writing of History in Nineteenth-Century Egypt. A Study in National Transformation* (Cairo: The American University in Cairo Press, 1984), p. 13. George Annesley, *The Rise of Modern Egypt. A Century and a Half of Egyptian History 1798-1957* (Edinburgh: The Pentland Press, 1994), chs 3 and 4. This section follows largely the account in Ingrid Nowel, "Das Leben von Giovanni Battista Belzoni". Introd. to G. Belzoni, *Entdeckungs-Reisen in Ägypten 1815-1819* (Köln: DuMont, 1982), pp. 11-17.

25   [John Barrow], "Belzoni's *Operations and Discoveries in Egypt*". *Quarterly Review* 24 (1820-21): 139-69, p. 162.

26   Cf. C. W. Ceram, *Gods, Graves and Scholars in Documents* (London:

Thames and Hudson, 1965), ch. 3; Bryan M. Fagan, *The Rape of the Nile. Tomb Robbers, Tourists, and Archaeologists* (New York: Charles Scribner's Sons, 1975), chs 6-15.

27   Though, when Belzoni tried to sell his authentic artefacts to the British Museum for £ 8000, the directors declined: they had just acquired the Elgin marbles for £ 35000 and were not disposed to involve themselves in further expenses; see Fagan, *The Rape of the Nile*, p. 243.

28   Prichard was an exception: he preferred to rely on reports of the original sites, where "the colours are preserved in a very fresh state". *Researches*, 2nd ed., 1: 320.

29   "Physical Evidences of the Characteristics of Ancient Races Among the Moderns". *Fraser's Magazine* 6 (1832): 673-79, quotation on p. 677 (original emphasis).

30   *Description of the Egyptian Tomb, Discovered by G. Belzoni* (London: John Murray, 1821), p. 12.

31   Jean-Jacques Champollion-Figeac, *L'univers. Histoire et déscription de tous les peuples anciennes. Egypte ancienne* (Paris: Firmin Didot, 1839), p. 30. How wrong the British observers were is revealed also in John Barrow's review that dated the bas-relief in the reign of Psamtik II (fl. 595-89 b.c.e.). See [Barrow], "Belzoni's *Operations and Discoveries in Egypt*", pp. 160-61.

32   See Chapter 8, below.

33   Prichard, *Researches*, 2nd ed., 1: 322.

34   William Hamilton, *Remarks on Several Parts of Turkey. Part I. Ægyptiaca, or some Account of the Antient and Modern State of Egypt, as Obtained in the Years 1801, 1802* (London: printed for T. Payne, Cadell and Davies, 1809).

35   Prichard, *Researches*, 2nd ed., 1: 323.

36   Fagan, *The Rape of the Nile*, p. 127.

37   Hamilton, *Ægyptiaca*, p. 51. According to modern historical researches it is impossible to say which elements of Egyptian culture were due to Ethiopian influences; cf. Geiss, *Geschichte des Rassismus*, p. 80.

38   Prichard, *Researches*, 2nd ed., 1: 323. A similar idea was put forward by Bunsen in the 1840s. He called it the "Ethiopian hypothesis". See *Memoir of Baron Bunsen*, 2: 66, 133.

39   Prichard, *Researches*, 3rd ed., 2: 227-32.

40   *Ibid.*, 1: 220. Cf. also his *Natural History of Man*, pp. 121-22.

41   The third volume of the *Researches* deals only with European nations, yet Prichard understood it as the first part of his treatment of European and Asiatic nations.

42   The Rajah's birthdate is not definitely ascertained. The year 1772 is given in the introduction of: M. A. Laird, ed., *Bishop Heber in Northern India. Selections from Heber's Journal* (Cambridge: Cambridge University Press, 1971), p. 8.

43   The name comes in various spellings. I have chosen to follow Ramohun Roy's biographer: B. N. Dasgupta, *The Life and Times of Rajah Ramohun Roy* (New Delhi: Ambika, 1980).

44   The account of his life relies on an article by an anonymous phrenologist: "On the Life, Character, Opinions, and Cerebral Development, of Rajah Rammohun Roy". *Phrenological Journal* 8 (1832-34): 577-603. Cf. also Lant Carpenter, *A Review of the Labours, Opinions, and Character of Rajah Rammohun Roy; in a Discourse, on Occasion of his Death, Delivered in Lewin's Mead Chapel, Bristol...* (London: R. Hunter, 1833).

45   "On the Life ... of Rajah Rammohun Roy", p. 584. Ramohun Roy has been seen as exemplifying anti-Hindu sentiments among the Indians which were diagnosed at the time as signs of a cultural "decomposing" of Indian society. Cf. Raymond Schwab, *La renaissance Orientale* (Paris: Payot, 1950), p. 208. Others attributed to him "the first Indian initiative for education after a Western pattern". See the introduction in: Laird (ed.), *Bishop Heber in Northern India*, p. 8.

46   These were his words, quoted in *ibid.*, p. 588.

47   See the anonymous review of Ramohun Roy's *Translation of an Abridgement of the Vedant. Monthly Review* 2nd s., 92 (1820): 173-77, p. 177.

48   Prichard, *Researches*, 3rd ed., vol. 4, note on p. 237.

49   Cf. Nicholas Wiseman, *Twelve Lectures on the Connexion Between Science and Revealed Religion*, 1: 220. For the "quasi-racist" structures of the Indian caste system see Geiss, *Geschichte des Rassismus*, pp. 49-53.

50   Prichard, *Researches*, 3rd ed., 4: 237. He also disclaimed the possibility of intermarriage between Brahmins and members of other Indian castes; see *ibid.*, p. 150.

51   Unfortunately, however, his fate was sealed in Bristol and perhaps by Prichard. In 1833 after a journey to France, the Rajah became feverish. His last weeks he spent in Bristol, where he was treated by Prichard's brother-in-law John Bishop Estlin and by Prichard himself. His treatment involved even a scandal, as another doctor publicly claimed that Prichard was guilty of malpractice. The allegation remained without any consequence, excepting Prichard's letter in which he severed all ties between him and the other doctor; see Richard Smith, "Manuscript Memoirs", p. 684.

52 Prichard, *Researches*, 3rd ed., 4: 237-38.

53 It was derived from a history of Ceylon by the physiologist and anatomist John Davy, brother of Humphry Davy and an army surgeon who published *An Account of the Interior of Ceylon* (1821). See: Prichard, *Researches*, 3rd ed., 3: 194; *idem*, *Natural History of Man*, p. 245.

54 Prichard, *Researches*, 3rd ed., 1: 247.

55 There were other tribes that did not form part of the "Europeans" and yet had settled in the same geographical regions. Prichard called these "Allophylians"; they corresponded, he said, by and large with that group of peoples – not necessarily belonging to one family of nations – which other writers (such as the famous Danish philologist Rasmus Kristian Rask) had termed "Scythians". Sometimes Prichard used the expression to describe the earliest known populations settling in Asia and Europe. At other times he employed it as a linguistic term. See Prichard, *Natural History of Man*, p. 185. *Idem*, *Researches*, 3rd ed., vol. 3, pp. 8-19; vol. 5, note on p. 27. Cf. note 110 in Chapter 8 below.

56 According to vol. 1 of the 1989 edition of the *OED*, the Alfuro (as they are spelled nowadays) are "a race or a group of races" [!] in Celebes and the surrounding islands, neither pertaining to the Malay nor to the Negrito populations in the area.

57 Prichard, *Researches*, 3rd ed., 1: 247. He acknowledged that not all peoples of the Earth fitted into this matrix. By the 1830s he had come to conceive of the existence of many aboriginal tribes who remained outside his ethnological taxonomy. See *ibid.*, p. 275.

58 Prichard, *Researches*, 3rd ed., 1: 261-62. Cf. Carl Ritter, *Die Vorhalle Europäischer Völkergeschichten vor Herodotus, um den Kaukasus und an den Gestaden des Pontus, eine Abhandlung zur Alterthumskunde* (Berlin: G. Reimer, 1820), p. 8. Nowadays the term "Turanian" represents no meaningful linguistic category. At Prichard's time, however, it was common currency in Germany. See Hartmut Bobzin, "Christian Carl Josias von Bunsen und sein Beitrag zum Studium orientalischer Sprachen". In *Universeller Geist und guter Europäer. Christian Carl Josias von Bunsen 1791-1860. Beiträge zu Leben und Werk des "gelehrten Diplomaten"*, ed. H.-R. Ruppel (Korbach: Wilhelm Bing, 1991), pp. 81-102, esp. pp. 92-93. There has been a dispute over the origins of the term "Turanian". Bobzin refers it to the German poet and Orientalist Friedrich Rückert. C. C. J. Bunsen, by contrast, claimed that it was used by Arnold Hermann Ludwig Heeren und the geographer Carl Ritter; see Bunsen, "On the Results of the Recent Egyptian Researches in Reference to Asiatic

and African Ethnology, and the Classification of Languages". In Christian Carl Josias Bunsen, Charles Meyer, Max Müller, *Three Linguistic Dissertations. Read at the Meeting of the British Association in Oxford* (from the *Report of the British Association for the Advancement of Science* for 1847) (London: Richard and John E. Taylor, 1848), pp. 254-99, see p. 296.

59 Beck, *Carl Ritter. Genius der Geographie*, p. 90.

60 See Beck, "Carl Ritter als Geograph". In *Carl Ritter – Geltung und Deutung*, pp. 13-36, p. 13.

61 Beck, "Carl Ritter als Geograph"; Ernst Plewe, "Carl Ritter. Von der Kompendien- zur Problemgeographie". In *Carl Ritter – Geltung und Deutung*, pp. 37-53.

62 Manfred Büttner, "Zur Beziehung zwischen Geographie, Theologie und Philosophie im Denken Carl Ritters". In *Carl Ritter – Geltung und Deutung*, pp. 75-91, p. 83.

63 Beck, *Carl Ritter. Genius der Geographie*, p. 93.

64 *Ibid.*, p. 76. For Ritter's cultural anthropology see also: Beck, "Carl Ritter als Geograph"; K. E. Müller, "Carl Ritter und die kulturhistorische Völkerkunde". *Padeuma* 11 (1965): 24-57.

65 Manfred Büttner, "Geographie, Theologie und Philosophie im Denken Carl Ritters", p. 83.

66 Peter Kremer, "Carl Ritters Einstellung zu den Afrikanern, Grundlagen für eine philanthropisch orientierte Afrikaforschung". In *Carl Ritter – Geltung und Deutung*, pp. 127-54, see p. 141. While Prichard relied heavily on Ritter, the latter also referred to Prichard's ethnology; see *ibid.*, note 30 on p. 145.

67 Prichard employed the term "Arian" first in his *Natural History of Man*, pp. 162, 165, 184. He always spelt it in the German fashion: with an "i". For the British career of the Aryan theory see Joan Leopold, "British Applications of the Aryan Theory of Race to India, 1850-1870". *English Historical Review* 89 (1974): 578-603 (note that Leopold did not name Prichard as one of the proponents of *Aryan* racialist theory). For the transformation of the term "Indo-Iranian" into the term "Aryan" see Hans Siegert, "Zur Geschichte der Begriffe 'Arier' and 'arisch'." *Wörter und Sachen* n.s., 4 (1941-42): 84-99.

68 Prichard, *Researches*, 3rd ed., vol. 2, note on p. 355.

69 Prichard, *Researches*, 3rd ed., 1: 280. For Owen see Adrian Desmond, *The Politics of Evolution. Morphology, Medicine, and Reform in Radical London* (Chicago: University of Chicago Press, 1992 (1989)); Dov Ospovat, *The Development of Darwin's Theory. Natural History, Natural Theology & Natural Selection 1838-1859*

(Cambridge: Cambridge University Press, 1981). For a different
appreciation see Nicolaas A. Rupke, *Richard Owen. Victorian
Naturalist* (New Haven: Yale University Press, 1994).

70 Prichard, *Researches*, 3rd ed., 1: 287.

71 Against all those anatomists asserting the contrary, Prichard cited
Owen's examinations of the skulls belonging to humans and simiae,
resulting in the conclusion that the "transition from mankind to the
simiae is much more gradual" than these anatomists assumed; see
Natural History of Man, pp. 113, 116-17; see also *idem, Researches*,
3rd ed., 1: 172, 280-89.

72 Prichard, *Natural History of Man*, pp. 107–8, 119; *idem, Researches*,
2nd ed., 1: 173-74; *ibid.*, 3rd ed., 1: 281ff.

73 Traditionally the Semitic peoples were deemed the most beautiful.
But, by the middle of the nineteenth century, some supporters of
Indo-European excellence referred Semitic features to the far East,
identifying the Chinese with the posterity of Shem. One example is
Prichard's disciple Robert Gordon Latham. See the review of
Latham's *Natural History of the Varieties of Man* (1850): "The
Natural History of the Varieties of Man". *Prospective Review* 6
(1850): 449-58, p. 453. This way of refusing the Semitic peoples
common ancestry with other Europeans belongs among the
foundations of late nineteenth-century antisemitism.

74 Prichard, *Natural History of Man*, p. 138.

75 Another criterion Prichard pursued was the shape of the pelvis. It was
adopted from M. I. Weber, Professor of Comparative Anatomy at
Bonn University; see his *Die Lehre von den Ur- und Racenformen der
Schädel und Becken der Menschen* (1830). Following Weber, Prichard
assumed that those peoples with "oval" skulls also displayed an "oval
shape of the pelvis". See Prichard, *Researches*, 3rd ed., 1: 330-33.
Having said this he did not further elaborate on the question.

76 Prichard, *Natural History of Man*, p. 138.

77 Prichard, "Abstract of a Comparative Review of Philological and
Physical Researches, as applied to the History of the Human
Species". *Edinburgh New Philosophical Journal* 26 (1838): 308-26,
quotation from p. 315.

78 Prichard, *Researches*, 3rd ed., 2: 233. He referred to Cuvier's article
on the dissection of the "Hottentot venus". For the significance of
that text see Londa Schiebinger, *Nature's Body*, pp. 164-72. Prichard,
for his part, apparently did not perceive the differences between the
sexes worthwhile to be discussed.

79 Léon Poliakov claimed that he was eulogizing the Aryans; Stuart
Gilman held him for a racial degenerationist; Reginald Horsman

declared that there was no difference between Prichard's "permanent" varieties and other writers' "races". Léon Poliakov, *Le mythe Aryen*, p. 240; Stuart C. Gilman, "Political Theory and Degeneration: From Left to Right, from Up to Down". In *Degeneration*, ed. Gilman and Chamberlin, pp. 165-98, esp. p. 186; Reginald Horsman, "Origins of Racial Anglo-Saxonism in Great Britain", p. 397.

80   The biologically grounded racial theory, developed in the nineteenth century, lasted well into the twentieth century, culminating in the racial ideology of the German National Socialists. In recent years there have been attempts to revivify pseudo-scientific notions of racial theory. Serious scholarship pursues two different strands: some authors assert the existence of three main racial groups (Caucasian, Mongoloid, Negroid); see: Geiss, *Geschichte des Rassismus*, p. 23. Others, by contrast, have approached the question through a systematic genetic analysis. Their investigations have yielded the result that it is useless to talk of "human races" unless one is prepared to take the existence of many thousands of races into account: specific genetic configurations can be discerned in various populations, but they are by far more diverse than racial theoreticians would have it. See L. Luca Cavalli-Sforza, Paolo Menozzi, Alberto Piazza, *The History and·Geography of Human Genes* (Princeton: Princeton University Press, 1994). Some scholars assert that "modern racism" began as early as the fifteenth century. Cf., e.g., Richard H. Popkin, "The Philosophical Bases of Modern Racism". In *Philosophy and the Civilizing Arts. Essays Presented to H. W. Schneider*, ed. Craig Walton, John P. Anton (Athens, Ohio: Ohio University Press, 1974), pp. 126-65. Arguments about periodization always end in splitting hairs. It seems to make sense, however, to distinguish between the so-called "scientific" racialism of the nineteenth century and earlier forms of racism. For a historical analysis of the terms "race" and "racism" see Robert Miles, *Racism* (London: Routledge, 1989). For a history of racism and racial theory see Michael Banton, *Racial Theory*; Jacques Barzun, *Race: A Study in Superstition*, rev. ed. (New York: Harper and Row, 1965); Michael D. Biddiss, ed., *Images of Race* (Leicester: Leicester University Press, 1979); Christine Bolt, *Victorian Attitudes to Race* (London: Routledge and Kegan Paul, 1971); Nancy Stepan, *The Idea of Race in Science: Great Britain 1800-1960* (London: Macmillan, 1982).

81   Prichard, *Researches*, 3rd ed., 1: 331. The quote applies to the form of the pelvis. For the skull see a similar quote in: *ibid.*, p. 285. For skin colour see *ibid.*, p. 343.

82   *Idem, Natural History of Man*, p. 473.

83 *Idem, Researches*, 3rd ed., 1: 248.

84 *Ibid.*, pp. 234-35. The parallels to similar ideas of Cesare Lambroso (1836-1909) are obvious, yet Prichard's notions had nothing to do with the concept of atavism.

85 Lawrence James, *The Rise and Fall of the British Empire* (London: Little, Brown and Co., 1994), p. 190.

86 Prichard, *Researches*, 3rd ed., 2: 347.

87 *Ibid.*, 3rd ed., 1: 215. Cf. Blumenbach, *Contributions to Natural History*, pp. 305-12.

88 Prichard, *Researches*, 3rd ed., 2: 346. In 1833 slavery had been abolished in *the British Empire* by Act of Parliament. Yet slaves employed in agriculture were forced to stay in "apprenticeship" until 1838.

89 The Mandingos are a large group of peoples living in the region of the Niger.

90 Prichard did not mean to say that these peoples had been "created" in Europe, but that they had invaded the continent long before the Indo-European migrations had taken place, cf. *Researches*, 3rd ed., 3: 284.

91 *Ibid.*, 2: 353-54. The words implicitly defied contemporary racialists and corrected the famous footnote of the sceptic David Hume (1711-76) who, in his essay "Of National Characters", had made the very opposite remark, claiming that only white peoples could become civilized, barbarian Tartars and Germans being culturally highly superior to people of colour. See David Hume, "Of National Characters". In *idem, The Philosophical Works*, 4 vols, ed. Thomas H. Green, Thomas H. Grose, 1882-86. Reprint (Aalen: Scientia Verlag, 1964), 3: 244-58, p. 252. For a judicious evaluation of that remark see Robert Palter, "Hume and Prejudice". *Hume Studies* 21 (1995): 3-23.

92 Cf. Jack B. Morrell, Arnold Thackray, *Gentlemen of Science. Early Years of the British Association for the Advancement of Science* (Oxford: Clarendon Press, 1981), pp. 283-86; George Stocking Jr, *Victorian Anthropology*, pp. 239-45.

93 See the introductory page in J. E. Gray, Thomas Hodgkin, J. C. Prichard, *Queries Respecting the Human Race, to be Addressed to Travellers and Others, Drawn up by a Committee of the British Association for the Advancement of Science, Appointed in 1838* (London: Richard and John E. Taylor, 1841).

94 Pritchard [sic], "Ethnology". In *A Manual of Scientific Enquiry Prepared for the Use of Her Majesty's Navy and Adapted for Travellers in General*, ed. John Herschel (London: John Murray, 1849), p. 424.

95 Hodgkin had urged Prichard that "an appeal should be made to the natural history section of the British Association". Quoted in Amalie

M. Kass, Edward H. Kass, *Perfecting the World. The Life and Times of Dr. Thomas Hodgkin 1798-1866* (Boston: Harcourt Brace Jovanovich, 1988), p. 390.

96   Stocking, *Victorian Anthropology*, p. 243.

97   Prichard, "Letter to Dr Hodgkin", pp. 56-57.

98   The Charrua, as they were commonly spelled, were a tribe of South American Indians who by 1910 were "almost extinct". See *Encyclopaedia Britannica*, 11th ed., vol. 5.

99   Pritchard [sic], "On the Extinction of Human Races". *Edinburgh New Philosophical Journal* 28 (1839-40): 166-70, p. 169.

100   *Ibid.* Charles Darwin expressed himself in almost exactly the same words: Darwin, *Voyage of the Beagle. Journal of Researches*, 1839, ed. Janet Browne, Michael Neve (Harmondsworth: Penguin Books, 1989), p. 322.

101   Prichard, "Horae Africanae". *The Friends' Monthly Magazine* 2, no. 13 (1830): 737-38 (my emphasis).

102   Cf. Boyd Hilton, *The Age of Atonement*.

103   Prichard, "Letter to Hodgkin", p. 57.

6

Linguistics and Politics in the Early Nineteenth Century: Prichard's Moral Philology

The French revolution, a watershed in so many respects, also left its stamp on languages. Jeremy Bentham, for one, held that what before the revolution might be considered philosophically a mere impropriety in language, turned from 1789 into an oral crime.[1] At the same time, the historical turn that brought about rising interests in the histories of nations was accompanied by a new thrust in philology. Amidst the scientific specialization of the early nineteenth century, the subject changed its character. Hitherto, it had been tied to classical studies and Biblical criticism; in the nineteenth century, it turned into a science whose pursuit was increasingly independent of religious considerations. Accordingly, the search for the ultimate origin of language became less important. With the demise of the Enlightenment concept of the uniformity of human nature, "universal grammar" gave way to a preoccupation with the grammatical structure of particular tongues. During the eighteenth century philologists had been obsessed with etymology; now they became increasingly concerned with the grammatical make-up of existing languages.[2] This chapter will explore how Prichard profited from what is described by historical linguists as the "modern" form of philology: he used it to claim that Hebrew was the God-given language and thereby to elucidate the truth of monogenesis. Maintaining the latter, he tried to establish that the major great language families were historically related to each other; going back thousands of years, he even alleged that the ancient Celtic languages formed the grammatical bridge between Sanskrit and Hebrew. In all these matters his arguments were rather fanciful, even in the opinion of his contemporaries. He hijacked the latest linguistic finds to bolster opinions that were rather foreign to, and sometimes the contrary of, the philosophy of language supported by the authors he quoted. Two of his major philological hypotheses were to stand the test of time: Prichard believed that the languages of Northern Africa were related to the so-called Semitic idioms, and he demonstrated that the Celtic dialects belonged to the Indo-European language family – both notions, as a matter of course, also formed part of his grand defence of monogenesis. The narrative of Prichard's pious philology will begin with a brief historical recapitulation.

The historico-comparative method that characterizes nineteenth-century linguistics was introduced by the orientalist Sir William Jones (1746-94). A High Court judge in Calcutta, he established the relationships between Sanskrit, Latin, Greek, and their linguistic offspring, all of which he grouped under the family of the Indo-European languages.[3] Deepening Jones's approach, the Dane Rasmus Kristian Rask as well as the Germans Friedrich and August Wilhelm Schlegel, Franz Bopp, Jacob Grimm and Wilhelm von Humboldt developed the historico-comparative method. Historians of linguistics regard this as a step towards modern linguistics, while at the same time characterizing it as a fundamentally Romantic conception.[4]

In the early nineteenth century it was remarked that, Jones apart, the British contribution to philology could not match that of the illustrious Germans.[5] British patriots noticed with regret the shortcomings of their country, though it was accepted that for the study of Sanskrit "only England could afford opportunity".[6] Later historians have attempted to find reasons for what had been perceived as British backwardness: in his important *The Study of Language in England*, Hans Aarsleff declared that the influence of Horne Tooke was responsible, lamenting in a rather Whiggish phrase the "deplorable state of philology in England" during the first two decades of the nineteenth century.[7] In his view, British allegiance to Tooke's method prevented English philology from modernizing itself. Aarsleff demonstrated that Tookian scholarship was genuinely utilitarian: an adherent of sensationalism, Tooke held that philosophical concepts such as that of right and wrong were questions of language and not of ethics. He thus engraved morality into language. Grammatical structures, by contrast, were no concern of his.[8]

There was, however, an eminent non-utilitarian author who adopted German linguistics during the supposed "dark ages" of British philology, and who is mentioned only in passing by Aarsleff: Dr Prichard.[9] As early as the 1810s, historico-comparative philology was one of the mainstays in support of his monogenism.[10] In his hands, this method became an instrument which buttressed the veracity of the Scriptures – something, for Prichard, no less "objective" than the "correct" results of the comparative historical method would be for a twentieth-century historian of linguistics. By way of a short introduction to Romantic linguistics we shall turn to

Prichard's philology, which will be illustrated through his treatment of the Hebrew language. For the role of the Semitic tongues was exceedingly controversial in the early nineteenth century. As we shall see, Prichard's attitude towards the Hebrew reflected his faithfulness to the Bible.

Romantic Philology

German Romantic philology tended to draw parallels between the cultural stages of a people and its tongue. Each language was seen as indicative of a particular spirit. It was a long-termist appreciation, bundling together several nations whose tongues shared in a common linguistic stem. Accordingly language development was not necessarily linked to the cultural rise and fall of a particular people. Franz Bopp's morphology of languages, for instance, focused entirely on the progress and decay of linguistic forms. His degenerationist language theory implied that the historical course of the Indo-European tongues led from the development of ever greater structural complexity towards subsequent dissolution.[11] While in the classical Indo-European languages verbs carried their pronominal denominations in themselves, later developments released the pronouns and turned them into individual particles which had to be added in every sentence.[12] Through the mist of historical language changes, Bopp tried to steer a path towards "the ultimate origin of grammatical forms".[13] Other German scholars, however, made not only diachronic, but also synchronic comparisons. The very idea of structural comparison invited value judgements as to which languages were particularly apt for introducing the mind to complex ideas. The understanding of language prevalent in the Romantic age implied an organicist philosophy: languages were considered as "living" bodies, whose laws of generation and decay could be discovered. They were intimately connected with the history of man.[14]

Here lies the reason why Prichard became interested in philology. In his zeal to prove the unity of mankind he had quickly discovered that the genealogical links between the peoples of the Earth could not be positively proved by physiological researches; and what little there were of historical records dating back to the first ages of mankind did not suffice conclusively to demonstrate monogenesis. What could be shown, however, were affinities among languages as well as among varying mythological, cultural, and religious outlooks. If languages could be related to each other, Prichard had learned from Sir William Jones, this was a sign that those who spoke them were of kindred origin.

In the first and, to a certain extent, also in the second edition of the *Researches*, Prichard cast his net of linguistic connections over the entire globe.[15] He was to grow more cautious, the more deeply he entered into the subtleties of linguistic history. Hardly had he acquired command of German than he read Friedrich Schlegel's *Ueber die Sprache und Weisheit der Indier* (On the Language and Wisdom of the Indians, 1808), being deeply impressed by its devout attempt to discover the roots of monotheism even in the polytheistic religion of the Indians.[16] By 1826 seminal philological works by Franz Bopp, Wilhelm von Humboldt and Jacob Grimm had been published, some of which Prichard took up. From then on, the framework of his philological views was established; new arguments, resulting from further reading and communications from friends and correspondents, were woven into the system.

Unlike the German linguists, Prichard used philology mainly as a historical tool, employing it to uncover the history of human descent, rather than the laws inherent in the growth and decay of languages. Always eager to discover linguistic affinities for ethnological purposes, he was more interested in classifying the *relationships* between them than in investigating languages themselves. Yet he fully adopted the distinction Friedrich Schlegel (1772-1829) had made in 1808. Schlegel divided languages according to their capability for inflections, by which he understood, in the words of Mária Tsiapera, "both the secondary parts adhering to the root to constitute the grammatical word and the alternation of root-vowels".[17] To give an example: the addition of the letters "ed" in the regular English past tense is as much an inflection as is the change of vowel in the word "wrote". Schlegel thought that languages could be divided into superior ones whose grammatical forms were expressed through inflections, and inferior ones which revealed grammatical specificities merely through the addition of other words. In this sense, the English future tense, such as in "will write", displays the lack of an inflection. Schlegel came up with a three-fold differentiation:

1. Monosyllabic languages consisted of words whose roots had only one syllable, and which were devoid of grammar. Schlegel's prime example was Chinese.
2. There were monosyllabic languages which expressed time, number, and person through inflections. These were, in his view, the most advanced languages; he called them "organic". The type was epitomized in the Indo-European idioms.
3. The third group included languages which engendered their

grammatical particulars not by means of inflection, but through the "agglutination" or addition of other word particles.[18] According to Schlegel, the Semitic tongues belonged to this group.

Prichard followed Schlegel in differentiating between inflective and non-inflective languages; he, too, worked from the assumption that the character of Chinese was monosyllabic.[19] For him, however, it was even more important that the Chinese "popular dialect" was related to other languages, namely the Mongol, German, and Celtic.[20] Keen to find affinities like these, Prichard had no interest at all in establishing cultural hierarchies based on linguistic excellency. This comes out very clearly in his selective quotations from Wilhelm von Humboldt's work on the Kawi language of Malaysia. Humboldt (1767-1835), the great humanist and Prussian reform minister of education, is another of those Germans on whom Prichard relied, as his own countrymen appeared increasingly swamped by soulless utilitarianism. He adopted Humboldt's remarks on the relations between thought and language almost word for word, so long as they contained positive views on the Chinese: "Chinese leaves the perception of these relations [of words and ideas expressed in grammatical forms] to be the work of the mind. Much greater exercise of the understanding is therefore called for in a conversation carried on in Chinese language than in the Sanskrit." The very "absence of all grammatical forms" in the Chinese "tends to enforce acuteness of the mind".[21]

Another revered figure was obviously Friedrich Schlegel. Some of his German peers were puzzled by Schlegel's deep romanticism, which drove him towards a Catholicism in which he hoped to find the depth his age seemed to deny a man of his sensibility. Prichard, however, either did not care about Schlegel's Catholicism or – living "out of the world" – simply had not heard about it. Schlegel's philology, nevertheless, was, and is, highly praised, and Prichard made extensive use of it. For Schlegel, the roots of words contained the philosophical potential of a language. "In the Indian and Greek languages", he wrote, "each *root* is actually that which bears the signification, and thus seems like a living and productive germ, every modification of circumstance or degree being produced by internal changes." This quotation is a perfect illustration of the organicist metaphor employed to explain linguistic characteristics. Respecting languages which did not fulfil organicist prerequisites, Schlegel maintained: "those languages, on the contrary, in which the

161

declensions are formed by supplementary particles, instead of inflections of the root, have no such bond of union: their roots present us with no living productive germ".[22] The disyllabic languages – those tongues, that is, whose verbal roots consisted not of one syllable but two – also fell into this category. These were the Semitic languages, including Hebrew: in its written form the Hebrew employs no vowels; verbal roots are made up of three consonants,[23] forming two syllables – hence the term disyllabic.

Denying that disyllabic languages were truly philosophical, Schlegel relegated Hebrew to a position of secondary value. Not that he was entirely dismissive: "the Hebraic lores and literature", he wrote, "are the body, whose soul is divine revelation".[24] But since the ancient Hebrews were living under oriental climatic conditions, he followed the traditional environmentalist criticism put forward by his intellectual forebear Sir William Jones and other eighteenth-century critics: Hebrew literature, being the product of the uncontrolled imagination that prevailed in hot latitudes, was lacking in refinement.[25] Hence Schlegel and Humboldt believed that language reached its culmination not in the Hebrew, but in the Indo-European tongues.

Some seventy years ago, Otto Jespersen pointed out that Schlegel was wrong and that the grammar of the Semitic languages was indeed based on the mechanisms of inflection.[26] In Prichard's time, however, those who subscribed to the system of inflective, agglutinative and synthetic languages tended to believe that the disyllabic character of the Hebrew implied its inferiority to monosyllabic languages, notably the Indo-European ones. This met with the approval of scholars who participated in the fashion of rampant Sanskrit-mania.[27] Prichard, by contrast, who upheld Biblical truths and cherished Hebrew as the tongue in which they had been expressed, consequently went out of his way to defend it. His concern for the Biblical languages engendered the most original features of his linguistic scholarship.

The Hebrew Dispensation

Prichard held that monotheism required a specific philosophical disposition of the mind. He was in harmony with Romantic correlations between mind and language in inferring that the Biblical Hebrew (its Talmudic form being generally considered as corrupted[28]) must have enabled the wandering shepherds of the ancient Israelites to express philosophical and religious concepts far superior to their rather rude life-style. "Perhaps the Semitic people", he suggested in 1836, "were the only race whose language displays a purer or more metaphysical conception" than that of the Greeks and Romans.[29]

His philology thus dovetailing with his ethnology, Prichard chose a linguistic terminology of his own: in his view the term "Semitic" was misleading. To all those who, like Prichard, referred the peoples of the world to the three sons of Noah – Shem, Ham and Japhet – the implication was that the Semitic languages were altogether distinct from the Hamitic ones. Prichard, by contrast, denied that this was the case. He cited the German Biblical critic and author of a Hebrew grammar, Friedrich Heinrich Wilhelm Gesenius (1786-1842), as the first scholar who had demonstrated that the so-called "Semitic" language family also included some Hamite tongues (which in turn were related to the Egyptian and gave rise to the modern African languages).[30] Hence the common choice of the term "Semitic" was unfortunate. "The Hebrew language", Prichard explained, "appears to have belonged to the Canaanitish or Hamite branch, the Syrian to the Shemite." In order to avoid confusion and be yet genealogically correct, he coined a term based on the geographical region where the respective languages were spoken. Hence, what other people called "Semitic" he chose to label "Syro-Arabian" idioms.[31]

To defend their philosophical status, he had to grapple with their disyllabic character. This had proved problematic for quite a few Biblical critics of the eighteenth century who wanted to assign Hebrew its due place among the great languages of classical poetry. The easiest way of solving the problem was to declare that Hebrew, too, was a monosyllabic language. This was what the German linguist and traveller Julius Klaproth (1783-1835) suggested. Even superficial knowledge, Klaproth contended, would be sufficient to recognize that the alleged disyllabic words were in fact composed of two individual ones.[32] A thorough investigation must yield the result that the original monosyllables of Hebrew roots were in fact nearly analogous to the respective words in Sanskrit.[33] This was an assertion which might have been very welcome to a linguistic monogenist. Prichard approved of Klaproth's linguistics in general;[34] he did not, however, embrace the idea that Hebrew was monosyllabic. Rather he quoted Wilhelm von Humboldt for support: "it appears on the whole to have been the opinion of M. de Humboldt ... that the Shemite language consisted in its original material of roots principally disyllabic". This was an exaggeration. Humboldt had simply said that the disyllabic Semitic tongues might have developed from a system in which monosyllabic and disyllabic roots had been mixed.[35] It was not the only occasion on which Prichard, keen to make his point, subtly misread another author.

What can be called his linguistic creed was set down in the fourth volume of the *Researches*, in a chapter called "Of the Syro-Arabian Nations".[36] Here we find a perfect illustration of the theological background of Prichard's philology; moreover, the chapter reveals his equivocal attitude towards the concept of civilization. It is, therefore, worth quoting extensively:

> Nothing in reality is more illustrative of the psychological difference between the Japetic and Shemite branch of our races than the conceptions which both have formed of the nature and attributes of the Divinity. ... *The Shemite people alone* appear to have possessed of old sufficient *power of abstraction to conceive the idea of a pure and immaterial nature,* and of a governing mind distinct from body and from the material universe. Their *conceptions were more pure and sublime, their sentiment of devotion more intense, their consciousness of guilt expressed itself in more significant and more definite acts,* than those of the Japetic nations ... . There is no particular in which the perfective character of the Shemite nations has been displayed more remarkably than in the singular character and construction of their language. ... the Shemite language, ... displaying in its very framework a deep conception and design, consists of disyllabic roots, of which the three consonants express the abstract meaning, the essential and leading sense or import, while all the relations of ideas to past and future time, to personal agency or passion, the possible or real, and even the differences of nouns and verbs, are denoted by changes in the interior vowels, changes *which the words themselves were obviously intended in their original formation or construction to undergo,* – a contrivance which implies a conception *and previous contemplation* of all that words when invented can be thought capable of expressing. ... The foundation of poetry among the Greeks, Latins, and Hindoos is, as everyone knows, rhythm and quantity, an arrangement of syllables producing a certain modification of sound, selected perhaps originally for the sake of harmony and a cadence pleasing to the ear, but in part designed to assist the memory in the long oral recitations practised before the invention of written signs. Far more intellectual and more indicative of reflection was the poetry of the Shemite nations.[37]

Familiarity with the writings of eighteenth-century scholars such as Robert Lowth and Johann David Michaelis proved fruitful for

Prichard. He bound up accepted teachings on poetical style with his personal views of the Hebrew grammar, and related the whole to the action of divine Providence. Even though he adopted the language classification developed by Schlegel, Bopp and Humboldt, he did not make the progressivist inferences drawn by the German authors. Although he followed the value system which placed "organic", "synthetic" and "inflective" languages above "analytic", "agglutinative" and "mechanic" ones, he did not share the prevalent philological opinion that the Indo-European was the most valuable of all languages. In the passage cited above, he explained that the Syro-Arabian tongues were constructed in such a manner as to predestine the Shemites for monotheism. He also made it clear that this was due to divine Providence, which had singled out one particular people for monotheistic revelation.

If Prichard's inferences were based on the widespread claim that languages were illustrative of the mental state of a people, this was due to the particular source he used in the context: his concepts of Hebrew were derived from Humboldt's philosophy of language. Quoting Humboldt, he found the particular quality of Hebrew in the fact that "the greater compass which the formation of roots by three consonants afforded" incited the habit of expressing "shades of meanings and the modifications of time and mode" through "changes of vowels", which in turn led to the conception of more elaborate roots, which lent themselves to such complicated mental operations.[38] To be sure, Humboldt did not think meanly of Hebrew, he simply perferred Indo-European languages. Prichard, by contrast, regarded the development of Sanskrit and other Indo-European tongues as an ambiguous process. On the one hand, polished perfection was obtained. On the other, disyllabism was given up and with it the capacity for higher spiritual attainments. Thus his views of civilization were also expressed through the medium of philology. Like civilized society, Indo-European languages were refined, yet not necessarily "moral".

Humboldt left no doubt that he considered Hebrew as inferior to Sanskrit: it was less "free" in its constructions. He granted inflections to Hebrew, but these were, in his system, of lesser value, since he (wrongly) believed that declensions as well as pronouns were expressed through additional letters instead of changes in the verbal roots. And what Prichard took as a strength of Hebrew – its resistance to compound words – Humboldt saw rather as a deficiency.[39] Prichard, however, did not quote him to this effect. He conceded that the Indo-European languages had great qualities, too; yet he insisted that the Hebrew was superior. It was true that the Indo-European tongues showed a tendency towards triliteral verbal roots. But in Sanskrit or Greek, its origination had to be "attributed to accident or to the unremediated and momentary efforts of the mind, and to the occasional development of a few original elements". It was the Semitic languages alone that displayed triliteralism in perfection: "the artifice of construction", Prichard wrote, "is so deeply inlaid in the very original elements of the Shemite language, and the principle of expression so refined and, if we may so speak, metaphysical, as to bear the appearance *of a premeditated plan*".[40] This remark suggests that he literally took Hebrew (or some parent-language) for the tongue God had given to His people.

Prichard's clear preference for the Syro-Arabian type of languages separated him from all those linguists who, in the Romantic era, pronounced the cultural supremacy of the Greeks over all other civilizations.[41] Around the turn of the century some European clergymen assumed that the New Testament had originally been written in Greek: much as the Septuagint was superior to the *Masorah*, Greek stood above the ancient Hebrew. Later in the nineteenth century Heinrich Heine was to say "that all men were either Jews or Greeks"; the critic Matthew Arnold named "Hellenism and Hebraism as the two points between which the human spirit must for ever oscillate"; Christian Carl Josias Bunsen, who was also an expert on early Christianity, declared that "everywhere the Semitic and the Japhetic mind assist and complete each other" (the latter being "nationally always the higher" and the Semitic being endowed with "the power of a great individuality").[42] Within this ideological dichotomy Prichard was clearly on the Hebrew side. And, while it became increasingly fashionable to deny the antiquity and influence of Hebrew,[43] he implied, as late as 1844, that it was closest to the language with which God had endowed mankind.

By that time such a claim would be perceived as fairly old-fashioned. It is true that Friedrich Schlegel revived hopes concerning the recovery of the First Language. He did not, however, attempt to suggest how research might bridge the abyss of time, going back to the antediluvian epoch.[44] In the previous century Gottfried Wilhelm Leibniz had already asserted that Hebrew was rather unlikely to be the primeval language. And so did the Scottish orientalist Vans Kennedy (1784-1846), another avid reader of European scholarship in the 1820s, in a voluminous work on Indo-European linguistics. Kennedy, a major-general in India who was knowledgeable in Continental philology, relied on the German Johann Christoph

Adelung (1732-1806), who had paved the way for the historico-comparative method, and his disciple Julius Klaproth.[45] Even the pious Sir William Jones had resigned himself to the supposition that the original language from which all others derived might be "irretrievably lost".[46]

Subscribing to the Biblical account of the Noachian Deluge, Prichard always preserved the basic distinction between Semitic (or Syro-Arabian), Hamitic, and Japhetic tongues. In view of the dispersion of languages, he believed that the events related in the story of the tower of Babel were involved in it.[47] Those among his readers, however, who were unwilling to rely on Providence to account for the development of languages, could content themselves with a more naturalistic explanation in the vein of eighteenth-century philosophizing. The greatest diversity of language was to be found among uncultivated peoples:

> Savage people, roaming about the banks of rivers, or the sea-shores, or wandering through forests in quest of a scanty subsistence, are necessarily divided into very small companies; in their almost solitary existence they have little use of speech, and their scanty vocabularies soon deviate from each other and lose all traces of resemblance.[48]

But it was not enough to show how the great variety of languages had come into being; in his endeavour to assert monogenesis with the Hebraic as the oldest cultural tradition, Prichard had to demonstrate that Hebrew and Sanskrit were related, or rather that Sanskrit had developed from Hebrew. Schlegel had insisted that it was impossible to show any affinities between the two language families. Notwithstanding the efforts of Gesenius and Georg Heinrich August Ewald, justifiably known as "the heads of the critical Hebrew school" who had introduced history into Hebrew grammar, there remained a huge gap separating it from Sanskrit.[49] It was in the original Celtic language that Prichard thought he had found a missing link connecting the two.

The Celtic Problem

In *The Eastern Origin of the Celtic Nations* (1831),[50] Prichard contradicted all those scholars who held that the Celts were originally distinct from other Europeans – a belief which corresponded to the widespread assumption that Celtic peoples were inferior. Some of the wildest disparagements were put forward by the Scottish antiquary and historian John Pinkerton (1758-1826), who dubbed the Celts "mere radical savages, not yet advanced even to a state of barbarism".[51] Another culprit was Cuvier whose attitude, for all his erudition, was, at best, ambiguous: in his *Leçons d'histoire naturelle*, he had omitted to mention Celtic in connection with the Sanskrit. To Prichard this seemed to indicate that "perhaps [he] regards them [the Celts] as Aborigines".[52] Being in part of Welsh extraction, Prichard had a personal interest in rehabilitating the Celts. He argued that their tongue was related to the Indo-European, and even claimed that it had special affinities to Sanskrit which no other Indo-European idiom possessed; in fact, it was the remnant of a language older than all other Indo-European idioms.

To make this point Prichard had to argue that once, in the remote past, Celtic had possessed proper pronominal inflections. Horne Tooke had asserted that all rude languages were devoid of pronouns, for unrefined civilizations required words for actions and things only. It had been Franz Bopp who argued to the contrary, asserting that pronouns led the historical linguist more deeply into the womb of time than any other grammatical form. Bopp also held that there had been an Indo-European language before Sanskrit, a language even more perfect than Sanskrit itself.[53] On the basis of an analysis of the pronominal suffixes of Celtic, adopted from Bopp, Prichard established an affinity not only to Sanskrit but also to Hebrew or Chaldaean.[54] This led him to a highly daring conclusion. "It must be allowed," he argued, "that the Semitic dialects constitute a very distinct department of languages, which can by no means be associated or brought into the same class with the Indo-European idioms." And yet, he went on, it would be wrong to deny all "traces of connection between the two classes". The "system of pronominal suffixes" was

> one point in which the Celtic, at the same time that it appears to be the least artificial and grammatically cultivated of the Indo-European languages, forms an intermediate link between them and the Semitic, or perhaps indicates a state of transition from the characters of one of these classes of languages to those of the other.[55]

Prichard's Celtic studies were endorsed as far as the connections to other Indo-European languages were concerned. By the latter half of the 1830s, Franz Bopp and Lorenz Dieffenbach in Germany, and Adolphe Pictet in France, established independently of Prichard the affinities between the Celtic and other Indo-European tongues.[56] Their publications won international fame. Prichard's was acknowledged only among his British peers, going through a second edition in 1857. At a meeting of the British Association for the Advancement of Science in 1847, the philologizing diplomat Bunsen paid homage to the achievements of recent Celtic researches. An erstwhile admirer of Prichard's learning, he had developed a few reservations.[57] Prichard, who attended the conference, was not even mentioned in Bunsen's paper.[58]

The merits of *The Eastern Origin of the Celtic Nations* notwithstanding, it was heavily criticized. The German orientalist, August Wilhelm Schlegel (1767-1845), brother of Friedrich, was quite dismissive. Prichard's error had been to choose Celtic derivatives of Latin words to prove original affinity: "he highlights the Latin verb *credo, credu* in Gallic, *credeim* in Irish. Could he have forgotten that this word, being the first of the formula of the creed, composed in Latin, which all neophytes had to learn by heart, must have impressed itself in the memory of the people?" Schlegel concluded "that the resemblance between a certain number of Gallic or Irish words and other Latin, Roman, Saxon, Scandinavian words cannot prove an original affinity with the Indo-European family".[59] The links between Hebrew and Celtic, in particular, Prichard's critics quickly discarded.[60]

But his monogenist project relied on these relations, and he went out of his way in their pursuit. The task, however, was much more complex in the 1830s and 1840s than it had been in 1813. Like Gesenius, the mathematician Francis Newman (1805-97), who spent some time in Bristol and was on good terms with Prichard, claimed relationships between African idioms and the Semitic.[61] Bunsen asserted that the Semitic and Egyptian were linked to the Sanskrit. Wilhelm von Humboldt argued that Sanskrit was connected to the Polynesian languages.[62] Referring to their finds, Prichard stipulated in 1847 that some of the greatest language families were related to the Indo-European idioms: "1. The idiom of the Shemite nations: 2. the languages of North-Eastern Asia, akin to the Turkish, Mongolian, and Tungusian: 3. The Coptic: 4. Several African languages".[63] Chinese was added to this happy union by virtue of "striking resemblances" between Chinese words and those of other Asiatic and European languages.[64]

Prichard's philological exploits were acclaimed by non-specialists. The influential Cambridge philosopher William Whewell, for instance, believed that his philology did for ethnology what geology had done for the history of the Earth: "to execute such a design as [Prichard's], we must combine the knowledge of the physiological laws of nature with the tradition of history and the philosophical comparison of languages".[65] Linguistic specialists, by contrast, tended to react differently: they admired Prichard's ethnology. In respect of his philological exploits, however, their praise was muted.[66]

In the 1830s Britain caught up with German philology. The chair of Oriental languages at the newly founded University of London was given to the orientalist Friedrich August Rosen who, having studied under Bopp in Berlin, personified German scholarship in England. By the 1840s, the independent scientific status of philology was institutionally cemented. In 1842, on the initiative of Connop Thirlwall, Thomas Arnold, and a group of scholars around Rosen, the Philological Society was founded.[67] Prichard did not, however, join.[68] By 1842 he had come to see himself as an ethnologist, rather than a philologist. Even though he admired Rosen's scholarship,[69] and could not possibly ignore influential figures like Bunsen's associates Hare, Thirlwall, and Arnold, it seems that his social relations were not extensive enough to make him automatically a member of the Society.[70] Moreover, he did not share the predilection for Anglo-Saxonism prevalent among its members. If his metaphysically oriented philologizing was rejected, it was in part because his defence of Hebrew was a lonely endeavour in a cultural environment increasingly obsessed with the Germanic and Aryan ancestry of the population of Northern Europe. In part it was also because philologists put ever greater emphasis on the secular aspects of their discussions.

Of course, Prichard was aware of this development that had started in the Higher Criticism of eighteenth-century Germany. And much as he profited from that liberal approach to the Scriptures, it yet paved the way for the infiltration of politics into linguistics.[71] So far we have been assessing the differing attitudes towards Hebrew as seen through Prichard's pious eyes. Yet his interest in philology was not confined to his concern with the origin of mankind and the unity of the human race. As we shall see he also involved himself in a later and rather different controversy. His appeal against racism was an analogue to his appeal against nationalism.

Nationalist Philology

Nationalism was stirring in the first half of the nineteenth century. Liberal nationalist scholars were turning towards history and philology as weapons in their fight against royal and aristocratic legitimism and imperial oppressors. In using history for their own ends they availed themselves of debates that had been going on for a long while. Thus, British and German readers of Tacitus had discovered their common descent from an ancient Germanic people that was invested with a particular love of freedom. The concept supported both Protestantism and an anti-absolutist position. According to Hugh MacDougall, in Britain that notion was employed from the seventeenth century when England moved "from a monarchically based society ... to a self-conscious nation dominated by landed and rising commercial interests".[72] Gradually, the Saxon tradition and good King Alfred replaced the earlier myth of King Arthur.[73] In the German territories, after the "liberation wars" against Napoleon's armies, liberal aspirations relied on references to the cultural excellency of the nation, philologists appropriating the past to bolster the invention of a Germanic tradition. Julius Klaproth, for instance, did not speak of the "Indo-European" languages, favouring the term "Indo-Germanic" instead.[74] This perspective helped to introduce a historical perception conveyed in the language of racial theory. From the middle of the century it became customary in Germany to emphasize the antagonism between Slavs and Germans as well as the notion that the "Aryans" were a particular people wholly distinct from, and superior to, other races.

In France, too, the historical discourse was snatched from the hands of *ancien régime* aristocratic debate. Harking back to the fifth-century invasion of the Franks, in the eighteenth century, Comte Boulainvilliers emphasized the Frankish origin of the French aristocracy at the expense of the Roman tradition (*Histoire de l'ancien gouvernement de la France*, 1727).[75] A century later this argument was to boomerang. From the 1820s, liberal bourgeois historians fought the French aristocracy with a historical arsenal and against the background of racial theorizing: juxtaposing the Frankish aristocracy against the original population, they concluded that the aristocracy had never ceased to be a minority consisting of foreign intruders.[76] In 1834 the historian Augustin Thierry described the antagonism: "we imagine that we are one nation, but we are two nations on the same land, two nations hostile in their memories and irreconcilable in their projects: one has conquered the other".[77] On one side was the nobility, descended from the Franks of Charlemagne, and on the other was the Third Estate, believed to have descended from the populace of ancient Gaul.[78] Thanks to the endeavours of the physiologist William Frédéric Edwards (1776-1842), the ensuing quarrel was set onto a biological footing. A naturalized Frenchman who had grown up in Jamaica, Edwards developed a physiology of racial characteristics to support political liberalism; he contemplated racial mixture and its effects, concluding that the Frankish race had not impressed its characteristics on the French population.[79]

Prichard was indifferent to French politics, but he felt obliged to intervene. In 1838 he visited the "Cwmreiggyddion", a Welsh festival in Llanover which was also attended by a delegation from Brittany. C. C. J. Bunsen, too, was present, noting that the French visitors were "zealous in the cause of their own and all cognate languages and antiquities". Moreover, "the Welsh and Bretons understood not each other's dialect".[80] The competition among the Celtic revivalists must have been considerable. If this in itself was not enough to call forth Prichard's comment, he clearly felt the need when he read a book by Augustin Thierry's brother Amédée who treated the Gauls and Welsh as if they belonged to different Gallic stems. Following a remark in Julius Caesar's *De bello gallico*, Thierry divided the French population into Gallic populations on the one hand, and Belgae or Cimbri, that is Germans, on the other hand. The British, he believed, were related to the latter.[81] What may be called Amédée Thierry's republican Celticism displeased Prichard because, in his view, the Frenchman was drawing dividing lines between peoples who actually belonged together. Prichard, too, distinguished between Belgic and Gallic Celts, yet he criticized Amédée Thierry for stating that the Belgae had nothing to do with the Gauls.[82] Equally, he accused British historians of driving a wedge between France and Britain by overemphasizing Britain's Anglo-Saxon traditions. The affinities between the Belgae and the British were undisputed. (On a political level Britain exerted her diplomatic powers in favour of Belgian independence from the Netherlands, gained in 1830.) Yet some historians considered the Belgae as a Germanic people.[83] This implied that they were very remote from the Gauls – and so were the descendants on both sides, the French and Britons. Prichard demurred, thinking it likely that "the Welsh or Britons" stemmed not from the Belgae, but "were a colony of the Celtic Gauls" and that hence contemporary Britons and Frenchmen were much more nearly related to each other than those historians believed.[84] Less than thirty years previously Prichard had been prepared to take up arms against Napoleon's France but, unlike many others who would be implacable in their enmity, he pleaded for a lasting peace, underlining that, from an ethnological point of view, the French and the Britons shared common ground.

The method by which Prichard tried to prove Amédée Thierry wrong was derived from Wilhelm von Humboldt. In 1821 Humboldt had shown that the Celts were not the first tribes to have arrived in Spain. A linguistic examination of the names of villages and other geographical landmarks yielded the result that Basque was not related to Celtic and that, as Prichard summarized it, "the Euscarian or Biscayan language was common to all the tribes of the Iberian race".[85] To the very same sort of exercise Prichard submitted the topographical names in France, Belgium, and Britain with the result that "the Celtic were the people of Gaul, and of Britain".[86]

Prichard's arguments were bound up with his ardent objections to what he considered artificial divisions among mankind. His theologically determined views predisposed him to defy the notion of cultural progressivism and of what may be termed patriotic philology. His book on *The Eastern Origin of the Celtic Nations* had aimed at closing the conceptual gap between Saxons and Celts. When the inner-French debate seemed to rekindle the antagonism between France and Britain he warned against the tendency to put politics on a historical-physiological footing. Abhorring racial arguments, in the European context as much as elsewhere, he observed with dismay how "races are made the groundwork of political coalitions, and a difference in stock and lineage becomes a plea for separation and hostility".[87] Prichard, too, subscribed to a notion of cultural hierarchy. But being grounded in Christian doctrines, it ran entirely against the ideas and stereotypes dominating the nationalist discourse that increasingly imbued political debates. His outburst at the Ethnological Society apart, he did not lecture his peers on what political causes they should support. His intellectual home, after all, was not the present but the distant past. When discussing Celtic place names, he illustrated his claims with an example which was meant to be immediately convincing: "any person who looks over a map of ancient Palestine, or one of Egypt, in which all the local terms are marked down correctly, would find no difficulty in recognising the Hebrew or Egyptian name wherever they appear".[88] In addition to Egypt and Palestine comes India – those are the three countries in whose past Prichard hoped to find the key to human history. To these we must now turn our attention.

Notes

1   Ross Harrison, *Bentham* (London: Routledge, Kegan Paul, 1983), p. 101.

2   For an acute delineation of that development see Michel Foucault, *The Order of Things*, p. 235.

3   For Jones see Garland Cannon, *Oriental Jones: A Biography* (London: Indian Council for Cultural Relations, 1964); *idem*, "Sir William Jones and Applied Linguistics". In *Papers in the History of Linguistics, Studies in the History of the Language Sciences* 38, ed. Hans Aarsleff,

Louis G. Kelly, Hans-Josef Niederehe (Amsterdam: J. Benjamins, 1987), pp. 379-89. According to Joan Leopold, the physician and Egyptologist Thomas Young was the first British author who used the adjective Indo-European "to designate Eurasian languages, including Semitic and Dravidian". See Leopold, "British Applications of the Aryan Theory of Race to India", p. 578.

4   See, e.g., Otto Jespersen, *Language. Its Nature, Development and Origins* (London: Allen & Unwin, 1949 (1922)); Holger Pedersen, *Linguistic Science in the Nineteenth Century*, trans. J. W. Spargo (Cambridge: Cambridge University Press, 1931); Hans Arens, *Sprachwissenschaft. Der Gang ihrer Entwicklung von der Antike bis zur Gegenwart*, 2nd enl. ed. (Freiburg, München: Karl Alber, 1969).

5   "Ethnology – The Unity of Mankind". "Report of the Seventeenth Meeting of the British Association for the Advancement of Science, Held at Oxford, in June, 1847". *British Quarterly Review* 10 (1849): 408-40, pp. 429-30.

6   *Memoir of Baron Bunsen*, 1: 89.

7   Hans Aarsleff, *The Study of Language in England, 1780-1860* (Minneapolis: University of Minnesota Press, 1983 (1967)), p. 112. John Burrow has pointed out that the English backwardness in philology had already been deplored by F. W. Maitland. Burrow, *A Liberal Descent, Victorian Historians and the English Past* (Cambridge: Cambridge University Press, 1981), p. 129.

8   Aarsleff, *The Study of Language*, p. 13.

9   *Ibid.*, p. 208. Prichard's role has been appreciated (though misjudged) in Arno Beyer, *Deutsche Einflüsse auf die englische Sprachwissenschaft im 19. Jahrhundert* (Göppingen: Kümmerle, 1981), pp. 73ff.

10 Prichard underlined the supreme role of philology in the pursuit of ethnology in various instances. See, e.g., *Natural History of Man*, p. 132; *idem*, "On the Relations of Ethnology to Other Branches of Knowledge" (Anniversary Address delivered at the Anniversary Meeting, 22. 6. 1847, of the Ethnological Society). *Journal of the Ethnological Society of London* 1 (1848): 301-29, p. 304.

11 See Oswald Panagl, "Figurative Elemente in der Wissenschaftssprache von Franz BOPP". In *Bopp-Symposium 1992 der Humboldt-Universität zu Berlin. Akten der Konferenz vom 24. 3.-26. 3. 1992, aus Anlaß von Franz Bopps 200-jährigem Geburtstag am 14. 9. 1991*, ed. Reinhard Sternemann (Heidelberg: Winter, 1993), pp. 195-207.

12 The notion that German itself was already a degenerate form had already been put forward by Herder; cf. Jespersen, *Language*, p. 29.

It was endorsed by August Wilhelm Schlegel; cf. Arens, *Sprachwissenschaft*, pp. 190-91. Humboldt too stated that the fertile principle of languages, their inflections, was more abundant in the youth of a language; see his *Prüfung der Untersuchungen über die Urbewohner Hispaniens vermittelst der Vaskischen* [sic] *Sprache* (Berlin: Dümmler, 1821), p. 282.

13 Mária Tsiapera, "Organic Metaphor in Early 19th Century Linguistics". In *History and Historiography of Linguistics. Papers from the Fourth International Conference on the History of the Language Sciences, Trier, 24.-28. 8. 1987*, ed. Hans-Josef Niederehe, Konrad Koerner, 2 vols (Amsterdam: J. Benjamins, 1990), 2: 577-87, p. 581.

14 The organicism of philology is discussed in some essays in Henry M. Hoenigswald, Linda F. Wiener, eds, *Biological Metaphor and Cladistic Classification: An Interdisciplinary Perspective* (Philadelphia: University of Pennsylvania Press, 1987). See also E. F. Konrad Koerner, "Toward a Historiography of Linguistics. 19th and 20th Century Paradigms". In *idem, Practicing Linguistic Historiography: Selected Essays* (Amsterdam: J. Benjamins, 1989), pp. 21-54.

15 Prichard, *Researches*, 1st ed., pp. 460-63; *ibid.*, 2nd ed., 2: 606-9.

16 *Ibid.*, 2nd ed., 2: 501-2. Prichard included a translation of passages from Schlegel's book in his *An Analysis of the Egyptian Mythology* (1819). See Chapter 7 below.

17 Tsiapera, "Organic Metaphor", p. 582.

18 The term "agglutinative" was coined not by Friedrich Schlegel, but by his brother, August Wilhelm Schlegel. See E. F. Konrad Koerner, "Friedrich Schlegel and the Emergence of Historical Comparative Grammar". In *idem, Practicing Linguistic Historiography*, pp. 269-90, see p. 280.

19 Prichard, *Researches*, 2nd ed., 2: 230; 3rd ed., 4: 404-5.

20 *Ibid.*, 3rd ed., 4: 481.

21 *Ibid.*, pp. 541-42. See Humboldt, *Über die Verschiedenheit des menschlichen Sprachbaus und ihren Einfluß auf die geistige Entwickelung des Menschengeschlechts*, 1836 (London: Routledge, Thoemmes, 1995), p. 324. Prichard had adopted Humboldt's thoughts regarding the interdependency between development of language and development (or absence) of letters; see his *Researches*, 3rd ed., 4: 542-43.

22 Friedrich Schlegel, *Ueber die Sprache und Weisheit der Indier: Ein Beitrag zur Begründung der Alterthumskunde*, 1808, ed. E. F. Konrad Koerner (Amsterdam: J. Benjamins, 1977), pp. 50-51. The English translation is quoted from: Tsiapera, "Organic Metaphor", p. 580.

23 This definition, though widely adhered to, is contested by some

linguists.

24   Thus Schlegel wrote in *Fragmente* (1812) cited in Joachim Dyck,
      *Athen und Jerusalem. Die Tradition der argumentativen Verknüpfung
      von Bibel und Poesie im 17. und 18. Jahrhundert* (München: Beck,
      1977), p. 91.

25   *Ibid.*, ch. 6.

26   Jespersen, *Language*, pp. 32ff; see also Tsiapera, "Organic Metaphor",
      p. 582. That the Semitic languages were inflective, too, had also
      been mentioned by Humboldt. Nevertheless, he considered them as
      imperfect compared to the Indo-European ones. Humboldt, *Über
      die Verschiedenheit des menschlichen Sprachbaus*, p. 307.

27   In 1823, in a letter to Humboldt, Schlegel deplored that "our
      countrymen are running wild talking about Sanskrit, without
      understanding it". See Wilhelm von Humboldt, August Wilhelm
      Schlegel, *Briefwechsel*, p. 153.

28   Maurice Olender, *Les langues du paradis. Aryens et Sémites: un couple
      providentiel* (Paris: Gallimard, Le Seuil, 1989), p. 57.

29   Prichard, *Researches*, 3rd ed., vol. 1, note on p. 199.

30   *Ibid.*, 3: 209.

31   *Ibid.*, 4: 547.

32   Julius Klaproth, "Observations sur les racines des langues
      sémitiques". In Andreas Adolf de Merian, *Principes de l'étude
      comparative des langues* (Paris: Schubart, Heideloff; Leipzig:
      Ponthieu, Michelsen, 1828), pp. 209-40, see p. 212.

33   Similar views had been advanced by Johann David Michaelis,
      Friedrich Heinrich Wilhelm Gesenius, and Johann Christoph
      Adelung. See Klaproth, "Observations", p. 209; Prichard, *Researches*,
      3rd ed., 4: 552-53.

34   Klaproth's *Asia Polyglotta* was particularly valuable for him. See
      Prichard, *Researches*, 2nd ed., 1: 2-3, 493; 2: 10, 30, 193; 3rd ed., 2:
      216; 3: 276; 4: 52. After the highly admired geographer Carl Ritter
      had declared Klaproth to be outdated, Prichard criticized Klaproth
      in cases where his findings did not conform to his own. See his
      Researches, 3rd ed., 3: 131, 398. Still, Prichard relied often and
      heavily on Klaproth.

35   *Ibid.*, 3rd ed., 4: 554. Cf. Humboldt, *Über die Verschiedenheit des
      menschlichen Sprachbaus*, pp. 396-97.

36   Prichard, *Researches*, 3rd ed., 4: 457ff.

37   *Ibid.*, pp. 549-51 (my emphases).

38   *Ibid.*, 4: 555. Cf. Humboldt, *Über die Verschiedenheit des
      menschlichen Sprachbaus*, pp. 307-15, esp. pp. 308-9. It is interesting
      to compare Prichard's praise for Hebrew with the words of Nicholas

Wiseman. While the former cherished Hebrew for its complexity, Wiseman followed eighteenth-century notions, celebrating its primitiveness: "the Semitic family, destitute of particles and grammatical forms suited to express the relations of things, stiffened by an unyielding construction, and confined by the dependence for words upon verbal roots to ideas of outward action, could not lead the mind to abstract or abstruse ideas; and hence its dialects have been ever adapted for the simplest historical narratives, and for the most exquisite poetry". Wiseman, *Twelve Lectures*, 1: 139.

39 Humboldt, *Über die Verschiedenheit des menschlichen Sprachbaus*, pp. 312-15.

40 Prichard, *Researches*, 3rd ed., 4: 555-56 (my emphasis).

41 The movement was greatly enhanced through the writings of Johann Christian Winckelmann. See Alex Potts, *Flesh and the Ideal. Winckelmann and the Origins of Art History* (New Haven: Yale University Press, 1994), p. 160. See also Martin Bernal, *Black Athena. The Afroasiatic Roots of Classical Civilization*, 2 vols (London: Vintage, 1991 (1987)), vol. 1; Raymond Schwab, *La renaissance orientale* (Paris: Payot, 1950).

42 Richard Jenkyns, *The Victorians and Ancient Greece* (Oxford: Blackwell, 1980), p. 69; Bunsen, "On the Results of the Recent Egyptian Researches in Reference to Asiatic and African Ethnology, and the Classification of Languages". In Christian Carl Josias Bunsen, Charles Meyer, Max Müller, *Three Linguistic Dissertations. Read at the Meeting of the British Association for the Advancement of Science in Oxford* (from the *Report of the British Association for the Advancement of Science for 1847*) (London: Richard and John E. Taylor, 1848), pp. 254-99, quotation from p. 270. Cf. Olender, *Les langues du paradis*.

43 See Edward Breuer, *The Limits of the Enlightenment. Jews, Germans, and the Eighteenth-Century Study of Scripture* (Cambridge, Mass.: Harvard University Press, 1996), ch. 3.

44 Koerner, "Friedrich Schlegel", pp. 277-78.

45 Vans Kennedy, *Researches into the Origin and Affinity of the Principal Languages of Asia and Europe* (London: Longman, Rees, Orme, Brown and Green, 1828), p. 216.

46 Jones, "Discourse the Ninth on the Origin and Families of Nations, delivered 23 February, 1792". In *idem, Discourses Delivered at the Asiatick Society 1785-1792*, ed. Roy Harris (London: Routledge, Thoemmes, 1993), pp. 185-204, quotation from p. 199. Cf. Cannon, "Sir William Jones and Applied Linguistics", p. 385.

47 Prichard, *Researches*, 2nd ed., 2: 593-94; *ibid.*, 3rd ed., 2: 225.

48   *Ibid.*, 2nd ed., 2: 611-12.

49   *Ibid.*, 3rd ed., 4: 552-53; Humboldt, *Über die Verschiedenheit des menschlichen Sprachbaus*, pp. 395-96. Ewald and Gesenius suggested relationships between Indo-European and Semitic verbal roots; cf. Beyer, *Deutsche Einflüsse auf die englische Sprachwissenschaft*, pp. 180ff.

50   Prichard, *The Eastern Origin of the Celtic Nations Proved by a Comparison of Their Dialects With the Sanskrit, Greek, Latin, and Teutonic Languages, Forming a Supplement to Researches into the Physical History of Mankind* (Oxford: S. Collingwood, 1831).

51   John Pinkerton, *Dissertation on the Origin and Progress of the Scythians or Goths, being an Introduction to the Ancient and Modern History of Europe* (London: John Nichols, 1787), p. 69. According to Demandt, Pinkerton was advancing "a sort of Indo-Germanic hypothesis", for he took Greeks and Romans to be of Germanic origin. See Alexander Demandt, *Der Fall Roms. Die Auflösung des römischen Reiches im Urteil der Nachwelt* (München: Beck, 1984), p. 132.

52   Prichard, *The Eastern Origin*, p. 19.

53   Francisco R. Adrados, "Bopp's Image of Indo-European and Some Recent Interpretations". In *Bopp-Symposium*, ed. Reinhard Sternemann, pp. 5-14, esp. p. 6.

54   Prichard, *The Eastern Origin*, pp. 107-8. Prichard remarked that in both Hebrew and Celtic the third person of the future tense equalled the root of the verb. As Kliger has shown, attempts to prove relationships between Celtic and Hebraic idioms were very old, employing a source as ancient as Flavius Josephus's *History of the Jewish War*. See Samuel Kliger, *The Goths in England. A Study in Seventeenth and Eighteenth Century Thought* (Cambridge, Mass.: Harvard University Press, 1952), pp. 291-93.

55   Prichard, *The Eastern Origin*, p. 191.

56   Franz Bopp, *Die Celtischen Sprachen in ihrem Verhältnisse zum Sanskrit, Zend, Griechischen, Lateinischen, Germanischen, Litthauischen und Slawischen* (Berlin: Dümmler, 1839); Lorenz Dieffenbach, *Celtica I. Sprachliche Documente zur Geschichte der Kelten; zugleich als Beitrag zur Sprachforschung überhaupt* (Stuttgart: Imle & Liesching, 1839); Adolphe Pictet, *De l'affinité des langues celtiques avec le sanscrit* (Paris: Benjamin Duprat, 1837).

57   By the 1840s, Bunsen held that mankind originated from Asia. Moreover, he extended the age of human existence to some 20,000 years. See Ursula Kaplony-Heckel, "Bunsen – der erste deutsche Herold der Ägyptologie". In *Der gelehrte Diplomat. Zum Wirken Christian Carl Josias Bunsens*, ed. Erich Geldbach (Leiden: E. J. Brill,

1980), pp. 64-83, esp. pp. 74-75. Stocking is mistaken in thinking that Prichard adopted Bunsen's extended time-scale; see Stocking, *Victorian Anthropology*, p. 75.

58   Bunsen, "Recent Egyptian Researches", p. 270. It was on that occasion that Prichard protected the young and talented Max Müller "most chivalrously against the somewhat frivolous objections of certain members, who were not over friendly towards Prince Albert, Chevalier Bunsen, and all that was called German in scholarship". Cf. Max Müller, *My Autobiography*, p. 204.

59   August Wilhelm Schlegel, "De l'origine des Hindous". *Transactions of the Royal Society of Literature of the United Kingdom* 2 (1834): 405-46, pp. 442-44. This statement was reiterated, a few years later, by William Donaldson who otherwise respected Prichard's contribution to philology; John William Donaldson, *The New Cratylus, or Contributions Towards a More Accurate Knowledge of the Greek Language* (Cambridge: J. and J. J. Deighton, 1839), p. 35.

60   [Richard Garnett], "Prichard *on the Celtic Languages*". *Quarterly Review* 57 (1836): 80-110, p. 85.

61   Francis William Newman taught at Bristol College. Even though he increasingly lost faith in the ability of philology to prove the unity of mankind, he delved extensively into linguistic comparisons between African idioms and Hebrew. It was to prove a fruitful approach: nowadays the Semitic and the African languages are comprised under the head of "Afro-Asiatic" idioms; see L. Luca Cavalli-Sforza, Paolo Menozzi, Alberto Piazza, *The History and Geography of Human Genes* (Princeton: Princeton University Press, 1994), p. 99. To the 4th volume of the 3rd edition of the *Researches* Prichard appended an essay by Newman: "On the Hebraeo-African Languages"; cf. also *ibid.*, pp. 587-88 and vol. 5, note on p. 27.

62   Prichard, *Researches*, 3rd ed., 5: 25-29.

63   *Ibid.*, note on p. 27.

64   *Ibid.*, 4: 481.

65   William Whewell, *History of the Inductive Sciences*, 3 vols (London: J. W. Parker, 1837), 3: 483.

66   Cf. Chapter 8 of my Ph. D. dissertation "James C. Prichard's Views of Mankind".

67   Aarsleff, *The Study of Language*, pp. 177-78, 211-63.

68   See the list of members in the *Proceedings of the Philological Society* 1 (1844).

69   Prichard, *The Eastern Origin*, p. v.

70   It is telling that the *Proceedings* of the Society between 1842 and 1848 did not refer to his books.

71 Cf. John Burrow, "The Uses of Philology in Victorian England". In *Ideas and Institutions of Victorian England. Essays in Honour of George Kitson Clark*, ed. Robert Robson (London: Bell, 1967), pp. 180-204; Hugh A. MacDougall, *Racial Myth in English History. Trojans, Teutons, and Anglo-Saxons* (Montreal: Harvest House, 1982).

72 MacDougall, *Racial Myth in English History*, p. 26, see also pp. 44ff. It is debatable, however, whether the oppression of the "Norman Yoke" that stood at the centre of these discussions, was perceived more in proto-nationalist than in legal terms. For the latter view see: J. G. A. Pocock, *The Ancient Constitution and the Feudal Law. A Study in English Historical Thought in the Seventeenth Century*, rev. ed. (Cambridge: Cambridge University Press, 1987 (1957)).

73 *Ibid.*, p. 37.

74 The term "Indo-German" has been attributed to the Danish geographer Conrad Malte-Brun (1775-1826). See Olender, *Les langues du paradis*, note 63 on p. 27.

75 Ruth Leners, *Geschichtsschreibung der Romantik im Spannungsfeld von historischem Roman und Drama. Studie zu Augustin Thierry und dem historischen Theater seiner Zeit*, Bonner romanistische Arbeiten 23 (Frankfurt, Bern: Peter Lange, 1987), p. 30.

76 Lionel Gossman, "Augustin Thierry and Liberal Historiography". *History and Theory*, Beiheft 15 (1976): 3-83; Michel Lémonon, "L'idée de race et les écrivains français de la première moitié du xixe siècle". *Die neueren Sprachen* 69 (1970): 283-92. Nowadays the debate about the Celts has been given a new twist: there are scholars who argue that the "Celts" are a cultural construct, yet another invention of tradition; see Simon James, "The Ancient Celts, Discovery or Invention?" *British Museum Magazine* 28 (1997): 18-23.

77 Quoted in Claude Blanckaert, "On the Origins of French Ethnology. William Edwards and the Doctrine of Race". In *Bones, Bodies, Behavior. Essays on Biological Anthropology, History of Anthropology* 5, ed. George Stocking (Madison: University of Wisconsin Press, 1988), pp. 20-55, see p. 25.

78 *Ibid.*

79 William Frédéric Edwards, *Des caractères physiologiques des races humaines considérés dans leurs rapports avec l'histoire: Lettre à Amédée Thierry* (Paris: Compère jeune, 1829), p 40. Edwards bolstered Amédée Thierry's opinion in emphasizing how few people were necessary to accomplish a conquest: 60,000 men could subdue Britain, but they would not be able to change the racial stock of the British. See his "Fragments d'un mémoire sur les Gaëls". *Mémoires de la société ethnologique* 2 (1845): 13-47, pp. 40-41. For a discussion of

Edwards's racial theory see Blanckaert, "On the Origins of French
Ethnology". For a contrary opinion that defends Edwards against
allegations of racialism, see Antje Sommer, "William Frédéric
Edwards, 'Rasse' als Grundlage europäischer Geschichtsdeutung?" In
Die Natur des Menschen, ed. Gunter Mann *et al.*, pp. 365-409.

80 *Memoir of Baron Bunsen*, 1: 473. For Welsh patriotism, see Gwyn A.
Williams, "Romanticism in Wales". In *Romanticism in National
Context*, ed. Roy Porter, Mikuláš Teich (Cambridge: Cambridge
University Press, 1988), pp. 9-36. Cf. also E. D. Snyder, *The Celtic
Revival in English Literature, 1760-1800* (Cambridge, Mass.:
Harvard University Press, 1923).

81 Cf. Sommer, "William Frédéric Edwards, 'Rasse' als Grundlage
europäischer Geschichtsdeutung?", p. 405.

82 Prichard, *Researches*, 3rd ed., 3: 54. Prichard has been vindicated by
modern scholarship.

83 Notably Francis Palgrave and John Mitchell Kemble, though his *The
Saxons in England, a History of the Anglo-Saxon Commonwealth*
appeared only in 1849, a year after Prichard's demise. Thomas
Arnold even maintained that the French themselves were at best
distantly related to the Celtic stem. See his *Introductory Lectures on
Modern History* (Oxford: John Henry Parker, 1842), p. 30.

84 Prichard, *Researches*, 3rd ed., 3: 54.

85 *Ibid.*, p. 112. For Humboldt's *Untersuchungen über die Urbewohner
Hispaniens*, see Jean Rousseau, "Les trois méthodes de la
comparaison chez Wilhelm von Humboldt". In *Papers in the History
of Linguistics*, ed. Hans Aarsleff *et al.*, pp. 461-64.

86 Prichard, *Researches*, 3rd ed., 3: 55; *idem*, "On the Recent Progress of
Ethnology". Anniversary Address for 1848 to the Ethnological
Society of London. *Edinburgh New Philosophical Journal* 46 (1848):
53-72, p. 72.

87 *Ibid.*, p. 71.

88 Prichard, *Researches*, 3rd ed., 3: 123-24.

7

The Uses of Mythology for the Study of History

Long before myth was characterized by Max Müller as a disease of language, it was regarded as a Janus-faced phenomenon testifying, on balance, less to the wisdom than to the folly of religious philosophizing. In the course of the eighteenth century the time-worn interpretation of myth as a select representation of historical and religious truths for the masses was toppled.[1] Instead mythology became seen as the outcome of uninformed, superstitious attitudes towards nature and religion. This Enlightenment interpretation gave a new tincture to theological approaches to mythologies, most notably that of the ancient Egyptians. Some Enlightenment critics aimed to compromise Scriptural tenets by calling them a copy of Egyptian traditions. Others regarded them as especially sublime folklore. At the same time Biblical scholars were fascinated by the Egyptian traditions, since the Pentateuch was seen to give a historical account of Egyptian–Hebrew cultural exchange. If the Egyptian priests were not endowed with some superior, hermetic knowledge – if, on the contrary, they were as superstitious as ordinary folk – then the encounter between Moses and the Egyptians needed to be examined afresh. Prichard attacked the problem in 1813 and, extensively, in an 1819 book on Egyptian mythology. As late as the 1840s he still considered his exposition as valid. This chapter will elucidate the structures which permitted such continuity in his thinking. Prichard was keen to establish ethnology as a "science". But his own approach to the subject was a thoroughly moral one and hence imbued by his value judgements. In the following we shall examine his contributions to Egyptian mythology as well as the moral premises from which they flowed. Finally, we shall connect the results of his culture studies to those of his physiological investigations.

Interest in ancient relics was given a great boost by Napoleon's expedition to Egypt in 1798-99: in the early 1820s, even the Bristol Institution was presented with two mummies by Thomas Garrard, the chamberlain of the city.[2] The pyramids and their contents were as great a mystery as hieroglyphics, whose secrets Jean-François

Champollion (1790-1832) and the physician Thomas Young (1773-1829), the scion of a Quaker family, who had studied in Edinburgh and in Göttingen, attending Blumenbach's lectures, were competing to unravel. Prichard threw his weight behind the latter, praising Young for having "ascertained the meaning of upwards of 200 characters, before Champollion entered into the investigation".[3] Young had also been the first to introduce British scholars to Adelung's early achievements in comparative language studies.[4] It was, not least, a matter of patriotic pride to support the English scholar.

One evening in January 1825 the lecture room of the Bristol Philosophical and Literary Society was packed: one of Garrard's mummies was being opened under Prichard's supervision. He suggested that "most ancient alphabets", like those of the Hebrews and Phoenicians, had derived from hieroglyphics. Pointing both to the elaborate method of embalming and also to Young's interpretations, he enlarged on the idea that the ancient Egyptians had believed in "resurrection" and life after death. At the close of the meeting the Revd William Daniel Conybeare burst out with the news that "a new work of M. Champollion, of the most important character, had been put into his hands a few hours since".[5] It was Champollion's *Lettre à M. Dacier*, containing the key to the hieroglyphs on the Rosetta stone.[6] We do not know whether Prichard was embarrassed about the fact that he had supported Young's erroneous conjectures.[7] In any case, Champollion's finds did not materially alter his views. These had been expressed in a book, published in 1819: *An Analysis of the Egyptian Mythology*, which deepened certain views set out in the first edition of the *Researches*.

Historical Truth and the Truth of Revelation

When *An Analysis of the Egyptian Mythology* appeared, it was regarded as an important treatise by all those of Prichard's contemporaries who were pious enough to endorse his theological considerations, yet secular-minded enough to be interested in heathen parallels to the scriptural account.[8] Within our history of Prichard's thought the book is seminal: more explicitly than in most other publications, he came near to discussing tenets which directly related to his religious outlook. Furthermore, the *Egyptian Mythology* helps us to understand his general attitude to universal history.

Prichard's aims in investigating Egyptian mythology were threefold:

a. Once more, to substantiate the concept of monogenesis.
b. To show how the doctrines of Revelation had been distorted

in pagan Egyptian culture.

c. To disclose "a clue" for the reconciliation of the long timescale of the Egyptian chronologies and the rather shorter scriptural chronology.[9]

The method he chose was to juxtapose Egyptian mythology to "the superstitions of the East".[10] Plenty of scholars before him had tried inconclusively to establish genealogical links between Greek and Egyptian or Indian and Egyptian cultures. In the mid-eighteenth century it was such a common subject that even the teenaged Edward Gibbon dabbled with "the origin and nature of the Gods of Polytheism": "the Dynasties of Assyria and Egypt were my top and cricket-ball: and my sleep has been disturbed by the difficulty of reconciling the Septuagint with the Hebrew computation".[11] By the early nineteenth century interest had somewhat subsided, leaving only a hard core of scholars to try their hand at it. Ultimately their efforts were fuelled by the same objective: how did Biblical chronology square with the rest of universal history?

Undeterred by the multifarious attempts of his predecessors, Prichard set out to show there was a kinship between Egyptian and Indian mythologies from which he deduced an intrinsic relationship. This in turn enabled him to compare Egyptian and Greek mythologies by means of substituting Indian for Egyptian data whenever the Egyptian relics were either obscure or conflicted with his monogenist views of mythology. In the course of his investigations, he took up many of the questions which had engaged generations of classical scholars before him, and which have been summarized by Arnoldo Momigliano: how polytheism came to replace primitive monotheism; what had been the relation between Mosaic law and the institutions of surrounding nations; and what sort of confirmation, if any, could be found for Hebrew and Christian truth in pagan texts.[12]

Egyptian Mythology was a big book, more than 500 pages long. At the age of 33 Prichard had mastered a huge array of sources, including pagan histories of antiquity, patristic writings, Biblical criticism, chronologies and mythographies from all ages, as well as the studies of many orientalists and Egyptologists. On the whole, he worked with the same body of literature upon which countless theologians, chronologists, and mythographers had exerted their minds. After an introduction on Egyptian theology and mythology, he plunged into a detailed discussion of individual Egyptian Gods and the philosophical doctrines of Egyptian esoteric learning. Then he attempted "to

185

illustrate the Egyptian Mythology, by comparing it with the superstitions of the East". He compared Egyptian and Hindu mythology as well as the role and significance of the individual gods in both systems. Finally, he explained the "exoteric", that is, the supposedly "popular" side of Egyptian idolatry: the custom of animal worship. This led to a disquisition on the relationship between the Mosaic legislation and Egyptian civil and religious laws. A discussion of chronology was appended as an independent text at the end of the volume. The book provided a historical evaluation and theological interpretation of mythology. Prichard was markedly indifferent to Egypt's merits as one of the first civilized nations: Egyptian science, culture and statecraft were not his concern.

Although there may be exceptions such as Walter Scott and Samuel Taylor Coleridge,[13] it is certainly true that, for most British literary Romantics, mythology simply represented the "corpus of past myth they had always drawn on for allusion or story".[14] Prichard himself was a perfect example of a theoretician who, in the words of Feldman and Richardson, strove to "recover in the mythological deeds of antiquity the detailed but disfigured history of all that happened among the Hebrew people".[15]

While most other British authors on mythology ignored the publications of German Higher Criticism, Prichard was drawn into its aura. In their Biblical studies Johann Salomo Semler (1725-91), Johann David Michaelis (1717-91), Ernst Friedrich Carl Rosenmüller (1768-1835) and many others discriminated between "the truth of revelation" and secular "historical truth". This attitude annoyed the strictly orthodox, but for a man like Prichard, who was prepared to consider some elements of religious faith as anthropological universals, German scholarship provided an approach which combined piety with historical insight.[16] In the 1830s Nicholas Wiseman (1802-65), the later Cardinal, explained this approach in the following words: "the Germans were laying the foundation of that system which, though not matured, so early, was the only true and solid method of proceeding."[17]

In the preceding chapter we saw how much Prichard's philology was influenced by German publications. Friedrich Schlegel, in particular, was a philologist who also involved himself in mythology. Prichard was so intrigued by his theories that he translated an entire chapter of Schlegel's *On the Language and Wisdom of the Indians* to include it in his *Egyptian Mythology*. In the light of his debt to German Romantic theory, it will be interesting to see how Prichard used the latest scholarship in order to sustain Biblical doctrines which the nineteenth century gradually relegated to the imaginative furniture of simple minds. Despite (or, rather, because of) his sympathy for Scripturalism, Prichard strove to defend mythological tenets against those scholars of his time who, like Georges Cuvier, dismissed Indian and Egyptian mythology as unhistorical and bogus.

The Mythological Background

Eighteenth-century Biblical criticism was pursued from two different angles: one was philological, while the other illustrated scriptural tenets "from analogous circumstances in the laws and government of other nations".[18] Johann David Michaelis, Christian Gottlob Heyne (1729-1812) and their pupils brought Biblical studies in line with other historical researches. There was a long-standing tradition which tried to tease historical truth – facts which fitted the scriptural account – out of mythological narratives, and to reconcile the Biblical and pagan chronologies. In late eighteenth-century Britain Sir William Jones[19] and Jacob Bryant[20] were among those who pursued this path.

It was through the writings of these two authors that Prichard was introduced to mythology. "Oriental" Jones endeavoured to explain how the various mythical traditions of exotic peoples could be referred to a single hypothetical common source. In 1785 he read his discourse "On the Gods of Greece, Italy, and India" to the members of the Asiatick Society of Bengal, trying to prove that the deities of these three cultures were construed in perfect analogy and in conformity to one universal pattern. Jones greatly approved of the findings of the classical scholar and mythographer Jacob Bryant (1715-1804), who also tried to demonstrate the historical account of the Deluge through similar events related in non-Christian mythologies. In the first edition of his *Researches*, Prichard noted that his own results were in agreement with those of Bryant, albeit "built on entirely different principles".[21] By then, however, the mythographer's fame was already on the wane – in 1815 the *British Review* brushed aside his merits altogether: "so much learning ... so completely thrown away".[22]

Extending his mythological studies to German authors, Prichard assimilated both Enlightenment Higher Criticism and Romanticism. One of the salient elements of German Romantic theory was the re-evaluation of mythology: critics saw their task as that of bringing out the essential poetic quality of ancient myths. Regarding the Scriptures this eighteenth-century "linguistic turn" had been introduced through a lecture of Robert Lowth, Bishop of London

(1710-87): *De Sacra Poesi Hebraeorum* (1741). This approach was taken up by many British and German scholars.[23] In the early nineteenth century their views were linked to Friedrich Wilhelm Joseph Schelling's transcendentalist philosophy, which led many Germans to regard "man" as "the great creative word spoken by the earth".[24] While Christian orthodoxy had referred the term "inspired" solely to those humans who had received the message of revelation, German Romantic critics considered poetry an outcome of inspiration – or as a particular way of making sense of the world. Johann Gottfried Herder, for example, defined myth as "a mode of knowing, a function of the imagination". Thus the mythological spirit was seen as influencing the present; the dividing lines between scriptural tenets and mythological imaginations became blurred.[25]

Prichard, however, who had no aspirations to being a bard or seer, turned to mythology for reasons of historical enquiry. The immediate spur prompting him to engage with Egyptian mythology, was the writings of Paul Ernst Jablonski (1693-1767). Between 1750 and 1752, the German oriental scholar had published *Pantheon Aegyptorum*. In three volumes, he had collated patristic and classical sources in order to describe "the sex worship" prevalent at the borders of the Nile.[26] He aimed at severing all links between Greek mythology, which he valued, and Egyptian worship, which he despised. When the Edinburgh philologist Alexander Murray (1775-1813) published an edition of James Bruce's *Travels to Discover the Source of the Nile*, he quoted from Jablonski's work. But the Scottish scholar misrepresented Jablonski's ideas, stating that the German had presented Egyptian culture as altogether indigenous. In the new edition of Bruce's *Travels*,[27] Murray added a commentary which, to Prichard, seemed to describe the Egyptians as "a race peculiar to Africa, and originally distinct from the posterity of Noah and of Adam". This ran counter to his deep-seated belief in the unity of mankind. It "contradicts", he wrote, "the testimony of the Sacred Records, the earliest memorials of mankind, and is at variance with the general observations that result from a survey of the organized world, and the distribution of species over the globe".[28] He undertook to set the matter straight and to show that Egyptian mythology – be it ever so "atrocious"[29] – was, indeed, not only connected to Greek mythology, but also to Indian traditions, and, for that matter, to Christian doctrines.

But it was not just Jablonski's book against which Prichard felt the need to argue. He also rejected that strand of eighteenth-century Egyptian scholarship which tried to depict an ascent from barbaric

ancient customs to true religion. The peculiarly barbarous side of
Egyptian mythology, namely animal worship, had been accounted for
in various ways. The French mythographer Charles de Brosses (1709-
77) interpreted it as a universal stage in the growth of religious
consciousness.[30] This notion was tied up with de Brosses's belief that the
origin of speech lay in the utterance of almost brutish original sounds.

A similar theory had been put forward by David Hume and
William Warburton (1698-1779), Bishop of Gloucester, who both
imagined that primitive languages were "concrete and pictorial
before they became abstract and ideational".[31] Warburton censured
the opinions of free-thinkers who asserted that the notion of the
future state was not given to man through revelation, but arose
independently, particularly in the philosophy of the Egyptians which
they considered as "universal and primordial".[32] At the same time the
clergyman contested the doctrines of the followers of the so-called
Hermetic tradition who assumed that the Egyptian priests were
possessed of some original knowledge which they strove to disguise
through the invention of hieroglyphics. Somesuch theories entailed
the possibility that Moses might have received his wisdom from those
priests rather than from God.

Warburton had no qualms about acknowledging that Moses
might have been given some sort of Egyptian education,[33] but the
prophet's role as divine legate, the future prelate insisted, had been
bestowed upon him directly by God. This argument was aimed at
Spinoza, who had had the temerity to maintain that the ancient Jews
possessed no idea of the immortality of the soul.[34] The point was later
taken up by Enlightenment critics such as Karl Leonhardt Reinhold
(1758-1823), seeking to bring Hebraic traditions into disrepute by
declaring the wandering tribes of the ancient Israelites unfit to
conceive of an idea as abstract as the after-life.[35] In *The Divine
Legation of Moses* (1738-41) Warburton cleverly undermined
Spinoza's idea by means of endorsing it: the very lack of reference to
the future state in the Pentateuch indicated that God himself had
established "a theocracy". There was no need for Moses to mention
the after-life since God himself was governing His people.[36] If the
argument smacked of casuistry, it was yet too ingenious to be
discarded as a mere trick.

Warburton held that hieroglyphics, for their part, did not contain
any hidden wisdom. They were merely a ruse of the priests who
wanted to make the populace believe that they were invested with
superior knowledge. This was proved by the fact that the hieroglyphs,
according to Warburton, were invented after the spread of

alphabetical writing. Moses had learned the alphabet from the Egyptians, and only later did the priests supplant it with their obscure symbolic hieroglyphs.[37] That explained the Egyptian worship of brutes: it had its source in the deification of local heroes which had been introduced by political leaders. Since their names were depicted in hieroglyphics of which only the priests knew the proper meaning, the populace came to take the signs for pictures of the deities themselves. It was the beginning of animal worship.[38]

The Divine Legation of Moses was the subject of a heated discussion which extended until the end of the eighteenth century[39] and secured the Bishop the epithet of "the great patron of freethinking".[40] Having read Warburton's tract, Prichard was convinced that the relationship between Moses and the Egyptians deserved further scrutiny. He was particularly dissatisfied with Warburton's ideas about language and Scripture: for Prichard these were divine gifts too. Being a creation of Providence, the first language had nothing to do with the Egyptians.[41] He wanted to rectify Warburton's theories as well as those of his sources. As he saw it, Moses had adopted only a very small number of religious rites from the Egyptians; moreover, the tenets of Egyptian mythology reached so far back into history that it did not seem altogether out of the question to find in Egyptian superstition the vestiges of a purer form of worship as it might have been preserved in the first generations subsequent to the Flood. So he set out to re-position the Egyptian religion within the historical development of mythology. He undertook to prove, first, that Egyptian mythology was linked to the Indian and Greek mythologies and, second, that it had preserved some core knowledge of Revelation.[42]

History and Myth in the Egyptian Mythology

As we have said, Friedrich Schlegel was tremendously important to Prichard because he provided a key not only to the understanding of Egyptian mythology but also to the method of explaining Egyptian tenets through their alleged Indian counterparts. Schlegel approached mythology as he did philology: "like language", it was "founded on an inner structure, a basic network whose constancy is indicative of a common origin, despite all external variations of development".[43] Thus, Schlegel was, in Prichard's eyes, not only one of the few authors who dealt with Hindu mythology; he even seemed to share his own argumentative thrust.[44]

Schlegel divided Indian mythology into four chronological eras. According to Prichard these were

1. the era of doctrines of the emanation and transmigration of souls, "which seem to be the foundation of the oldest system of philosophy prevalent in the East"
2. the age of "Astrolatry, including the barbarous worship of nature, of the visible elements, and heavenly bodies"
3. the epoch dominated by "the dogma of two principles, or of the warfare between light and darkness, between the good and evil genius"
4. the age "in which the doctrines or representations of the Eastern schools acquire a more refined and metaphysical description".[45]

Briefly, the four stages theory of religious development was this: emanation and metempsychosis was followed by pantheism, which gave way to "hylozoism" (the deification of visible elements), which was finally superseded by the veneration of heroes as incarnations of the gods (euhemerism).[46] While Schlegel despised the fourth stage, which he equated with pantheism, he exalted the earliest of these epochs. The view that all souls were "emanations", that is, flowing "from one soul of the universe"[47] was, in Schlegel's eyes, at once deeply pious and philosophical: "the system of emanation is seen in the most favourable point of view, when we contemplate it as the doctrine of restitution. From the divine origin of man, it takes occasion to remind him of his restoration, and to set before him a reunion with the divinity."[48] Emanation was related to metempsychosis or the doctrine of transmigration of souls, which in turn linked up with the notion of the resurrection of the soul. It involved belief in some form of universal judgment after death and subsequent redemption or damnation.[49] Schlegel read Christian doctrines into Indian mythology. And, even though he disliked pantheism, at least the earliest stages of Indian philosophy he regarded as being permeated by truly Christian notions: "this law of progressive debasement and regular deterioration, and the sentiment of inward sorrow and remorse connected with the consciousness of guilt and the expectation of death, are the foundations of the oldest sagas".[50] In previous chapters we have encountered Prichard's preoccupation with guilt – as his publication on Egyptian mythology shows, the theme was present as early as 1819.[51]

Schlegel shared one of Prichard's central beliefs, namely, the notion that the most ancient religions, like the earliest language, had been pure and pious: mythological tenets were not the starting point of a development which led to monotheism, as de Brosses had seen it, rather they were degenerate, "corrupted" versions of true religion. Prichard wrote:

> The earliest faith was pure and simple, exhibited comprehensive and exalted conceptions of the Deity, and contained the most awful and impressive sanctions of morality. In subsequent periods it appears to become continually more depraved and sensual.[52]

William Warburton had explained the propensity for the Christian religion as a capacity which developed in the course of civilization. "The Doctrine of the *Metempsychosis*" seemed to signify "a *moral Designation of Providence*."[53] For Prichard, this exegesis was only half the truth: emanation and metempsychosis were not just parts of providential typology, but rather significant elements of the "holier belief" which characterized the early ages of mankind.[54] Subsequent civilization, by contrast, merely served to disguise and distort revelation: it did not make for a better understanding of its doctrines. For Prichard, ill-founded philosophy was, if anything, rather more pernicious than primitive ignorance: "the first step of corruption of this simple form of theology", he wrote, "seems to have been the attempt to adorn it with the figments of philosophy, according to that style of philosophizing that was suited to the genius of the age". The genius, Prichard thought, was low, but so were the efforts of philosophers – whoever they were, be they pagan priests or Spinoza. One instance exemplifying his disdain was the primeval "doctrine that the world was created by the voluntary agency of the Supreme".[55] This idea, Prichard said with a view to pantheism, was apparently "not enough to satisfy curiosity, and we find it often blended with some fanciful analogies derived from natural processes that are daily observed".[56] As Prichard saw it, Egyptian philosophers helped to blur the purity of the complex, abstract truth of Revelation.

After he had established the nature of Indian religion and mythology, Prichard proceeded to compare the Egyptian and the Indian gods. Since Egyptian polytheism displayed superstitions which appeared grosser than those of the Indian system, it was only "in more recondite parts of the Egyptian mythology ... that we trace any resemblance to the older doctrines of the Hindoos, respecting the creation of the world, and the emanation of subordinate beings from the essence of an eternal spirit".[57] He addressed five major principles: the existence of a supreme god; the notion of a religious triad comparable to the Trinity of God the Father, the Son, and the Holy Ghost; the occurrence of the Deluge; the doctrine of a future state; and the existence of the soul. These will be outlined in the following paragraphs.

Both the Egyptians and the Hindus believed in "a Deity, in the sense in which that word is understood among Christians and European philosophers in general": the creation as well as the end of the world lay in the hands of a powerful individual being.[58] The idea that the Egyptians had a notion of the Trinity was not Prichard's alone: in the seventeenth century the German Jesuit polymath Athanasius Kircher (1602-80) had stipulated the same;[59] the idea resurfaced in Friedrich Schlegel's interpretation of the Indian notion of emanation. It was Schlegel from whom Prichard gleaned that Egyptian and Indian traditions contained "a triple personification", representing "the generative, the destructive, and the restoring powers of nature".[60] Prichard was at pains to avoid the impression that he was attempting to relate this "obscure tradition" of the Egyptians to the "Divine Nature and the modes of its subsistence, which distinguish Christian theology".[61] But his denial could hardly conceal the point that, in a historical sense, this was exactly what he had in mind.

It was well known that pagan mythologies included the notion of catastrophes brought about by fire and floods. The latter events were akin to the Biblical story of the Deluge. "Fortunately ... for the history of mythology", wrote Prichard, "the same dogma may be traced in the antiquity of several nations, who, if they obtained it not from Egypt, certainly derived it from some common source."[62] The comparison between the respective stories of the Greek philosophers, in particular the Stoics, and those of the Vedic tradition proved the intimate relation between Egyptian and Indian teachings. Finally there was the doctrine of the future state and the immaterial soul. To demonstrate the Egyptian belief in the existence of the soul Prichard referred to the Pythagoreans whose accounts he deemed "more particular" than the obscure hints entailed in Egyptian mythology.[63] Thus the three systems of the Greeks, Hindus, and Egyptians "afford an outline that may unite the different fragments of their doctrine into an uniform and not wholly unconnected system".[64] Christian doctrines, that is, permeated the oldest known systems of mythology, which, therefore, displayed "not only speculative philosophy; but a system of religion in the proper sense" of the term. Like Indian mythology, Egyptian religion "contemplated in the Deity, not merely the author of the universe, but a moral governor of the world, whose dispensations were so arranged as to reward the virtuous and take vengeance on the guilty".[65]

Traditionally, the starting point for pagan mythological studies had been the question as to how idolatry had come into the world. There were three standard responses: it was seen as proof of religious corruption; alternatively, it was taken to derive from reverence for distinguished individuals (this was the euhemerist explanation to which Warburton adhered); or, thirdly, it was assumed that religious tenets developed from worship of the elements or physical forces, to the notion of individualized gods.[66] Prichard's approach was based upon the first response. But he turned the argument around: instead of following up the development of idolatry, he looked for the survival of monotheistic vestiges.[67] Animal worship and pantheism, for him, were the outcomes of ignorance and bad philosophy. As a result, over time, common people could no longer distinguish between the Creator and His works: they confused cause and effect. Thus polytheism came into being, and the habit of praying to natural forces, as people were taking, for example, a river for a deity.[68]

Prichard's insistence that "the religion of the first ages" as well as "the consciousness of guilt and the expectation of death" had framed "the whole national and personal character" of most diverse peoples, amounts to the assumption of a religious sense ingrained in human nature.[69] We have encountered it already when discussing his philosophy of the human mind and its delusions. This concept was the residue of Revelation present in human conscience. Thus, Prichard's later notions concerning the feeling of "gloom" were foreshadowed as early as 1819, although he had not yet expounded his concept of the psyche.

Was Prichard himself plagued by feelings of guilt? Was his dissatisfaction with philosophical casuistry and utilitarian egoism more than the moral accusations pious people of all ages have thundered against their less pious neighbours? Given the lack of personal testimony, there is no definite answer to these questions. It is, however, significant that his theory of mythological history closely reflects his judgment upon the age he lived in. Indeed, the results of his studies delineated in the preceding paragraph were informed by religion, so as to lead him into circular thinking: he chose his own criteria of comparison, that is, the main Christian doctrines; then he projected them back onto ancient pagan mythologies. Where Egyptian mythology defied this operation, Indian traditions came into play. At the end, he sternly concluded that the existence of the main Christian doctrines in the earliest stages of all ancient mythologies proved that they all had sprung from one common source.[70] The existence of Christian traces in pagan religions was central to the *Analysis of the Egyptian Mythology* in two respects: it was the core of Prichard's hypothesis, and it was, at the same time, the proof through which he showed the historical account of Genesis to be correct. Thus, by using Genesis, he demonstrated the truth of Genesis.

Of course, Prichard acknowledged that the after-life was not the only characteristic of the institutions he investigated. The Pentateuch itself abounded with prescriptions concerning the civil institutions of the Hebrew polity. These, too, he believed were useful when it came to comparing Egyptian traditions to those of the Israelites. He probed into those institutions from a functionalist viewpoint that aimed to find instances of cultural diffusion.

Civil Institutions in Mythology

In the previous chapter, we saw that Prichard was extremely interested in the Celtic language family. One of the reasons for his optimism concerning the possibility of uncovering its links to primeval human idioms lay in the widespread tendency to compare the Celtic institution of the Druids to the Hindu caste system. The antiquarian William Stukeley (1687-1765) had already conjectured that Kircher's Trinitarian theory was applicable not only to the Egyptians but also to the Celts.[71] Stukeley maintained that the Celtic Druids had received Abraham's religion from Phoenician priests who had, at the time of the Patriarchs, established a colony in Britain. By the nineteenth century this theory struck most scholars as quite fanciful, but at the end of the eighteenth century it still found quite a few adherents.[72] Prichard probed further into this tradition. A caste system, as it was to be found in India, which differentiated the strata of a population into priests, warriors, and peasants or herdsmen, could be discerned in Celtic traditions as well as in Egyptian relics.[73] In 1826 he even surmised that Wotan might be historically linked to Buddha. As with the Egyptians, the superior castes of the Celts had subjected the populace to servitude, rendering them "little better than slaves".[74]

In *Egyptian Mythology*, civil institutions also came into focus. Since the seventeenth century, Egyptian scholarship had been asking whether Moses' familiarity with Egyptian customs had influenced the laws he had given to the Israelites. When Prichard took up the subject, he considered both its theological and its socio-political aspects. Theologically, he did not discover any similarities between Egyptian doctrines and those which the Jewish law-giver put in place. Even if the Egyptians had retained elements of the faith "of the patriarchs", it was unlikely that the Hebrew captives had adopted them from their Egyptian masters, the former being a nomadic people, "the simple and unvaried tenour of whose existence precludes all great innovations in manners and sentiments".[75] Prichard as a matter of course followed the eighteenth-century view that non-refined society was more natural than its civilized counterparts.

If the religion of the Hebrews was not influenced by the Egyptian example the same was true for their political customs. Following the teachings of Michaelis, Prichard affirmed that their political system was unique to them. Unlike the Egyptians who "consigned the lower castes, with their posterity, to a state of perpetual servility and abject degradation", the Hebrews did not know a hereditary hierarchy: their prophets, Prichard wrote, "were men raised up from any tribe, without distinction, and the most illustrious were not descended" from the high echelons of the Levite family.[76] In making these points, he opposed himself to British comparative theology, set out by John Spencer (1630-95)[77] and emulated by Warburton, which saw many parallels between Egyptian and Mosaic legislation. For Prichard this was untenable, if not intolerable. Spencer historicized the origins of the Mosaic codex, referring many of its laws to Egyptian customs. That was the beginning of a protracted debate about Moses' role as legislator.[78] Thanks to Spencer the idea gained ground that Egyptian civilization and religion were considerably older than those of the Hebrews. In his *Canon Chronicus* (1672) John Marsham (1602-85) argued that Egyptian culture preceded Moses by some 900 years.[79] Modifying Spencer's teachings, Warburton drew many parallels between the religious tenets of the ancient Israelites and Egyptians. He saw no theological danger in the fact that Egyptian culture might have been more developed than that of the Hebrews: faith had nothing to do with civilization.[80]

Prichard endorsed the notion; in other respects, however, Warburton's historical approach seemed to go too far. Prichard's contribution to the debate was based on the crucial prerequisite that the greater part of the Jewish dispensation was primeval. Only on this condition could the notion of global cultural unity be reconciled to the idea that the monotheism of the Old Testament was the foundation of metaphysics. Or, as Prichard's admirer, the Hebraist Daniel Guildfort Wait (1789-1850), put it in a book published in 1823: "notwithstanding the antiquity of the Egyptian hierarchy, we have shewn, that the Israelitish institutions are not to be referred to *their* school, but rather to the Patriarchal remains re-modeled and enlarged at the delivery of the law of Mount Sinai".[81] Only in respect of the doctrine of the future state did Prichard fully agree with Warburton. It was a point Michaelis had made as well: Moses had no need to mention the "invisible world" as he "had declared, in the outset, that God had promised to govern Israel as its immediate sovereign, with temporal rewards and punishments". Moses not only dispensed with the Egyptian hereditary class system, but also ensured that the entire population had equal access to learning and religious understanding.[82]

We have come to see Prichard as a conservative who yearned for the patriarchal order of the *ancien régime*, loathing the political radicalism that gained ground during the 1830s.[83] It should, therefore, appear striking that he seemed to adopt rather liberal, or even egalitarian, views when discussing the Mosaic polity. At second glance, however, the apparent radicalism dissolves. Everything he said about the civil and social constitution of the Hebrew polity was derived from Michaelis, Professor of Philology at the University of Göttingen, who was soon to achieve recognition in Britain as the chief authority on Moses.[84] Much has been made of the freedom of enquiry prevalent at Göttingen University in the second half of the eighteenth century,[85] and Michaelis was one of the protagonists of this spirit. Having studied under Robert Lowth, he assimilated the latter's teachings on the poetical genius of the Hebrew. In addition he was a self-professed disciple of Montesquieu whose social "laws" he applied to the Hebrew polity.[86] Given the atmosphere at Göttingen, Michaelis's *Commentaries on the Laws of Moses* was not particularly radical – although it was more daring than Prichard's excerpts suggest. Prichard's own political position is therefore revealed not so much in those passages which he quoted, but in those which he omitted.

Michaelis pursued social analysis with much more enthusiasm than Prichard. For Michaelis, the pastoral state of the Mosaic polity implied that "there was no *Bourgeoisie*, or distinct class of Citizens". He conceived of Moses as the first democrat in history: "this equality of all citizens, without a class of nobles, properly so called, could not but give the Israelitish state a democratic tendency; and we need not wonder that on such a foundation, Moses should have established a democracy, and not a monarchy".[87] In his introduction prefixed to his translation of the *Commentaries*, the clergyman Alexander Smith distanced himself from Michaelis's "political castles in the air".[88] Prichard, for his part, needed no such political disclaimer – he simply omitted what he disliked. If he embraced the notion of equality among the ancient Israelites, this was because the immediate rule of God made worldly hierarchies unnecessary. "Peers of the realm must needs be", Edward VI had long ago been lectured, "but the poorest ploughman is in Christ equal with the greatest prince there is."[89] The idea was a commonplace of Christian piety, it appealed especially to Quaker sensibilities. But

Prichard certainly did not wish to lend the concept of democracy credence enough as to quote the relevant passage in the *Commentaries*. On the contrary, when describing Prichard's medical outlooks we have come across his censorious remarks on the Poor Law reforms and the expression of his hankering after what he called the "liberality of former generations" that had made use of "the patriarchal gift of tenths" to alleviate hardship. In the "present age", by contrast, he could perceive but "sordid penury"[90] – modern times and their social institutions did certainly not commend themselves to the doctor; he had no reason to follow Michaelis's subtle social criticism.

The only true parallels between Egyptian and Mosaic regulations that Prichard allowed concerned elements of ceremonial law. He was particularly intrigued by the custom of circumcision. This had been a long-standing practice among the Egyptians. But Prichard was far from claiming that Moses, being used to Egyptian rites, had adopted the custom because he did not know any better. Nor, for that matter, did Prichard agree with Warburton who stated that "the Pagans might indulge themselves in the Imitation of Jewish rites".[91] Instead, he followed Michaelis who presented the introduction of circumcision as pragmatic expediency. An awareness that all government had to rest in "the habits and character of the people whom it was designed to controul [sic] and edify" induced Prichard to believe that Moses had adopted circumcision as a rite "connected with some idea of purity" from the Egyptians. Michaelis suggested that, in Egypt, it had been only the priests who were circumcised.[92] For Prichard this seemed to explain why the custom had sacral connotations for the Hebrews when introduced by Moses.

This example brings us to another aspect of Prichard's thought that requires examination: the question of his Biblicism. Some historians who know his writings well have suggested that he was increasingly obliged to shed Biblical tenets: science, they have alleged, triumphed over belief. His attitude towards the Bible, W. F. Bynum has claimed, "became increasingly flexible".[93] An examination of his comments on the scriptural account of natural history, however, suggests another conclusion: Prichard's beliefs in scriptural doctrines did not change all that much. He never was a rigid literalist; but those teachings he had embraced as a young man tended to characterize his faith until his dying day.

Prichard's Attitude Towards the Bible

In their time, an Athanasius Kircher or a Jacob Bryant pursued comparative mythological historiography with great zeal. It was accepted that the history of the globe could be accommodated within the scriptural doctrine of an Earth no older than some 6000 years. But by the beginning of the nineteenth century, geological theory had undermined this approach. As a result, even defenders of the faith henceforth admitted that the world was much older than the Bible apparently stated: the six-day period of Creation could be understood allegorically, each day signifying an entire epoch.[94] Prichard happily accepted those theories that read some six million years into the six days of Creation.[95] After all, the Mosaical account was open to interpretation just as any other ancient historical source.[96] At the same time, however, he took it for granted that, during the early stages of the Earth's existence, Providence had materially interfered with the course of events:

> In the first ages of the world events were conducted by operative causes of a different kind from those which are now in action; ... this sort of agency continued to operate from time to time, as long as it was required, that is, until the physical and moral constitution of things now existing was completed, and the design of providence attained.[97]

This assumption allowed for several miraculous occurrences, including the Fall, the story of the Tower of Babel, the Flood and Noah's Ark.[98] Even early in his career Prichard was defending the theory that the six days of Creation represented six extended epochs in the history of the Earth.[99] The idea was theologically unproblematic since its scope was confined to the era before the creation of human kind. The same applied to the notion, publicized by Georges Cuvier, that there had been not one but several catastrophes, or "revolutions in nature", which wiped out those species living at the time, thus preparing "the earth for supporting new tribes of organized creatures".[100] Prichard had no qualms about extending the age of the world beyond scriptural doctrine, nor did he have any compunction about giving his own interpretation of the Deluge. In the second edition of the *Researches* he deviated from the Linnaean conjecture that all existing land-animals "descended from a stock that was preserved in Noah's Ark".[101] There was plenty of evidence in the fossil record that many animal species were peculiar to the past histories of certain landmasses only: their bones and fossils were found, for example, in America and Australia, but not in the area between Egypt and Persia. In a section titled "Comparison of the preceding Remarks with the History of Mankind and the Deluge, contained in Genesis",[102] Prichard concluded that not every species

199

extant at the time of the last Deluge had survived the catastrophe in Noah's Ark: by the time of the Flood human kind had not yet spread across the globe, and when Noah built the Ark only those animals were saved which coexisted with humanity. "Mankind", he suggested,

> escaped by the means which are recorded in the sacred, and in many profane histories, and with them were saved the stock of animals peculiar to the region in which before the flood they had their dwelling, and of which they, and most of the early domesticated animals, are in all probability the native inhabitants.[103]

Prichard was not quite sure whether the Deluge was universal, though "geological Phaenomena, and a variety of considerations, render it most probable" that it was. There was no doubt, however, that not all species were saved. Those that were not essential to mankind were, in a "partial creation" after the Deluge, replaced by new orders, better adapted to the new surroundings. Genesis, he wrote, "refers to the stock of animals peculiar to the region inhabited by men before the deluge, which were, perhaps, chiefly the domesticated kinds, and the clean, or those used for sacrifice in the patriarchal institutions".[104] Much as he loathed utilitarianism, his own understanding of the sacred history could itself be quite utilitarian: "it was of no importance for men to be informed at what era New Holland began to contain kanguroos, or the woods of Paraguay anteaters and armadilloes".[105] In the final analysis, in other words, it did not matter when these animals had come into existence, before or after the Flood; it did not even matter whether a Deluge had actually taken place in Australia.[106]

For Prichard, it was not a retreat from the truth of the Scriptures to assume a partial creation. Even though he adopted the idea only in the 1820s, after having assimilated Cuvier's interpretation of the fossil record, it did not imply a major reorientation: the very fact that, as early as 1816, he regarded the six days of Creation as a metaphor, shows that his scriptural concerns were confined to human history. He never held that speculating on pre-diluvial rocks and extinct species amounted to impinging on theology. There are, indeed, only two instances in which his change of mind can be seen as detrimental to his personal allegiance to scriptural doctrine: by 1847 he no longer assumed that Moses had written the whole of Genesis the "first portions", he surmised, must have been compiled by a number of unknown authors.[107] And he came to doubt in the longevity of the Patriarchs.[108]

Compared to the body of scriptural tenets Prichard did adhere to, these deviations were anything but crucial. As early as 1819 he noted that, when Moses was composing Genesis, he was not inspired by the "dictates of immediate revelation".[109] As will become clear below, his doubts as to the longevity of the Patriarchs were bound up with the case of monogenesis. Another example which has been advanced as a proof of Prichard's retreat in the face of scientific evidence concerns the Biblical chronology.[110] As we will presently see, however, this subject underlines his adherence to tradition rather than contradicting it. Confronted with the necessity of presenting natural history in such a manner as to leave enough time for animals and human populations to develop their particular physical features, he restructured the Biblical timescale.

Egyptian Chronology

Prichard's remarks on chronology constitute an appendix to his *Analysis of the Egyptian Mythology*. Although not strictly related to the subject of mythology, it was included as he thought he had "discovered a clue" to solve, once and for all, the discrepancies between the Biblical timescale and other records.[111]

For many centuries, chronology had involved the most intricate problems of theology.[112] Scriptural chronology was thoroughly ambiguous, the accounts of the Hebrew Masorah, the Greek Septuagint, and the "Bible-Chronology" of James Ussher (1581-1651), Bishop of Armagh, contradicting each other (in addition there was also the so-called Samaritan version of the Pentateuch which Ussher had brought to the attention of European scholarship).[113] Following the conventional understanding of the Septuagint, some 5400 years had elapsed between the creation of the Earth and the birth of Christ; following the Masoretic text, however, the interval was 1440 years shorter.[114] Moreover, Biblical chronology differed considerably from numerous other chronological accounts, those of the Egyptians and the Indians being considerably longer than their Christian counterparts. The two most important Egyptian computations were the account of Manetho, the Egyptian priest and historian of Egypt (fl. 280 b.c.e.),[115] and the historical work of the Greek philosopher Eratosthenes (ca. 276-194 b.c.e.) who served as the director of the great library in Alexandria.

In medieval times, it was commonly believed that some 4000 years had passed between the creation of the world and the birth of Jesus. Later authors modified the figure, the range reaching from 3947 to 5868 years.[116] Theoretical warfare raged between those who, like Bishop Ussher, based their computations on the Hebrew text and those who preferred the chronology of the Septuagint.[117] Isaac Newton, following the latter, was one of many authors who tried to reconcile the Egyptian and Biblical chronologies: he declared that Osiris, Bacchus, Sesostris, and Sisa were merely different names for one single person, namely, the lawgiver who had introduced civilization in Egypt, roughly two generations before the Trojan war.[118] In Newton's view this sufficiently explained the greater Egyptian timescale. But since his computation was based on the assumption that the Egyptian dynasties were more recent than even Scripture allowed, Bishop Warburton rejected it.[119]

During the seventeenth century and throughout the eighteenth, John Marsham (1602-85) was widely accepted as authoritative in Britain. Having stipulated the antiquity of Egyptian civilization he forced it back into the Biblical timescale. In his interpretation, ancient Egypt was divided into several kingdoms. Not being aware of this basic fact, Ma netho had just added up their respective chronicles, having one kingdom follow another instead of seeing that they belonged to the same epoch: the Egyptian timescale, therefore, appeared more extended than it actually was. Prichard presented his own speculations on chronology as a refutation and replacement of this theory. Theologically satisfying as it was, he realized that there was no historical proof available to affirm it.[120]

Setting out to solve the question of chronology, Prichard started not so much from the viewpoint of absolute figures and numbers of years, but in terms of the chronological relations between historical events – a practice common at the time.[121] He had two main tasks: to bring the historical accounts of the Egyptian Manetho and of the Greek Eratosthenes into line, and to reconcile scriptural with Egyptian chronology. In response to the first problem he argued that both scholars had conflated the records of different cities, which led them to assign varying names to the same kings. Manetho's timescale was exorbitant because, as Prichard suggested, he had counted prefects and provincial governors as kings, thus adding several imaginary Pharaonic reigns to the historical records.[122] If this solution was comparatively easy, the reconciliation of scriptural and Egyptian chronologies proved far more difficult.

When Abraham visited Egypt – according to the Septuagint around 2000 b.c.e. – the Egyptian polity was already thriving.[123] But how far back did its history actually reach? Prichard believed that Manetho – being a priest – "must be supposed to have possessed the most accurate information". He himself drew upon Enlightenment philosophy and Higher Criticism to bolster traditional beliefs. It was well known that the Bible contained different accounts of one and the same event. Most conspicuously there were those passages which referred in one version to God by the name of "Elohim", and in another by the tetragram (YHWH).[124] Prichard assumed that similar overlapping narratives might be found in the history of Manetho. On the assumption that the priest had committed minor errors and that later transcribers of his chronology had shown "carelessness in copying", he managed to ascribe accounts of two different conquests of Egyptian territory to the same era, namely the age of the Hebrew Shepherd Kings, the Hyksos, who invaded Egypt in the seventeenth century b.c.e.[125] As Manetho at one point referred to the Hyksos as "captives", the Jewish historian Flavius Josephus identified them as the Hebrews of the Egyptian captivity. If both were the same, then, Prichard argued, Manetho's timescale was longer than history allowed – there were no parallel kingdoms, as Marsham and Scaliger had suggested, but parallel narratives.[126] Prichard toyed with names and numbers until pagan and Biblical chronologies were successfully correlated. The Exodus had taken place in 1619, he concluded, and the Egyptian monarchy was founded between 5043 and 4792 before Christ.[127] That left enough time, between 4792 and creation of the world, for the Flood, and the development of society.

How are we to assess Prichard's reading of Egyptian mythology? Modern scholarship tends to believe that the Shepherd Kings, i.e. the tribe of the Hyksos, and the Hebrew tribe of Exodus are identical. This identity, however, is not of a historical but of a mythical nature. There is no historical foundation of the "Egyptian captivity" and the story of Exodus, yet over time narrative traditions turned the conquerors into captives: Jan Assmann has perceptively described how the memory of the Hyksos invasion inspired the story of Exodus.[128] Of course, Prichard had no inkling of this, he simply wanted to prove the Pentateuch right, to adapt pagan chronologies to that of the Bible. The thrust of his argument was deeply conservative. Still, his endeavours were original insofar as he took Manetho's records seriously, which in turn enabled him, in his capacity as ethnologist, to treat Egyptian traditions as at least a semi-reliable source. His *Egyptian Mythology* presupposed and sustained the notion that there was a core of historical truth in pagan lore, whereas a man like Cuvier dismissed Egyptian as well as Indian mythologies as products of pure fantasy.[129] Not least to bolster his monogenist doctrine, Prichard had to assume a different attitude. Otherwise, the whole project of using mythology to prove the genealogical parentage between Egypt and India would have been impossible, and that would have jeopardized the unity of mankind.

Add One Thousand Years to the Age of the World

The reception of the *Egyptian Mythology* was ambiguous. The theologically moderate *Monthly Review* as well as the Cambridge Hebraist Daniel Guildfort Wait were impressed by it.[130] But to those uninterested in the theological implications of Egyptian history, it seemed excessively permeated by religious considerations, while some defenders of Christian orthodoxy considered it as too free-spirited. "We are at a loss what to say about this book", the *British Critic* grumbled: the attempt "to blend all religions in one" was "mystical nonsense".[131] That organ understood itself as an orthodox Christian journal. More liberal-minded reviewers were equally puzzled, though for other reasons: "a labyrinth of numbers and names", was the verdict of August Wilhelm Schlegel, the German orientalist: Prichard was no better than "the harmonists who in the preceding centuries have tried in vain to reconcile the contradictions between so-called profane history and the sacred tradition".[132] Schlegel did not single out Prichard for blame: British scholarship, he remarked, was as yet not emancipated from paying tribute to religious doctrine.[133] All the same, Schlegel thought it worthwhile to translate Prichard's treatise, the German version appearing in 1837.

That decade saw a new wave of chronological speculations. Prichard himself, however, came back to the topic only in 1847. This time it was not part of mythological interpretation, but of anthropology. His opinions on human nature were often challenged. One objection, in particular, appeared troubling: in 1846 the *New Quarterly Review* pointed out that Prichard could sustain his notion of climatic influence on skin colour only at the expense of scriptural chronology.[134] By then it was generally assumed that a change of skin colour in any given race, if possible at all, could be brought about only over a long period of time. Referring to the paintings found in Egyptian tombs, the American doctor Samuel George Morton and the classical scholar John Kenrick (1788-1877) were two amongst others who stipulated that there had been several distinctly different human types as early as 1000 to 1500 years b.c.e.[135] Either they had been created as such – as many Scripturalist polygenists believed, or the world was older than 6000 years: anyone wanting to prove that these different complexions had been induced by climate, had to envisage a timespan since Creation long enough for the Egyptians to divide into white, brown, and black varieties.

Prichard acknowledged the problem. A thousand years or so

between the era of the Noachian Deluge and these Egyptian works of art were not long enough for such a significant development.[136] On the authorities of German authors such as Michaelis, Baron Bunsen, and the orientalist and theologian Ernst Friedrich Carl Rosenmüller (1768-1835), he explained that scriptural chronology was incomplete. The Bible was historically accurate as far back as ten centuries before the birth of Christ. How many years human history went back before that date, however, was largely a matter of speculation:

> the Hebrew chronology may be computed with accuracy to the era of the Building of the Temple [under Solomon ca. 966-26 b.c.e.], or at least to that of the Division of the Tribes. In the interval between that date and the arrival of Abraham in Palestine it cannot be ascertained with exactness, but may be computed with a near approximation to truth. Beyond that event we can never know how many centuries nor even how many chiliads of years may have elapsed since the first man of clay received the image of God and the breath of life.[137]

Speaking of chiliads of years was a bit of a rhetorical flourish which Prichard could afford since he had "only to consider the chronology of the Bible as far back as the origin of the human race".[138] In fact he argued that the Bible had "omitted" merely a few generations, and had instead exaggerated the longevity of the Patriarchs. It was not his aim to declare the history of mankind to be measured in millions of years; he thought it sufficient to consider "one or two thousand years [as] the period of time supposed to have intervened between the Deluge of Noah and the origin of the great Asiatic monarchies" – such as the Assyrian empire or Babylon which flourished from 1137 b.c.e.[139] (Yet, none of those realms was older than the Hebraeo-Chaldean tradition.)[140]

At first sight, Prichard's "note on chronology" appended to the fifth volume of the *Researches* looks like a concession to secularizing trends. He was in need of more time. But instead of resigning himself to the notion that human history far exceeded the Biblical timescale, he merely extended it by several hundred years which he, moreover, procured through Biblical exegesis. Through some sophisticated manipulations he managed verbally to uphold the short Biblical timescale – following Michaelis, he declared the Masorah to be more reliable, although it was, on the whole, much shorter than that of the Greek version. Ironically it was precisely this preference in the text used which provided Prichard with a large chunk of the required amount of years: the Masorah admitted a considerably greater interval "between the age of Abraham and the Exode" than the Septuagint. Since Prichard had admitted that the Biblical compilers had no revelation on the subject of chronology,[141] he was free to tamper with the time scales offered by the various Biblical versions. Thus he argued that "generations have certainly been omitted in the early genealogies".[142] It was, Prichard said, due to a "custom" prevailing "among those who devoted their care to the preservation of national archives", the archives in question being those of the "Ante-Abrahamitic genealogies". By blaming their "first recorder" and correcting his supposed errors, Prichard enlarged Biblical chronology without departing from it. This was in itself a deed almost as miraculous as the miracles of the Scriptures.

This amendment in his chronological interpretation went hand in hand with Prichard's new conviction – gained from the writings of the orientalist and theologian Ernst Friedrich Carl Rosenmüller – that pre-Abrahamitic humans were not endowed with exorbitant longevity.[143] In early modern times it was assumed that the posterity of Noah attained a vast old age – and thus had sufficient time to engender an equally vast number of offspring.[144] This would account for the growth in the Earth's population. But it was not of help in explaining the development of different human varieties. That process required not just time, but also the succession of many generations. Hence Prichard maintained that several generations had been "omitted in the early genealogies".[145]

Prichard began his comment upon chronology in 1847 with frank words: "I might have avoided the discussion, had it not been pointed out as one which is necessary for the support of my argument, and for establishing the probability of the main conclusion that all mankind are the offspring of one family."[146] This declaration is decisive: if he had to choose between maintaining the foundations of Genesis on the one hand, and comparatively trifling chronological details on the other, he opted for the former. It was the specific problem of the origin of human varieties – not some notion of scientific objectivity – which led him to discard Biblical tenets. When Prichard began his studies of pagan mythology and chronology, he did so in order to sustain the unity of mankind. His last words on the subject were written in the name of the same objective. Over the years, his interpretation of Egyptian and Indian mythology changed as little as his views about the beginnings of human history.

Scientific Scripturalism

For clergymen like Conybeare or Buckland, it was natural to pursue science from the perspective of the Divine dispensation. If the physician Prichard did the same, this was apt to create problems that arose not from scientific developments but from those in theology. While the natural theology school that received such a boost in the 1830s with the publication of the *Bridgewater Treatises* was safely allied to utilitarian considerations and the expression of British national interest, Prichard's works upheld the authenticity of the religious world-view. While positivism arose endowing the appeal to science with yet greater currency than it had before, Prichard's attempts to reconcile science to the Scriptures afforded consolation to many who did not entirely agree with the flourishing doctrine of progress. His works were not written for the "angry young men" teaching at the newly founded University College London. It is, by contrast, characteristic that Nicholas Wiseman paraphrased Prichard's natural history of mankind with a degree of enthusiasm as if it had been an appendix to the Pentateuch.

In this and the previous chapter it has been maintained that Prichard employed Higher Criticism and philology, those "modern" disciplines emanating from the traditional philology, to buttress his ethnology and inscribe the natural history of mankind in universal history connecting the vicissitudes of the mundane to the transcendental. German Higher Criticism had been introduced to delimit the sphere of the miraculous. But in Prichard's hands the distinctions it drew between Biblical myth and "reality" were used to highlight those scriptural doctrines which, Prichard believed, might be vindicated as proper historical facts. He availed himself of the insights gained through Higher Criticism in order to turn the Scriptures into a history book. And he, therefore, distinguished between miracles and their more worldly explanation, all the while asserting that it was no threat to religion to prefer the latter.[147]

Prichard himself professed his belief in scriptural miracles on the grounds of something he considered as a natural law: he did not conceive the world as infinite, hence there must have been a beginning when it was created. By virtue of the uniqueness of that event, it was legitimate to call it "supernatural". That being granted, it was easy to comprehend that "in the first ages of the world events were conducted by operative causes of a different kind from those which are now in action". But, he stated in 1826, "our confidence in the continuance of the present order of things having been established by the uniform experience of so many ages", it was natural that mankind increasingly lost the capacity to envisage the occurrence of supernatural events. And what in earlier epochs would not be seen with disbelief, was over time regarded with growing "scepticism".[148] In 1837 Prichard repeated that he, for his part, found "no difficulty in admitting" miracles, as they happened "in an age when so many events must have occurred which were out of the present course of nature".[149] Thus he presented belief in scriptural miracles as an attitude that was rather more scientific than disbelief.

It was this attitude which informed his approach towards mythology: as mythological traditions dated from remote epochs that were still nearer to the time of Creation, they comprised some authentic memories of that age. Prichard, therefore, examined mythology in the light of historical evidence. His studies reveal his belief in a historical development that led from purity to religious corruption. The same was true for his notion of the history of language. Interestingly, he did not regard these deteriorations as resulting from some transcendental law of history; the cause he made responsible for moral decline was rather concrete and man-made: false philosophizing and the pursuit of selfish interests corrupted first religion and then language until the idioms of the world were so far removed from the Hebrew original that their very structure had lost the philosophical capacity to prepare the mind for understanding monotheism.

The physical history of mankind as Prichard conceived it, by contrast, put a lot less emphasis on degenerative processes, tending, on the contrary, to the assumption of a physical improvement accompanying the ascent of civilization. Where these two contradictory movements met, there was a paradox: civilization was physically desirable, but bad for the mind and soul. For it brought about not just the abject perversion of human fellow-feeling, but in extreme cases also lunacy. The ambiguity inherent in the concept of civilization has troubled the world ever since mankind possessed historical consciousness. The problem in Prichard's case was that he wanted it both ways. In its infancy mankind was endowed with supreme understanding of the duties it owed to the Creator – in the nineteenth century there was no doubt that Christianity was the religion of the light. In the last event, the state of rudeness, without which there was no physical history of mankind deserving that name, had no proper place on Prichard's timescale. He devised many hypotheses, but did not try to bring them all into a logically consistent system, accounting for the rise or the decline of nations, physical features, languages, and mental endowments. In this lies both the weakness and the strength of his approach. On the one hand it saved him from the erroneousness those systems are liable to, on the other it deprived his theories of clarity as he attempted to establish laws fitting to all the evidence he came across. The result was all but conceptual chaos.

George Stocking pointed out that, in ethnological terms, Prichard was a diffusionist.[150] Witness his idea of linguistic unity: no language had arisen on its own, they all were related to each other, having developed one out of the other: Hebrew engendered the Celtic languages, which in turn were linked to the Sanskrit. Regarding the inbred moral sense, and the universal notion of monotheism, the matter was rather different. In his researches on mythology and in his linguistic studies, Prichard did his best to show that these concepts were ingrained in the human consciousness. In this sense, the evolutionist theorizing shared alike by Scottish Enlightenment thought regarding the origins of society and, later, by Tylorian ethnology, was not present in Prichard. Instead he supported the notion of, to put it in the terminology of common-sense philosophy, innate faculties, or of an anthropological fact, to say it in modern terms. In my final chapter, which will attempt a summary of Prichard's agenda and achievements, other striking parallels between his thought and that of later Victorian anthropology will be demonstrated. Were the latter echoes of Prichardian tenets due to diffusion or did they arise of their own accord?

Notes

1 This point was emphasized by Martin Bernal, *Black Athena*, vol. 1, chs 3 and 4. For a more comprehensive and reliable account see Frank E. Manuel, *The Eighteenth Century Confronts the Gods* (Cambridge, Mass.: Harvard University Press, 1959), ch. 2; Paolo Rossi, *The Dark Abyss of Time*, trans. Lydia G. Cochrane (Chicago: University of Chicago Press, 1984), pp. 236-50.

2 See Richard Smith, "Manuscript Memoirs", p. 646.

3 See the entry for 6 January 1825 in "Abstracts of Papers, & c Read Before the Philosophical & Literary Society Annexed to the Bristol Institution. Beginning with the Paper Read at the Evening Meeting on 6th January 1825". Compiled by the Philosophical and Literary Society. MS. B 12361, Bristol Central Library.

4 Arno Beyer, *Deutsche Einflüsse auf die englische Sprachwissenschaft*, p. 63.

5 "Abstracts of Papers", see the entry for 6 January 1825.

6 Jean-François Champollion, *Lettre à M. Dacier, Secrétaire Perpétuel de*

l'Académie royale des inscriptions et belles-lettres, relative à l'alphabet des hiéroglyphes phonétiques... (Paris: Firmin Didot, 1822). Despite this report, it is rather unlikely that it should have taken three years before Bristol learned of Champollion's publication of 1822.

7   In 1834 Prichard gave three lectures "on Egyptian Mummies, Egyptian antiquities, and the Rosetta Stone" at the Bristol Institution. Smith, "Manuscript Memoirs", p. 644. Prichard co-authored the lectures with G. T. Clark. Their contents are lost. In his other writings he mentioned the Rosetta stone only once, in respect of a question of secondary importance.

8   See below.

9   Prichard, *An Analysis of the Egyptian Mythology: To which is Subjoined a Critical Examination of the Remains of Egyptian Chronology* (London: John and Arthur Arch, 1819), pp. ii, v, vii. (A second edition appeared in 1838.)

10   *Ibid.,* p. 221.

11   Edward Gibbon, *Memoirs of My Life,* ed. Georges A. Bonnard (London: Nelson, 1966), pp. 104, 43.

12   Arnoldo Momigliano, "Ancient History and the Antiquarian". In *idem, The Classical Foundations of Modern Historiography* (Berkeley, Los Angeles: University of California Press, 1990), pp. 1-39, see p. 22.

13   For Coleridge's familiarity with German Higher Criticism, see E. S. Shaffer, *"Kubla Khan" and the Fall of Jerusalem. The Mythological School in Biblical Criticism and Secular Literature 1770-1880* (Cambridge: Cambridge University Press, 1975). For Scott see A. Dwight Culler, *The Victorian Mirror of History* (New Haven: Yale University Press, 1985), esp. pp. 28, 58; Thomas Preston Peardon, *The Transition in English Historical Writing, 1760-1830* (New York: Columbia University Press, 1933), ch. 8.

14   Burton Feldman, Robert D. Richardson, *The Rise of Modern Mythology 1680-1860* (Bloomington: Indiana University Press, 1972), p. 365.

15   *Ibid.,* p. 171.

16   See Walter Sparn, "Vernünftiges Christentum. Über die geschichtliche Aufgabe der theologischen Aufklärung im 18. Jh. in Deutschland". In *Wissenschaften im Zeitalter der Aufklärung,* ed. Rudolf Vierhaus (Göttingen: Vandenhoeck & Ruprecht, 1985), pp. 18-57. Breuer has pointed out that until 1750 British Biblical scholarship was well ahead of that in Germany; see Edward Breuer, *The Limits of the Enlightenment. Jews, Germans, and the Eighteenth-Century Study of Scripture* (Cambridge, Mass.: Harvard University Press, 1996), p. 92.

17 Nicholas Wiseman, *Twelve Lectures*, 2: 196.

18 Thus the German Scriptural scholar Johann Gottfried Eichhorn,
    quoted by A. Smith in his introduction to: John David Michaelis,
    Commentaries on the Laws of Moses, trans. Alexander Smith, 4 vols
    (London: Rivington, Longman, Hurst, Rees, Orme, and Brown,
    1814), 1: xx.

19 Cf. Sir William Jones, "On the Gods of Greece, Italy, and India". In
    idem, *Works*, 6 vols (London: G. G. and J. Robinson, 1799), 1: 229-
    80. See also: Feldman, Richardson, *Modern Mythology*, p. 268;
    Manuel, *The Eighteenth Century Confronts the Gods*, p. 275; A. Leslie
    Willson, *A Mythical Image: The Ideal of India in German Romanticism*
    (Durham, NC: Duke University Press, 1964), pp. 38-43.

20 Jacob Bryant, *A New System; or an Analysis of Ancient Mythology
    Wherein an Attempt is Made to Divest Tradition of Fable and to Reduce
    the Truth to its Original Purity*, 3 vols (London: T. Payne, 1774-76).
    See also: Manuel, *The Eighteenth Century Confronts the Gods*, pp.
    274-75.

21 Prichard, *Researches*, 1st ed., p. 558.

22 "Townsend *on the Character of Moses as an Historian*". *British Review*
    6 (1815): 26-50, p. 32. Cf. also Stocking, "From Chronology to
    Ethnology", pp. xliif., lxvif. By 1826 Prichard had adopted the same
    attitude; in passing he referred to Jacob Bryant's "learned dreams".
    Prichard, *Researches*, 2nd ed., 2: 167.

23 Cf. Wolf-Daniel Hartwich, *Die Sendung Moses* (München: Wilhelm
    Fink Verlag, 1997), ch. 3; Rudolf Smend, "Lowth in Deutschland".
    In *idem*, *Epochen der Bibelkritik* (München: Chr. Kaiser Verlag,
    1991), pp. 43-62.

24 Thus the writer Joseph Görres, quoted in: Mareta Linden,
    Untersuchungen zum Anthropologiebegriff des 18. Jahrhunderts (Bern:
    Herbert Lang, 1976), p. 299.

25 *Ibid.*, pp. 227, 199. For Herder see Georg C. Iggers, *The German
    Conception of History: The National Tradition of Historical Thought
    from Herder to the Present* (Middletown, Conn.: Wesleyan University
    Press, 1968).

26 Cf. Feldman, Richardson, *Modern Mythology*, p. 249; Manuel, *The
    Eighteenth Century Confronts the Gods*, p. 259.

27 James Bruce, *Travels to Discover the Source of the Nile in the Years
    1768, 1769, 1770, 1771, 1772, and 1773*, 3rd ed., 8 vols, ed.
    Alexander Murray (Edinburgh: A. Constable, Manners & Miller,
    1813).

28 Prichard, *Egyptian Mythology*, note on pp. ii-iii.

29 Prichard referred this term to Egyptian animal worship, not to

Egyptian mythology on the whole. See Prichard, *Egyptian Mythology*, p. v.

30   Charles de Brosses, *Du culte des dieux fétiches, ou Parallèle de l'ancienne religion de l'Egypte avec la religion actuelle de Nigritie* (1760).

31   For Hume see "Prichard *on the Egyptian Mythology*". *Monthly Review*, 2nd s., 92 (1820): 225-42, p. 228. For Warburton see Manuel, *The Eighteenth Century Confronts the Gods*, p. 249; Rossi, *Abyss of Time*, p. 242.

32   Rossi, *Abyss of Time*, p. 238. My explanation of Warburton's theory is greatly indebted to Rossi's lucid account.

33   William Warburton, *The Divine Legation of Moses demonstrated, on the Principles of a Religious Deist, from the Mission of the Doctrine of a Future State of Reward and Punishment in the Jewish Dispensation*, 2 vols (London: Fletcher Gyles, 1738-41), 2: 356. Cf. Rossi, *Abyss of Time*, p. 244.

34   Rossi, *Abyss of Time*, p. 236.

35   Hartwich, *Die Sendung Moses*, p. 35.

36   Warburton, *The Divine Legation*, p. 236.

37   Rossi, *Abyss of Time*, pp. 244-45. Warburton was right: only in the age of the Ptolomies were hieroglyphics used as a secret code; see Jan Assmann, *Moses the Egyptian. The Memory of Egypt in Western Monotheism* (Cambridge, Mass.: Harvard University Press, 1997), pp. 107-9.

38   Cf. Stocking, "From Chronology to Ethnology", p. xlii; Prichard, *Egyptian Mythology*, p. 48.

39   Arthur William Evans, *Warburton and the Warburtonians. A Study in Some Eighteenth-Century Controversies* (Oxford: Oxford University Press, 1932), pp. 294-306.

40   B. W. Young, *Religion and Enlightenment in Eighteenth-Century England. Theological Debate from Locke to Burke* (Oxford: Clarendon Press, 1998), p. 183.

41   Prichard, too, believed that the Egyptian priests retained hieroglyphics to satisfy their sense of secrecy; see his *Egyptian Mythology*, p. 415.

42   Since Greek pantheism was regarded as the legacy of Egyptian mythology, Prichard also devoted many pages to proving that "the rites and attributes, and even many of the names, of the Grecian gods, may have been originally derived from a mythology, founded on very different principles from the deification of men". In the context of this chapter, however, there is no room to dwell upon the Greek side of the problem. For the quotation see Prichard, *Egyptian Mythology*, p. 49. As Burrow has remarked, Prichard's aims were

212

common among scholars at the time. See John Burrow, "The Uses of Philology in Victorian England". In *Ideas and Institutions of Victorian England. Essays in Honour of George Kitson Clark*, ed. Robert Robson (London: Bell, 1967), pp. 180-204, see p. 190.

43 Friedrich Schlegel, *Ueber die Sprache und Weisheit der Indier*, pp. 90-91.

44 Prichard, *Egyptian Mythology*, p. 223.

45 Prichard, *Egyptian Mythology*, pp. 223-24. The fourth stage Prichard deliberately put into a better light than Schlegel had done. For Schlegel, it was signified by the abject system of pantheism. Prichard had no sympathy for pantheism, but the researches which Henry Thomas Colebrooke had carried out after the publication of Schlegel's book had shown pantheism to be present even in the first epoch of Indian mythology. Since Prichard shared Schlegel's praise for the early system of Indian religion, he was obliged to show some indulgence towards pantheism. The other amendment Prichard applied to Schlegel's theory of mythological epochs concerned the second stage of the struggle between light and darkness: this principle, crucial to the philosophy of Schelling, had no particular appeal for Prichard, wherefore he omitted it from his list of the four ages. Prichard, *Egyptian Mythology*, pp. 253-54, 262.

46 *Ibid.*, pp. 262-63.

47 Quoted in *ibid.*, p. 208; cf. Schlegel, *Ueber die Sprache und Weisheit der Indier*, p. 101.

48 Prichard, *Egyptian Mythology*, p. 233; for the German original see Schlegel, *Ueber die Sprache und Weisheit der Indier*, p. 110.

49 Cf. *ibid.*, pp. 89-153, esp. pp. 95-96. Cf. also Willson, *A Mythical Image*, pp. 199-220; Feldman, Richardson, *Modern Mythology*, pp. 352-53.

50 Prichard, *Egyptian Mythology*, p. 231. Cf. Schlegel, *Ueber die Sprache und Weisheit der Indier*, p. 101.

51 Nowadays, Schlegel's *On the Language and Wisdom of the Indians*, published in 1808, is interpreted in the light of the religious struggle which led to his conversion to Catholicism in the very same year. Cf. Willson, *A Mythical Image*, p. 93.

52 Prichard, *Egyptian Mythology*, p. 296.

53 Warburton, *The Divine Legation*, 2: 346 (original emphases).

54 Prichard, *Egyptian Mythology*, p. 257. Prichard had mentioned metempsychosis in 1813; see *idem, Researches*, 1st ed, p. 343. But at that time, he had not described the theological background of the doctrine. The universality of metempsychosis had already been stipulated by Buffon who held that "the same metaphysical religion

diffused itself over every quarter of the globe". Prichard must have been elated to find references to the same tenet in authors as diverse as Buffon and Schlegel. See Buffon, *Natural History, General and Particular*, trans. William Smellie, 9 vols (Edinburgh: printed for William Cleech, 1780), 9: 390.

55   Prichard, *Egyptian Mythology*, p. 297.

56   *Ibid.*, pp. 296-97.

57   *Ibid.*, pp. 265-66.

58   *Ibid.*, pp. 293, see also *ibid.*, p. 291.

59   Momigliano, "Ancient History", p. 22. For Kircher see Erik Iversen, *The Myth of Egypt and its Hieroglyphs in European Tradition*, 2nd ed. (Princeton: Princeton University Press, 1993), pp. 94ff.

60   Prichard, *Egyptian Mythology*, pp. 84, 270. The same sort of superstition "decorated and reduced to a system of mystical representations", he added, "appears to have been the popular religion of the most cultivated nations of antiquity"; see *ibid.*, p. 34-35.

61   *Ibid.*, p. 295, see also p. 84. The respective Indian gods are Brahma, Vishnu and Siva, this triad being a common trope. See Willson, *A Mythical Image*, p. 42.

62   Prichard, *Egyptian Mythology*, p. 189.

63   *Ibid.*, pp. 193, 294-95, 14.

64   *Ibid.*, p. 217.

65   *Ibid.*, p. 294.

66   These alternatives are stated in "Prichard's *Analysis of Egyptian Mythology*". *British Critic*, 2nd s., 14 (1820): 55-69, p. 59.

67   This approach was not new. According to Neo-Platonist theories put forward by Plutarch, Plotinus and, later, the Cambridge Platonist Ralph Cudworth, polytheist learning bore secret testimony to monotheism. See Jan Assmann, *Monotheismus und Kosmotheismus. Ägyptische Formen eines 'Denkens des Einen' und ihre europäische Rezeptionsgeschichte* (Heidelberg: C. Winter, 1993); *idem, Moses the Egyptian*, ch. 6.

68   Prichard, *Egyptian Mythology*, p. 34 (the same notion can be found in Warburton).

69   *Ibid.*, p. 296.

70   He thus performed for Egypt what Schlegel had done for India. Both found proto-Christian beliefs in ancient mythologies. But while Schlegel was content with establishing their existence in early Indian religion, Prichard first proved that they suffused Egyptian religion as well and then corroborated the doctrine of monogenesis from his discovery.

71   William Stukeley, *A Letter from Dr. Stukeley to Mr. Macpherson, on*

his Publication of Fingal and Temora (1763); quoted in Momigliano, "Ancient History", p. 24. For a history of views on the Druids, see A. L. Owen, *The Famous Druids. A Survey of Three Centuries of English Literature on the Druids* (Oxford: Clarendon Press, 1962).

72 See Jon Mee, *Dangerous Enthusiasm. William Blake and the Culture of Radicalism in the 1790s* (Oxford: Clarendon Press, 1992), pp. 92-93, 99. The concept of a Phoenician visit to Scotland was also mentioned in Friedrich Schlegel, *Ueber die Sprache und Weisheit der Indier*, p. 112. For sixteenth-century ideas of early Scottish-Egyptian relations, see William Matthews, "The Egyptians in Scotland: The Political History of a Myth". In *Viator. Medieval and Renaissance Studies* 1 (Berkeley, Los Angeles: University of California Press, 1970), pp. 289-306.

73 For Prichard's views on the Celtic tradition see his *Researches*, 2nd ed., 2: 117, 170. See also *idem, The Eastern Origin of the Celtic Nations*, p. 16; *idem, Researches*, 3rd ed., 3: 175, 403, 460-61. For Egypt see *idem, Egyptian Mythology*, p. 397 (the similarity between the Indian caste system and the ancient Egyptian stratification of society Prichard deemed to be "striking").

74 Prichard, *Researches*, 2nd ed., 2: 175, 170. This rather critical attitude towards Celtic customs modifies the image of Prichard as a Celtic revivalist: he aimed at rehabilitating the Celts, but he did not idealize their traditions.

75 Prichard, *Egyptian Mythology*, pp. 406-7.

76 Prichard, *Egyptian Mythology*, pp. 408-10.

77 In 1685 Spencer, master of Corpus Christi College, Cambridge, published *De Legibus Hebraeorum Ritualibus et Earum Rationibus Libri Tres* in which he asserted that the Hebrews had adopted many details of Egyptian legislation.

78 See Jan Assmann, *Moses the Egyptian, passim.*

79 *Ibid.*, p. 92.

80 Cf. Rossi, *Abyss of Time*, p. 243.

81 Daniel Guildford Wait, *Jewish, Oriental, and Classical Antiquities; Containing Illustrations of the Scriptures, and Classical Records from Oriental Sources* (Cambridge: printed by J. Smith for the University, 1823), p. 295 (original emphasis). Prichard was acquainted with Wait; they had probably met in 1809 at Oxford. In 1819 Prichard commended Wait's erudition, but the latter's publication came too late for him to comment on it. See Prichard, *Egyptian Mythology*, note on p. 131. For Wait see *DNB*, vol. 5.

82 Prichard, *Egyptian Mythology*, pp. 412, 415. For Michaelis see *idem, Commentaries*, 3: 45-47.

83   Cf. Chapter 1 above.

84   Cf., e.g., the entry on Moses in *The Penny Cyclopaedia*, ed. The Society for the Diffusion of Useful Knowledge, 27 vols (London: Charles Knight and Co., 1833-43), vol. 15, pp. 439-46, see p. 439.

85   Robert S. Leventhal, "Language Theory, the Institution of Philology and the State: the Emergence of Philological Discourse 1770-1810". In *Papers in the History of Linguistics*, ed. Hans Aarsleff *et al.*, pp. 349-63, esp. p. 358.

86   Michaelis, *Commentaries*, 3: 1, 25-28. For the Levites see 1: 251-62. Cf. also Hartwich, *Die Sendung Moses*, pp. 64-73. Rudolf Smend, "Aufgeklärte Bemühungen um das Gesetz. Johann David Michaelis 'Mosaisches Recht'". In *idem, Epochen der Bibelkritik*, pp. 63-73.

87   Michaelis, *Commentaries*, 1: 206, 225.

88   *Ibid.*, 1: xxi. Smith's disdain aimed also at Michaelis's speculations on the question why Moses had no interest in inciting a commercial spirit in his people: intercourse with other nations would have exposed the Hebrews to idolatry. Moreover, the Israelites were not supposed to indulge in "foreign luxury". For Smith, luxury and commerce were not ungodly. See *ibid.*, 1: 215-16.

89   This sentence of Hugh Latimer's is quoted in Peter Vansittart, *In Memory of England. A Novelist's View of History* (London: John Murray, 1998), p. 10.

90   See Richard Smith, "Manuscript Memoirs", p. 622. Quoted in Neve, "Science in Provincial England", p. 289.

91   Warburton, *The Divine Legation*, 2: 335.

92   Prichard, *Egyptian Mythology*, pp. 417, 426. Cf. Michaelis, *Commentaries*, 3: 76. August Wilhelm Schlegel later rejected Prichard's assertion that in Egypt only the priests were circumcised. Apparently, Schlegel was unaware of Prichard's source. See Schlegel, "Vorrede". In Prichard, *Darstellung der Aegyptischen Mythologie verbunden mit einer kritischen Untersuchung der Ueberbleibsel der Aegyptischen Chronologie*, trans. L. Haymann (Bonn: Eduard Weber, 1837), pp. i-xxxiv, see p. xxiii.

93   Bynum, "Time's Noblest Offspring", p. 94.

94   Cf. Norman Cohn, *Noah's Flood. The Genesis Story of Western Thought* (New Haven: Yale University Press, 1996), p. 110.

95   Prichard, *Researches*, 3rd ed., 5: 555. He relied on *Philologia sacra* (1776) by the German philologist Johann-August Dathe (1731-91).

96   *Ibid.*, 2nd ed., 2: 595.

97   *Ibid.*, 2: 593-94.

98   *Ibid.*, 3rd ed., 1: 98-102; *ibid.*, vol. 2, note on p. 225; cf. also Chapter 3 above.

99 Prichard, "On the Cosmogony of Moses…". *The Philosophical Magazine* 46 (1815): 285-92, p. 287.

100 Prichard, *Researches*, 2nd ed., 1: 83-84. Cf. also *ibid.*, 3rd ed., 1: 102.

101 *Ibid.*, 2nd ed., 1: 81.

102 *Ibid.*, 1: 81-89.

103 *Ibid.*, 1: 82

104 *Ibid.*, 3rd ed., 1: 99; for his notion of a partial creation, see *ibid.*, p. 101.

105 *Ibid.*, 2nd ed., 1: 82-83.

106 Note that Prichard formulated this opinion years before Robert Jameson published an article in the *Edinburgh New Philosophical Journal* in 1831 which dealt with fossils of giant kangaroos recently found in Australia, proving that the flora and fauna of the region had existed for much longer than had been thought. Cf. Browne, *The Secular Ark*, p. 97.

107 *Ibid.*, 3rd ed., 5: 562. Moses' role as divine penman had been questioned since the seventeenth century; see Breuer, *The Limits of the Enlightenment*, p. 82.

108 Prichard, *Researches*, 5: 570.

109 Prichard, "A Critical Examination", p. 2.

110 Stocking, "From Chronology to Ethnology", p. xcvii.

111 Prichard, "A Critical Examination of the Remains of Egyptian Chronology". Appended to *idem, Egyptian Mythology*, pp. vi-vii, note on p. 49.

112 For discussions of chronology see Iversen, *The Myth of Egypt*; Heinrich Meyer, *The Age of the World. A Chapter in the History of Enlightenment* (Allentown, PA: Muhlenberg College, 1951); J. D. North, "Chronology and the Age of the World". In *Cosmology, History, and Theology*, ed. W. Yourgrau, A. D. Breck (New York: Dover; London: Constable, 1977), pp. 307-33; Rossi, *Abyss of Time*, pp. 145-52; Martin L. Rouse, "The Bible Pedigree of the Nations of the World". *Journal of the Transactions of The Victoria Institute, or, Philosophical Society of Great Britain* 38 (1906): 123-50.

113 Ussher's account is important as, in 1701, its chronology was inserted into the Bible of King James. See Cohn, *Noah's Flood*, p. 95. For the Samaritan version see Breuer, *The Limits of the Enlightenment*, pp. 81-83.

114 Rossi, *Abyss of Time*, p. 145.

115 Manetho's history survives in patristic texts and in Josephus Flavius's *Contra Apionem*.

116 Meyer, *The Age of the World*, p. 29.

117 Rossi, *Abyss of Time*, pp. 145-49.

118 Iversen, *The Myth of Egypt*, p. 102.

119 Warburton, *The Divine Legation*, 2: 206-81, esp. p. 207. Cf. Rossi, *Abyss of Time*, p. 244.

120 Prichard, "A Critical Examination", p. 96.

121 See Ian Jenkins, "'Contemporary Minds'. Sir William Hamilton's Affair with Antiquity". In *Vases & Volcanoes*, ed. Ian Jenkins, Kim Sloan (London: British Museum Press, 1996), pp. 40-64, see p. 45.

122 Prichard, "A Critical Examination", pp. 97ff.

123 Cf. Prichard, *Researches*, 1st ed., p. 432.

124 *Idem*, "A Critical Examination", pp. 160, 128. For the difference between Elohim and "Jehovah" – as he put it – Prichard referred to Michaelis's pupil Johann Gottfried Eichhorn.

125 Prichard, "A Critical Examination", note on p. 52, pp. 79-80. See also *ibid.*, pp. 85-86. To demonstrate the identity of the Shepherd kings and the Israelites Prichard cited the renowned liberal and anti-Catholic Göttingen orientalist Georg Heinrich August Ewald (1768-1835). For the historical background see Manfred Görg, *Die Beziehungen zwischen dem alten Israel und Ägypten. Von den Anfängen bis zum Exil* (Darmstadt: Wissenschaftliche Buchgesellschaft, 1997), pp. 20-21.

126 Prichard, "A Critical Examination", p. 68.

127 *Ibid.*, pp. 80, 89. The year 1619 was not generally accepted: many, if not the majority, of Prichard's contemporaries dated the Exodus at 1491 b.c.e.

128 See Assmann, *Moses the Egyptian*, ch. 2, esp. p. 40.

129 Georges Cuvier, *Discours sur les révolutions de la surface du globe, et sur les changemens qu'elles ont produits dans le règne animal*, 3rd rev. ed. (Paris: G. Dufour and Editions d'Ocagne, 1825 (1812)), p. 211.

130 "Prichard *on the Egyptian Mythology*". *Monthly Review*, 2nd s., 92 (1820): 225-42. Wait thought the book was "one of the best and most elaborate inquiries into the subject, that has appeared of late years". See Wait, *Jewish, Oriental, and Classical Antiquities*, p. xi.

131 "Prichard's *Analysis of Egyptian Mythology*", p. 55.

132 Schlegel, "Vorrede". In Prichard, *Darstellung der Aegyptischen Mythologie*, p. xxxii. Schlegel's criticism did not dissuade Prichard from his chronological computation. In 1837 he gave a short summary of the contents of his *Egyptian Mythology*. In that context he even referred to "the assent given by M. Schlegel to my conclusions". See Prichard, *Researches*, 3rd ed., 2: 219-20. Later he admitted having expressed himself "somewhat too decidedly" in that respect. See *ibid.*, p. 370.

133 Schlegel, "Vorrede", p. xxxii.

134 "Prichard's *Physical History of Mankind*". *New Quarterly Review* 8

(1846): 95-134, see p. 134. The same criticism was put forward in "Physical History of Mankind". *Prospective Review* 3 (1847): 355-69, see pp. 361-62.

135 Cf. Prichard, *Researches*, 3rd ed., 5: 552. For John Kenrick see his *An Essay on Primeval History* (London: B. Fellowes, 1846), pp. xi-xii, 20.

136 *Ibid.*, pp. 552-53.

137 *Ibid.*, p. 570, see also pp. 555-56. It was commonly held that the years back to ca. 970 b.c.e. did not pose a major historical problem. Cf. *Memoir of Baron Bunsen*, 1: 562.

138 Prichard, *Researches*, 3rd ed., 5: 555.

139 *Ibid.*, p. 554.

140 In 1847 Prichard still insisted that the Bible was more accurate than the histories of "Indian and Egyptian fabulists". *Ibid.*, pp. 554, 570.

141 *Ibid.*, p. 557. Following German learning he doubted whether Moses himself was the author of the Bible, though "even if the introductory chapters of Genesis were not written nor even compiled by Moses, this would not necessarily impugn their canonical authority". *Ibid.*, p. 563.

142 *Ibid.*, p. 569.

143 *Ibid.*, p. 570.

144 See, e.g., Matthew Hale, *The Primitive Origination of Mankind, Considered and Examined According to the Light of Nature* (London: printed for William Shrowsbery, 1672), pp. 145, 169.

145 Prichard, *Researches*, 3rd ed., 5: 567-68, quotation from p. 560.

146 *Ibid.*, p. 553.

147 For the dispersion of languages after the fall of the Tower of Babel, see Prichard, *The Eastern Origin*, p. 11; *idem*, *Researches*, 2d ed., 2: 594; *ibid.*, 3rd ed., vol. 2, note on p. 225. For the Ark, see note 85 in Chapter 3 above.

148 Prichard, *Researches*, 2nd ed., 2: 594.

149 *Ibid.*, 3rd ed., vol. 2, note on p. 225.

150 Stocking, "From Chronology to Ethnology", p. lix.

8

Conclusion:
Prichard's After-life

John Stuart Mill said famously that every Englishman was "by implication either a Benthamite or a Coleridgian", the one representing utilitarian realism and efficiency, the other a penchant towards theories of German Idealist philosophy and German Romanticism.[1]

Mill's astute observation may serve as our starting point for an assessment of Prichard's career and significance. The truth is that Prichard's views did not coincide with those of either Bentham or Coleridge. Although he believed in rewards and punishment and an order of Creation which was good because it was regular, he rejected the mechanistic world-view that he called "utilitarian". We have seen that he relied heavily on German Romantic theories of insanity as well as on German Romantic linguistics and German Biblical criticism. Yet he stopped short of embracing the transcendentalism generally associated with the philosophy of the epoch. Elisabeth Jay has remarked that "the Romantic movement as such had passed the Evangelicals by". Prichard for his part snatched from it what he could use – but nothing more.[2] If Thomas Preston Peardon was right in stating that "the growth of a nationalist outlook, the spread of Whig views, and the appearance of romanticist histories ... constitute the three most important trends of the early nineteenth century", it is easy to understand why Prichard dug his heels in against the new spirit.[3] His indifference to aesthetics has been addressed in the first chapter. His highly sceptical attitude towards secular philosophy has been mentioned in Chapter 7. He had little respect for the Herderian vision of history and shows no sign of ever having read Hegel. As has been shown in Chapters 5 and 6, Biblical criticism was turned by Prichard into a tool for theological conservatism.

Prichard's religious doctrines did not permit him to embrace Romanticism. In Peter Allan Dale's blunt description, the latter entailed the "effort to find in poetry and art an alternative means for doing what religion and philosophy traditionally had done".[4] In its preoccupation with beauty and poetry the post-Kantian Idealist movement, Dale maintains, unwittingly demolished its own theological basis. Prichard, by contrast, was never in danger of doing likewise. Within his post-Quaker, evangelical framework, the "eternal, invisible church" assumed a supreme position,[5] and this was a commitment which he did not dilute by diverting it into artistic channels. The human predilection for culture and embellishment was not even mentioned by Prichard. Reversing Feuerbach's dictum, it could be said that, for him, *all anthropology was theology*, as he took the universal belief in life after death for a sign of the uniformity of human nature and the truth of revelation. Unlike Schlegel or Coleridge, he did not take up the speculative potential of contemporary ideas. Schlegel's philosophy of language was imbued by *Naturphilosophie*. Coleridge too developed a dialectics of nature, juxtaposing peoples whom he identified with "thesis", "antithesis", and "synthesis".[6] None of this can be found in Prichard. Equally he did not subscribe to the Romantic veneration of the "people" as the bearer of the spirit of history.

Duncan Forbes and John Burrow have described the elements of racial and nationalistic theory that can be found in the views of Whig Anglican historians.[7] Prichard's interest in peoples, by contrast, was that of a natural historian, at times that of a sociologist, but he was dismissive of the patriotic enthusiasm for tracing the historical forefathers of his "race", present in so many of his contemporaries, including Bunsen and Jacob Grimm, Thomas Arnold and the philologist John Mitchell Kemble, Guizot and Thierry. During the nineteenth century, the notion of race was employed to set up a new hierarchy among mankind where previously social status had served as classifying principle.[8] Prichard, however, in many respects continued to rely on eighteenth-century concepts, calling, for instance, upon the notion of caste or status to account for human physical diversities and the relationship between living conditions, external appearance and mental development. He believed that the upper classes generally tended to have a fairer skin than the lower orders, since they lived more civilized lives. And if the lower orders of "our countrywomen" had no "invincible repugnance to the Negro race", this was because they were lacking in civilized refinement apt to pervert the natural constitution.[9]

These and similar observations left open the question of how the human varieties were related to each other and how one variety had developed into another. Instead of formulating a consistent theory of hereditary change, Prichard side-stepped the problem, putting ever greater emphasis on the significance of psychology and inbred human instincts: a universal human psychological frame seemed to vouchsafe the unity of mankind.

Interestingly, he was not explicitly concerned with rising industrialism or the plight of the working classes. His aim was to sustain the unity of the human species while admitting its variability. It was only in this context that anthropological notions of class achieved prominence in his work. Prichard's insistence on social status as a category of natural classification was striking at a time of blossoming racial theories, enthusiasms for phrenology, physical anthropology, geographical determinism, and eugenics. It was the theoretical sheet-anchor of his conservatism, and belonged as much to the eighteenth-century context of social theory as to his own age. Since Prichard did not travel he had only very limited first-hand experience of foreign tribes.

Deliverance from Utilitarianism

In its various adumbrations utilitarianism was pervasive in late eighteenth-century and early nineteenth-century British thinking: according to John Stuart Mill, Anglican natural theology was suffused by "utilitarian doctrine".[10] Scottish Enlightenment social science also drew an analogy between the ends in nature and moral ends. Moreover, British national character was itself considered as utilitarian: in 1839 the Revd William Donaldson maintained that "we have all of us a bias towards the practical and immediately profitable, generated by our mercantile pursuits, which make all of us, to a certain extent, utilitarians".[11] Yet, by the 1830s Benthamite Utilitarianism had fallen into disrepute among strict Anglicans and the politically conservative-minded because it supported political radicalism. Against what had become the "deadly heresy" (Mill) of utilitarianism, German metaphysics was taken up by those who regarded its speculativeness as a lesser evil than home-grown materialism and political radicalism.[12]

Richard Jenkyns has described "the distinctive tone in English life which we call Victorian" more broadly as a consequence of the anti-utilitarian critique of British literati striving to free moral truth from the fetters of utilitarian expediency.[13] At Trinity College, Cambridge, the classical scholars Connop Thirlwall and Julius Charles Hare as well as the natural philosopher William Whewell pitted German metaphysics against the evil of utilitarianism.[14] Coleridge railed against "utilitarian notions of education" and Archdeacon Paley's praise of expediency.[15] Thomas Carlyle, too, sought "deliverance from the fatal incubus of Scotch or French philosophy, with its mechanisms and Atheisms".[16] For Prichard himself, the pernicious word was also allied to the doctrines of the parson Thomas Robert Malthus. When he railed against "a so-called utilitarian age whose scarcely disguised principle is to crush out of existence or drive out from the table of nature those who have not the strength and energy to scramble for their places",[17] he implicitly scorned Malthus who had claimed that at "nature's mighty feast" no places were laid for the poor. Nature, Malthus stated, told the poor man

> to be gone, and will quickly execute her own orders, if he does not work upon the compassion of some of her guests. If these guests get up and make room for him, other intruders immediately appear demanding the same favour. The report of a provision for all that come, fills the hall with numerous claimants. The order and harmony of the feast is disturbed...[18]

For Prichard, the social framework which Malthus's vision implied was nothing short of derisible. In that he was not alone. While Malthus had done away, as it were, with the optimistic Enlightenment Jacobinism of the 1790s, the bleak prospect his population theory offered called for mediation. A. M. C. Waterman has described the "Christian political economy" resulting from those efforts: Malthus's economics that contemplated the struggle for subsistence as lying beyond rational behaviour, would be welded to Paley's "theological superstructure". Other tenets were added: "the doctrine that inequality is both inevitable and beneficent would be greatly amplified, the futility of legislation to achieve economic goals explained, and the validity and importance of private charity reinforced."[19] The charitable half of Waterman's Christian political economy obviously appealed to Prichard, but he was not willing to compromise it by taking Malthus seriously.

Against this background, Prichard's turning to German authors – some of whom were all but unknown in Britain – is less surprising. If he was early in appreciating German learning, the development of British philosophy proved his instincts sound. By the 1840s Germanic scholarship had become something akin to a household term. It is reflected in Prichard's foreword to *The Natural History of Man*: in his dedication to Baron Bunsen he praised the Germans as the "most learned" of all, "a nation among whom my researches have ever been more favourably estimated than among my own utilitarian countrymen".[20]

In rejecting the drab views of his "utilitarian countrymen"

Prichard found himself in growing company. Yet, whilst Dickens, John Ruskin and Thomas Arnold fought it, not least of all in the name of poetry, it was in the cause of morality that Prichard repudiated utilitarianism,[21] using German philosophy as a way of linking Scottish common-sense doctrines to his spiritual concerns. Moreover, he needed theoretical assistance to annihilate phrenology which was the subject of many discussions of the British medical establishment and became increasingly fashionable.[22] In Chapter 2 we saw that Thomas Hancock's theories assumed the role of mediator between common-sense philosophy and German medical theory, enabling Prichard to conceive of the moral sense as a faculty that was prone to disease and largely independent of the brain. He thereby aimed to undermine the phrenologists' theory which came so very close to the assertion that the brain was the organ of the soul; and Prichard's notion of man's moral conscience, which was addressed in Chapter 3, shifted the emphasis to man's inward moral nature, complementing his notion that the integuments – hair, feathers, and skin colour – had no significance for natural classifications.

This preference for internal over external characteristics was in line with the insistence of Quakers and Evangelicals alike that faith was a question of inner conviction rather than of formal observance. It also squared with Prichard's opinion, discussed in Chapter 2, that temporal hierarchies constituted a superficial, albeit necessary, outward order. Among the ancient Hebrews, the invisible church of the faithful had been properly established with God as the supreme ruler. There had been no need for a worldly government, all men were equal under the rule of God. The more distant mankind became from that state, the more order and survival had to be promoted by other means. A sense of moral demerit had, therefore, been implanted into man's conscience. Prichard stressed that this sentiment, being prevalent in all humans, was a strong indicator for the unity of mankind. It had not only a religious but also a worldly rationale: anxiety and foreboding were part and parcel of man's ability to anticipate (and cater for) future material wants; at the same time they were liable to produce mental perturbation, subjecting the individual to insanity. It was these products of the moral instinct implanted in the human fabric which unified his anthropology and his theory of insanity. All the theorists of instinct, Greta Jones has stated, "began their work with an explicit renunciation of utilitarianism and the tabula rasa".[23]

To many of his contemporaries Prichard appeared increasingly old-fashioned. Boyd Hilton has shown that, "after 1850", the evangelical occupation with guilt and the atonement was superseded by an emphasis on the Incarnation of God the Father in God the Son.[24] Religion became, as it were, emotionally more comfortable. Prichard, by contrast, was still haunted by a theology of guilt and atonement and not in step with the imminent shift in religious perceptions. His reluctance to embrace most of the philosophies characteristic of Romanticism and the early Victorian age corroborated the impression of many reviewers – demonstrated below – that his ideas were not only conservative but also somewhat outdated. In some respects he was more a man of the eighteenth century than of the nineteenth. While he rejected late eighteenth-century primitivism[25] and spurned the *Idéologue* assumption that a "primitive tribe" might progress "of itself from barbarism" to civilization,[26] his ideas of historical development and the role the environment played in shaping external human appearance were inspired by Scottish Enlightenment philosophy. His concept of marital choice – what later was called sexual selection – drew on the notion that the environment had an oblique influence on the formation of a people (namely, by determining the level of civilization). Familiarity with Scottish teachings also enabled Prichard to appreciate similar foreign theories such as the humoralism of the Nasse school, Ritter's geography, and Alexander von Humboldt's environmentalist researches.

Prichard's appreciation of civilization was ambiguous: as long as it was not complemented by Christianity, the existence of basic arts, such as the faculty of language and "the use of fire, of artificial clothing, of arms, and the art of domesticating animals" did not mean very much: all of these could be lost if circumstances were unfavourable. This notion culminated in the assertion that these cultural attainments were "variable traits of human action". Because they were subject to change they were not of much value for ethnological classification.[27] In the 1840s this notion was augmented with speculations concerning the reversal of acquired characteristics. In a sudden turn against the analogical argument, Prichard claimed that such reversal was possible only in animals, but not respecting the higher attainments of mankind.

The second crucial aspect of his views on civilization was his belief that primitive tribes achieved a more civilized stage only through the influence of more refined peoples. This viewpoint of radical diffusionism did not justify imperialism, but it certainly gave legitimacy to missionary activities. Prichard stressed that his theory did not apply only to contemporary savages, but also to the former primitive population of Europe. When dealing in the third edition of the *Researches* with "the history of the nations of Asia & Europe" he aimed to show that Europe owed its civilization to the influx of other nations from the east – he supported, in other words, the doctrine of diffusionism: "these races", he wrote to Thomas Hodgkin, "were & probably would have remained but for the communication of external aids, in a state of Society – as Barbarous as that of the most Savage Africans".[28] Despite his use of the term, Prichard did not bolster a theory of race, nor did he pave the way for racial degenerationism. Individuals or even whole populations might deviate towards the type of another human variety, but this was due to external circumstances and ensuing changes in the mental constitution – it had nothing to do with an inbuilt tendency to degenerate. There is an element of environmental determinism in Prichard's theory, yet what distinguished him from outspoken theories of racial determinism supported by later physical anthropologists, was his belief that the natural history of human development was in a constant flux: a state of degeneration must not be considered as fixed, for improvement was always within reach. As Christian outlooks gradually ceased to permeate anthropological teachings, the theory of degeneration arose – in part as the result of the desire to make sense out of a world which appeared to many out of joint. The social hierarchy being under threat, a racial hierarchy was put into its place. Prichard's ethics, by contrast, were still so deeply rooted in Christian teleology and a Christian notion of paternalism that racial theory was not an option for him. The year of his death, 1848, witnessed a number of attempts to terminate the old European orders by means of revolutionizing them. Although most of these efforts were doomed, the year was a watershed, terminating what may be called the world in which Prichard had felt at home. "1848", wrote Eric Hobsbawm:

> marked the end, at least in western Europe, of the politics of tradition, of the monarchies which believed that their peoples (except for middle-class malcontents) accepted, even welcomed, the rule of divinely appointed dynasties presiding over hierarchically stratified societies, sanctioned by traditional religion, of the belief in the patriarchal rights and duties of social and economic superiors.[29]

Not just Prichard's politics, but also his research style was quite different from those of the rising generation of physical anthropologists. Racial theoreticians such as William Frédéric Edwards and Robert Knox emphasized that they missed no opportunity to search people's faces for their genuine racial features, Edwards travelling for the purpose through the south of France, Italy and Switzerland, and Knox looking "attentively at the population of Southern England".[30] On their way through Ireland the ardent craniometer John Beddoe and his company would regularly pretend to quarrel about the relative sizes of their heads. "The unsuspecting Irishmen", Beddoe remembered with a smirk, "usually entered keenly into the debate, ... eagerly betting on the size of their own heads, and begging to have their wagers determined."[31] Such a hands-on approach was not Prichard's thing, his adventurousness usually being satisfied in his study rather than on the road.

A "Powerful Authority"

Although he had been publishing since the 1810s, Prichard first truly achieved fame during the 1830s, no doubt thanks to his prominent role in the British Association and other learned societies which provided him with a proper platform for publicizing his views. After 1842 the Ethnological Society of London gave him a forum to reach people beyond the medical audiences Prichard mostly addressed, but living in provincial Bristol meant that he was always liable to be marginal. His ambition allowed him to accomplish much, but his fame never quite transcended the comparatively narrow circles within which he moved, and after his death he passed quickly into semi-oblivion.

Nonetheless, people as diverse as Bunsen, William Daniel Conybeare, Alexander von Humboldt, and Nicholas Wiseman respected and endorsed Prichard's arguments for the unity of mankind.[32] Even Robert Chambers, author of the scandalous *Vestiges of the Natural History of Creation*, mentioned him favourably.[33] The first edition of the *Researches* had been greeted as a work "of much amusement and information" by the *Monthly Review*.[34] The *British Critic* was mainly concerned with its theological virtues.[35] But subsequent editions received a more mixed response. As the *Researches* grew longer, reviewers found the work more difficult to analyse, one author simply resorting to the verdict that it was "not susceptible to abridgement".[36]

The third edition was deemed "a vast store of highly interesting facts and speculations".[37] Yet Prichard's attempts to convince through a coherent argument seemed to founder through the sheer bulk of the material he presented. "He occupies himself wholly with the collection of ethnographical matter", the *Prospective Review* complained, "the primary object appears almost to have vanished from his view."[38] Some reviewers completely mistook his purposes.

Despite his efforts to disprove the Caucasian hypothesis, the *British Quarterly Review* concluded that his "craniological division of mankind corresponds, in most respects, with the geographical classification of Baron Cuvier".[39] The *New Quarterly Review* meant well when it wrote "that the value of the work before us by no means depends on the question whether the writer has or has not proved, either that man is one species, or that this species descends from one pair. It is in fact a storehouse of information concerning the whole controversy."[40] One can imagine, however, that Prichard threw his hands up in despair at such a well-intended but patronising remark.

Nevertheless, during the thirties and forties his books were still widely and positively, if imprecisely, reviewed. The third edition of the *Researches* was considered as "superior",[41] as "a masterly-drawn scheme",[42] "an exceedingly valuable contribution",[43] "as a work of reference and authority in its own department, we know of none that can compete with it";[44] in short, it was a "classical work"[45] by a "powerful authority".[46] The prevailing view became that Prichard was an upholder of traditional doctrines. The *New Quarterly Review* stated: "the results at which he arrives may be described as (in the general) *conservative*; that is, they are mostly in favour of older rather than newer views".[47] The *British and Foreign Medical Review* praised the *Researches* for being "undertaken and executed in the spirit of former days, when men devoted their lives to the prosecution of one subject" and were "thinking of the attainment of truth alone".[48]

Nobody could ignore the great amount of labour and learning Prichard had invested. Therefore, "as a work of reference", the *Researches* and *The Natural History of Man* were valuable. Many reviewers endorsed his claim that physiognomy was a corollary of civilization, and that manners did not only make the man, but also human variety.[49] At the beginning of his career, Prichard's Biblicism was not unusual for an early nineteenth-century Anglican. But as the evangelical fervour of the early nineteenth century waned, his unchanging faith appeared outmoded. His insistence on monogenesis met with increasing exasperation. Reflecting new geological thinking, by the 1840s, the *New Quarterly Review* and the *Prospective Review*, amongst many, were beginning to criticize the brevity of Prichard's timescale. He had been so desirous to stick to Biblical chronology that he seemed to ignore developments in the study of biology. "Conservatives", said the Unitarian *Prospective Review*, "occasionally become the greatest destructives."[50]

Arguments rarely hinged on theology alone. The theory of hybridization was often attacked. The monogenist William Benjamin

Carpenter conceded in the *Edinburgh Review* that there were "many who maintain that the limits of hybridity are much wider than Dr. Prichard supposes".[51] The *New Quarterly* altogether rejected the benefits of intermixture: "Dr. Prichard overrates the hardihood of mixed races".[52] The *North British Review* even maintained that "on the whole, other races keep distinct from the true Negroes".[53] Other objections were raised against Prichard's hypothesis of the uniformity of the animal economy: to the *North British Review* it was evident that intermixture between human races produced a "generally short-lived hybrid".[54] Opinion was clearly turning against Prichard's endorsement of interbreeding.

It is significant that the harshest strictures were expressed in the 1840s. "On reviewing the whole argument", the *New Quarterly* stated,

> we cannot shake off a feeling that the result might have been attained *with far less effort.* For what have we proved? that men have actually descended from common parents? No: but that they may have so descended; out of which is educed (by the author) the idea of "common species".[55]

Writing in *Blackwood's Magazine* in 1844, William Robert Grove (1811-96), a judge and man of science, shared this new tone of scepticism: "differences in external condition may effect remarkable changes in tribes of human beings, and yet the collective body may be made up of different races".[56] A future president of the British Association and an influential member of the Royal Society, Grove was an important representative of scientific opinion.[57]

Views from Abroad

If most British reviewers of the 1840s were willing to accept at least some aspects of Prichard's argument, French observers tended to judge more critically. As early as 1824 the polygenist Julien-Joseph Virey dismissed Prichard's monogenism: the idea that black populations might engender white varieties appeared ludicrous to him. And Prichard's claim that all humans were prone to the same diseases was in his opinion unfounded.[58] In 1829 William Frédéric Edwards rejected Prichard's idea that civilization might exert an influence on human physiognomy, maintaining that human diversities "may be explained more naturally by reference to the mixture of races".[59] Gustave d'Eichthal spoke for most members of the Société Ethnologique de Paris when he criticized Prichard's religious stance and his environmentalism: according to d'Eichthal, the Briton had underrated the importance of racial diversity.[60] Writing in the 1850s, Arthur de Gobineau (1816-82), who told the history of Europe as the history of racial developments, mocked Prichard as "a mediocre historian and even more mediocre theologian", who was not interested in knowing the truth, but only in serving his deluded philanthropic ideals.[61] By then, ethnological investigations were routinely carried out from the perspective of physical anthropology, while the religious foundations of monogenism were discounted. Paul Broca (1824-80), a surgeon and anthropological writer, looked at Prichard's "Biblical viewpoint" without enthusiasm and rejected the argument of hybridity.[62] Even a man like Jean Louis Armand de Quatrefages (1810-92) who supported monogenism classified mankind into black, white and yellow races. "Unfortunately", wrote Quatrefages, Prichard had failed to do the same, due to a lack of familiarity with the natural sciences, and the "natural method" Quatrefages considered as the basis of racial classification. His criticism notwithstanding, the Frenchman paid some credit to Prichard who had seen the necessity to rally "all the resources provided by the different branches of learning" behind his ethnological endeavour. Therefore, he "deserved a place among the founders of anthropology".[63]

It was not only French anthropological writers who were dismissive of the scriptural argument. We have seen that August Wilhelm Schlegel regretted what he considered as Prichard's pitiable theological orthodoxy. Writing to Schlegel, Wilhelm von Humboldt observed that Prichard had an incomplete knowledge of mythological sources.[64] After having met Prichard in 1838, Bunsen praised the former's ability to combine ethnographic-philological researches with "the physiological element".[65] If Prichard's combination of traditionalist morality and progressive scientific methods appeared increasingly old-fashioned, he was not alone in his thinking that way. Bunsen, too, aspired to a grand unifying synthesis, hoping to find confirmation for his view "which I have held and followed up throughout my life, ... that the human race possesses *one* language, and the ancient history of the world lies deposited in the speech of subsequent nations".[66] But Bunsen's theology was more idiosyncratic, he did not shy away from ideas that Prichard would not have touched with a barge-pole. Thus he held complex views on the growth of languages and that of nations, believing that "a new language cannot originate without the dissolution of an ancient nationality".[67] He envisaged a time scale for human history of up to 20,000 years, traced the origins of mankind to Asia, and applied to the growth of languages Robert Chambers' idea that the development of the human embryo went through several stages of what formerly had been called the "chain of being". "All our languages", he wrote, "have at one time been *Chamitic*; as the human embryo passes through a period of fish-existence."[68] As Prichard did not contemplate the implications of early nineteenth-century secular philosophy, his philological history was comparatively uneventful. It was considered simple ethnographic philology. This was the opinion many German scholars adopted. As long as there were no doubts as to the validity of that method, Prichard's fame was assured, in Britain as well as abroad.

In the 1840s a German edition of the *Researches* appeared.[69] People like Bunsen and the philologist Max Müller in whose thought, as John Burrow has put it, "the idea of 'God' came to replace the notion of historical development", could agree with Prichard.[70] As time went on, however, philosophical speculations on the links between races and languages superseded his Scripturalism. Prichard had built his approach towards philology and mythology upon Genesis. His monogenism went hand in hand with diffusionism as he believed that mankind, when spreading across the globe, had also spread its customs and manners. His successors, by contrast, found "survivals" in mythology rather than the spirit of Revelation. Mythology turned into a linguistic "disease".[71] Müller (who himself was accused of conflating science and religion) deplored that ethnology and language studies "suffered most seriously from being mixed up together".[72]

While French and German authors tended to criticize the Christian undergirdings of Prichard's science, Americans had other fish to fry. American reviews clearly reflect the prominence of the slavery issue. William Frederick van Amringe (1791-1873)[73] criticized what he called Prichard's "speculative analogy". In his view "the anatomical and physiological structure and functions of the different races of men are sufficient to constitute distinct species".[74] Skin colour was of tremendous importance, the argument of hybridity fanciful nonsense: "it has been a favourite theory with some visionary philanthropists, that intermarriages of the different species would be highly favourable to the race; but we have never heard of any of them who was willing to commence the practice in their own families".[75] The example of ant colonies, Van Amringe stated, proved that slavery was a natural institution.[76] In his book we find all the elements characteristic of nineteenth-century scientific racialism, including scepticism towards racial mixture as well as the assertion that some races were not fit to survive.[77]

Even more disparaging were Josiah Clark Nott (1804-73) and George R. Gliddon (1809-57). Living in Mobile, Alabama, the former was a surgeon, well known in the American south; the latter was an archaeologist, adventurer, and representative of an insurance company; he was of English descent and came to live in America after he had served as American consul at Cairo. In 1854 they edited their influential *Types of Mankind*.[78] In the introduction it was pointed out that the monogenism of Blumenbach and Prichard had hitherto been attacked from a theological point of view; they, by contrast, would use scientific facts to expose its flaws.[79] Prichard, "the grand orthodox authority with the advocates of a common origin for the races of men", was credited with having published "one of the noblest monuments of learning". Yet, his Scripturalism precluded him from a sound grasp of the natural history of man:

> the constant changes of his opinions, his "special pleading", and his cool suppression of adverse facts, leave little confidence in his judgment or his cause. ... We behold him, year after year, like a bound giant, struggling with increasing strength against the records which cramp him, and we are involuntarily looking with anxiety to see him burst them asunder. But how few possess the moral power to break through a deep-rooted prejudice![80]

Prichard had failed: Nott and Gliddon were amused by his "extraordinary performance" of asserting the truth of the Pentateuch while denying "its genealogies; ... its chronology; ... all its historical and scientific details".[81] "One of the main objects of this volume", they continued, "is to show, that the criterion-point, indicated by Prichard, is now actually arrived at; and that the diversity of races must be accepted by Science as a *fact*, independently of theology, and of all analogies or reasoning drawn from the animal kingdom."[82] Like Van Amringe, they believed in the existence of several human races, they rejected environmentalism as well as the argument of hybridity, and prophesied the extinction of the "Negro" race.[83]

What distinguished scientific racialism from earlier assertions of polygenism is its final departure from theology and, in particular, the renunciation of the consanguinity of European and Semitic peoples. Nott and Gliddon dismissed both. In their view, white races were "Japhetic", yellow races "Shemitic".[84] Accordingly, those later Egyptian dynasties, who by others were associated with Semitic nations, were considered as an "amalgam of foreign (chiefly Asiatic) stocks".[85] Denying genealogical links, so prominent in Prichard's ethnology, between the Semitic and Japhetic nations, Nott and Gliddon discarded the theory of the Eastern origin of the European nations.[86] The type of racism they promulgated was based not simply on anatomy, but also on philology and archaeological relics.[87] Summing up what appears to us as an imperialist doctrine of racialism, they wrote:

> The World now advances in civilization more rapidly than in former times, and mainly for the substantial reason that the higher types of mankind have so increased in power that they can no longer be molested by the inferior; and the white races, or Iapetidae, have commenced the career of oriental conquest, and already "dwell in the tents of Shem".[88]

An Ongoing Tradition?

This opinion was not unique to American slave-holder society. Prichard's own former disciple, the ethnologist and amateur philologist Robert Gordon Latham (1812-88), professed similar opinions shortly after the teacher's death. While upholding monogenism and the notion that mankind originated in "intertropical Asia",[89] he denied that the ancestors of the Europeans had come from as far as India: "all the theories suggested by the term Indo-Europeans must be either abandoned or modified".[90] He equally rejected the idea that Semitic peoples were related to the Indo-European stock.[91]

Undermining Prichard's attempts to include the Celts among the Indo-Europeans, Latham remarked that "the Celts have a skull of their own just as they have a language".[92] He believed that the anthropologist ought to concentrate on physical appearance.[93] Despite his monogenism and a certain reticence towards the term "race", he made much use of the latter, contemplating laws of racial mixture and enlarging on the concept of "pure" races.[94] This was something Prichard had never done.[95] He had weighed the effects of intermarriage against those brought about by migration. But only very rarely did he refer to "purity of race". And he did not assign any particular cultural significance to the concept itself. On the contrary, he believed that intermixture was a healthy process. Latham, by contrast, distorted the doctor's views when he wrote: "from what I collect from Prichard, purity of blood is the rule rather than the exception".[96] Quite unlike Prichard, an approach to the topic of race couched in a chemical terminology of blood mixture, amalgamation, or fusion was typical of nineteenth-century scientific racialism. The advantages and disadvantages of pure and mixed blood respectively stood at the heart of the foundation texts of racialism: Charles Hamilton Smith's *The Natural History of the Human Species* (1848), Robert Knox's *Races of Men* (1850), Nott and Gliddon's *Types of Mankind* (1854), and Joseph Arthur de Gobineau's *Essai sur l'inégalité des races humaines* (1853-55).

We have seen above that many reviewers found Prichard's greatest merits in his ability to amass so much material. As the example of Latham shows, his theories were easily distorted. It is no accident that Prichard's Bristol colleague John Addington Symonds muddled up the doctor's account of skull formations in his obituary address of 1850.[97] When Henry Mayhew suggested that London's poor displayed the prognathous physiognomy of "vagabond" races, he referred his readers to Prichard's physical description of nomadic peoples.[98] In 1868 the ethnologist Richard King maintained that the ethnographer had gradually turned into a polygenist himself, alleging "that Dr. Prichard had at one time contended for the unity of the human race, but that latterly he had changed his opinion, and said that as a philosopher he could not agree to that opinion, but that as a Christian he must".[99] There is no evidence to support this seemingly tendentious opinion.[100] What the quotation illustrates, however, is the prominence of polygenism during the 1860s. Even the break-through of Darwinism did not beckon the demise of polygenism; rather to the contrary. As late as 1887 Quatrefages stated that, tacitly or implicitly, "the polygenists confuse *species* and *race*".[101]

The Father of British Ethnology?

This book has explored Prichard's opinions on all aspects of the emergent disciplines of anthropology and ethnology. In his endeavour to assess human nature he dealt with the philosophy of mind, with ethnology, physical anthropology, psychology, and the historical sciences in so far as they contributed to the natural history of man. The thrust of his arguments changed remarkably little during the forty years of his intellectual career. His religious commitments determined not just his opinions, but also his procedures. Though a notable traditionalist, Prichard was not simply backward-looking.[102] In his ambition to reconcile science and religion he made himself familiar with the latest trends of early nineteenth-century science, using liberal-progressive disciplines such as German comparative philology and Higher Criticism to bolster his own viewpoints. He realized, of course, that he did not manage to convince the world of monogenism; he might have noticed that his adversaries rejected his

235

doctrines as the prejudiced opinions of an anachronistic philanthropist. The fact that quite soon after his death even his followers began to distort his views would have reinforced his rather disenchanted views upon all things merely human.

In its infancy physical anthropology had been, as George Stocking put it, "nourished in the shadow of Cuverian comparative anatomy and the phrenological movement".[103] After Prichard's death, ethnology's turn towards physical anthropology intensified. Skull measurements were carried out according to the cephalic indices developed by the Swedish anatomist Anders Retzius (1796-1860) and others. Theories of arrested development and congenital moral deficiencies held sway. As Britain explored the politics of informal Empire, analogies were being drawn between "savage" peoples and retarded individuals in civilized societies. Both the Anthropological Society and even the Ethnological Society of London abounded with members whose interests were focused on "racial" distinctions.

In the 1850s and 1860s Prichard's *Researches* and the *Natural History of Man* were still rather widely read. Indefatigably, his intellectual heir Latham continued collecting ethnographic information, thus upholding the spirit of Prichardian ethnography. The archaeologist Daniel Wilson (1816-92), who was to become Professor of History and Literature at Toronto University, drew on Prichard's works for details concerning Scotland's past.[104] Alfred Russel Wallace (1823-1913), an admirer of Malthus and also of Chambers's *Vestiges of the Natural History of Creation*, merely used Prichard's data to interpret them in the light of Chambers's doctrines.[105] John Ferguson McLennan (1827-81) who dealt with the development of society rather than with ethnology *stricto sensu*, read in the *Researches* when contemplating "the divisions, the movements, and the progress of mankind".[106] When compiling material for a prize essay on "the origin of the English nation" offered by the Welsh National Eisteddfod,[107] the physician John Beddoe (1826-1911), consulted the *Researches*. But when his *Races of Britain* finally came out in 1885 he had removed all references to Prichard; one of the very few traces Prichard left in Beddoe's writings was the latter's usage of the term "Allophylian".[108] It is true that the term "Allophylian" gained some prominence in Britain. But it seems that nobody really knew what it meant. Daniel Wilson held that to refer to "the early races, which we describe loosely as primitive, or as aboriginal or primeval, Dr. Prichard has suggested the conveniently indefinite term 'Allophylian'".[109] Others believed that it was a linguistic category.[110]

Survivals: Signs of Decline or of Progress

As a matter of fact, Prichard's writings influenced the mainstream of British ethnology, Edward B. Tylor himself being well versed in Prichardian ethnography. According to George Stocking, Tylor (1832-1917) asked at least initially the same questions as Prichard. But as his ethnography unfolded against the background of Darwin's evolutionary time scale he could not possibly come to the same conclusions.[111] Prichard's diffusionist ethnology followed as a matter of course from, and proved his, monogenism. Tylor, by contrast, developed an evolutionary ethnology that centred on the discovery, and explanation, of survivals – those relics of customs and beliefs that once had made sense, but over time as society developed had lost their meaning.[112] Nonetheless, Tylor in more than one sense took up Prichard's mantle, if wearing it in a quite different fashion. For, in a sense, Prichard's ethnology, too, culminated in what may be called a doctrine of survivals. Yet while Tylor considered them as the rudiments of more barbarous epochs, Prichard's "survivals" were the residues of a more perfect age, consisting in those relics of monotheism which pagan myth-makers and civilized philosophers had not managed to destroy. Tylor's theory of survivals was progressive, Prichard's theory of "corruption" was degenerational.[113]

George Stocking has described the methods of "evolutionary titans, seated in their armchairs", who "culled ethnographic data from travel accounts to document their vision".[114] According to Stocking, who himself presides over the Olympus of anthropological historiography, Prichard's and Tylor's ethnology was in certain respects of a piece: both practised their science not just from similar armchairs, but also on the basis of the same set of sources.[115] Like Prichard, Tylor was brought up as a Quaker and his central ethnological research interest was tied to the subject of religion. Yet while Prichard had based the unity of mankind on the argument of universal psychology which culminated in the universal attitude towards a supreme Being, Tylor took the universality of belief as a starting point for his doctrine of evolutionary ethnology: all human populations, he believed, passed through a number of developmental stages that led from animism towards the abstract notions of revealed faith. Yet, Tylor did not stop here. Whilst the very title *Researches into the Early History of Mankind and the Development of Civilization* (1865) shows his affiliations with Prichard's thinking, he gradually turned towards Positivist philosophy, relegating religion to the early stages of human development later to be superseded by the age of science.[116]

To the extent that evolutionary ethnology was built on foundations Prichard had laid, it may be said that its systemic aversion to racial thinking owed something to Prichardian morality. Tylor himself, the banker and ethnologist Sir John Lubbock, and McLennan all rejected the concept of race because evolutionary ethnology – unless it was modified – implied that all human varieties went through the same sort of development.[117] When Tylor took over the editorship of the *Notes and Queries on Anthropology, for the Use of Travellers and Residents in Uncivilized Lands*, published by the British Association for the Advancement of Science in 1874, he succeeded to a task Prichard had fulfilled in the 1840s.[118]

On the whole, the prevalence of religious motivations among Victorian ethnologists is striking: like Tylor, William Robertson Smith (1846-94) who began his career as a Biblical scholar, Alfred Cort Haddon (1855-1940) who joined the Torres Straits expedition, and James G. Frazer (1854-1941), author of the *Golden Bough*, came from strong religious backgrounds. And although Frazer lost the faith he preserved "a life long habit of reading about religious belief".[119] Andrew Lang (1844-1912) and the Revd Robert Henry Codrington (1830-1922), both critics of evolutionary ethnology, searched independently for, as Codrington put it, "the common foundation, if such there ¡be, which lies in Human nature itself, ready for the superstructure of the Gospel".[120] Probably, the problems of "primitive religion" intrigued Victorian ethnologists more than any other, more than marriage patterns and questions of kinship.

As evolutionary anthropology itself grew embattled – fighting a revamped version of diffusionism, refined notions of racialism, and methodological criticisms – Prichard's memory receded. Once anthropology and ethnology organized themselves as disciplines, Prichard's ethnographical works were seen, like the Bible, as source books, but neither ethnologists nor anthropologists would consider it worthwhile to engage with his theories. When he was cited, as in the works mentioned above, in Gobineau's *Essai* or in John Lubbock's *The Origin of Civilisation and the Primitive Condition of Man* (1870) it was only for factual evidence.[121] By the 1880s, when Prichard was quoted it was in context not of anthropology but its history.

In his own books Tylor did not cite the *Researches* or the *Natural History of Man*, but in his entry on anthropology in the *Encyclopaedia Britannica* he paid tribute to Prichard, treating him as "founder of British ethnology" and as one who had long since disappeared from the scene.[122] The *Dictionary of National Biography* endorsed Prichard's knowledge, though it did not highlight specific achievements. "Had he not divided his energy" between philology and ethnology, wrote the psychiatrist Daniel Hack Tuke, "he would doubtless have achieved results in one of them that would have entitled him to a place among the greatest men of science". Yet Tuke conceded that Darwin's "doctrine of development rehabilitates his discussion of the races of man as varieties of one species" – thus, continuing the history of misunderstandings, the myth of Prichard as the precursor of Darwin was born.[123] Prichard's research interests, however, were entirely different from those of Darwin: he went back in time to prove the common origin of mankind, while the latter's narrative worked its way up from the past, sketching the tree of evolutionary development. Prichard abhorred Malthus, while Darwin found him stimulating. Moreover Darwin's work, like that of Herbert Spencer, Tylor and many others, is marked by a singular absence of explicit reference to Prichard.[124] Nonetheless, Tuke was not entirely mistaken, and if Darwin's own thinking implied a unitary origin of mankind, he and Prichard harboured similar considerations for native populations whom they pitied for their fate at the mercy of European colonists.

As even those who read Prichard's books were reluctant to quote him or excised references to his works from their books, it might be tempting to regard Prichard as a specimen doomed to extinction. It is, indeed, true that his science did not fit the mind-set of the second half of the nineteenth century and later scientific preoccupations. It is not helpful to represent him as anticipating any major theory prevalent after his death. Stocking refers this mainly to the different time scales within which Prichard and Tylorian ethnologists were operating.[125] While this is certainly true, it is only one aspect of the great divide that separates Prichard from later generations: it was not his mode of thinking, nor his intellect, nor his reading that made him unfit for intimate discourse with late Victorian minds, but his moral stance and, in particular, his specific attitude towards religion. Where later Victorians would observe their own doubts with horror, Prichard attempted to prove that Scripturalism was perfectly scientific. Where the Victorians strove to separate science from philanthropy, Prichard pursued both from the same pulpit, or rather armchair. British philanthropy, of course, continued to thrive, supporting abolitionism in other countries, and promoting the interests of native peoples, but it was characteristic of Prichard's age that this went hand in hand with scientific enquiry.

These differences marked a shift in general attitudes; they also point to a specific side of Prichard's character: a certain naivety. Prichard knew his books, and he knew Bristol but he did not know much else. This helps to account for the credulity he displayed towards the information he received. In a nutshell it may be said that Prichard's first-hand knowledge of the world was derived from intimate experience of two institutions only: universities and mad-houses. It would not be surprising had he had a notion that the world was a mad place, yet this would not drive him to the brink of desperation as he knew of another world that promised both atonement and redemption.

What applied to his anthropology and ethnology was also true for his medicine and his philosophy of mind. His concept of moral insanity has very little to do with what a later generation made of it. While in this term the adjective "moral", for Prichard, had ethical, religious, and behaviouristic connotations, its meaning was later reduced to the notion of "psychopathy".[126]

The other topic that survived was his insistence on the universality of human "psychology". It was in Germany that this idea was adopted and reiterated. Adolf Bastian (1826-1905), who in 1873 was made extraordinary Professor of Ethnology in Berlin, underlined the links between psychology and ethnology and demanded that the latter ought to focus on "the mental life of peoples". According to Klaus-Peter Koepping, Bastian envisaged "a connection between psychology and culture history": ethnology's task was to find "the psychological laws of the mental development of groups".[127] Through Bastian – who had read Prichard – some idea of psychological unity akin to Prichard's own notion reached C. G. Jung whose concept of archetypes harked back to Bastian's comparative psychology.[128]

This peculiar genealogy of thought – even though the full meaning of Prichard's ideas got lost on the way – bolsters the case this book has sought to make: Prichard was not a sort of anthropological Pre-Adamite. The very fact that he appeared a worthy anachronism some thirty years after his death – a distant "father" to a science – supports the suggestion that the scientific formulations to which he was driven by virtue of his religious convictions, came to be at odds with their time. From today's viewpoint, his scientific opinions and his humanitarianism seem to be remarkably in tune with many present-day sentiments.

Prichard's views of "race", indeed, have more in common with the anti-racialism of the latter half of the twentieth century than with the theories of race of the intervening century. And his idea that historical philology provided a key to the classification of human populations might be compared not only to the endeavour of Sir William Jones but also to that of a group of twentieth-century geneticists, headed by L. Luca Cavalli-Sforza.[129] At the end of the nineteenth century, Max Müller offered this perceptive assessment:

His careful weighing of facts and difficulties went out of fashion when the theory of evolution became popular, and every change from a flea to an elephant was explained by imperceptible degrees. He dealt chiefly with what was perceptible, with well-observed facts, and many of the facts which he marshalled so well, require even now, in these post-Darwinian days I should venture to say, renewed consideration.[130]

Notes

1   John Stuart Mill, "Coleridge". In J. S. Mill, Jeremy Bentham, *Utilitarianism and Other Essays*, ed. Alan Ryan (London: Penguin, 1987), pp. 177-226, quotation from p. 180.

2   Elisabeth Jay, *The Religion of the Heart. Anglican Evangelicalism and the Nineteenth Century Novel* (Oxford: Clarendon Press, 1979), p. 146.

3   Peardon, *The Transition in English Historical Writing*, p. 253.

4   Peter Allan Dale, *The Victorian Critic and the Idea of History* (Cambridge, Mass.: Harvard University Press, 1977), p. 255.

5   The term is derived from Frank M. Turner, "The Crisis of Faith". In *idem, Contesting Cultural Authority. Essays in Victorian Intellectual Life* (Cambridge: Cambridge University Press, 1993), pp. 73-100, see p. 78.

6   Trevor H. Levere, *Poetry Realized in Nature. Samuel Taylor Coleridge and Early Nineteenth-Century Science* (Cambridge: Cambridge University Press, 1982), p. 115.

7   Duncan Forbes, *The Liberal Anglican Idea of History* (Cambridge: Cambridge University Press, 1952), pp. 67-71; John Burrow, *A Liberal Descent, Victorian Historians and the English Past* (Cambridge: Cambridge University Press, 1981).

8   This has been shown by Michael Biddiss with respect to the racial theory of Gobineau; see Biddiss, "Arthur de Gobineau (1816-1882) and the Illusions of Progress". In *Rediscoveries*, ed. John A. Hall (Oxford: Clarendon Press, 1986), pp. 27-45, esp. p. 41.

9   Prichard, *Researches*, 2nd ed., 1: 128-29.

10   John Stuart Mill, "Whewell on Moral Philosophy". In Mill, Bentham, *Utilitarianism and Other Essays*, pp. 228-70, quotation from p. 232.

11   John William Donaldson, *The New Cratylus, or Contributions Towards a More Accurate Knowledge of the Greek Language* (Cambridge: J. and J. J. Deighton, 1839), p. 3.

12   Mill, "Whewell on Moral Philosophy", p. 232. For an analysis of the utilitarian side of natural theology see A. Dwight Culler, *The Victorian Mirror of History* (New Haven: Yale University Press, 1985), p. 22.

13   Richard Jenkyns, *The Victorians and Ancient Greece* (Oxford: Blackwell, 1980), p. 30.

14   Philip F. Rehbock, *The Philosophical Naturalists*, p. 25; Nicolaas Rupke, *The Great Chain of History*, p. 265.

15   Levere, *Poetry Realized in Nature*, pp. 87, 214. For utilitarianism in Paley's natural theology see D. L. LeMahieu, *The Mind of William Paley. A Philosopher and his Age* (Lincoln: University of Nebraska Press, 1976). For the prevalence of utilitarianism in the *Bridgewater Treatises* see Frank M. Turner, "Cultural Apostasy and the 'Foundations of Victorian Intellectual Life". In *idem, Contesting Cultural Authority*, pp. 38-72, see p. 47.

16   Quoted from Adrian Desmond, *Archetypes and Ancestors*, p. 43.

17   See Richard Smith, "Manuscript Memoirs", p. 622. Quoted in Neve, "Science in Provincial England", p. 289.

18   Thomas Robert Malthus, *An Essay on the Principle of Population: A View of Its Past and Present Effects on Human Happiness, With an Inquiry into our Prospects Respecting the Future Removal of the Evils which it Occasions*, 2nd ed. (London: J. Johnson, 1803 (1798)). Note that Prichard's invective against Malthus was part of his comment on the Poor Law reforms; cf. Chapter 1 above.

19   A. M. C. Waterman, *Revolution, Economics and Religion. Christian Political Economy, 1798-1833* (Cambridge: Cambridge University Press, 1991), p. 150.

20   Prichard, *Natural History of Man*, p. v.

21   Cf. Jenkyns, *The Victorians and Ancient Greece*, p. 245.

22   See Roger Cooter, *The Cultural Meaning of Popular Science*, pp. 19ff.

23   Greta Jones, *Social Darwinism in English Thought: The Interaction Between Biological and Social Theory* (Brighton: Harvester Press, 1980), p. 135.

24   Hilton, *The Age of Atonement*, p. 299.

25   For primitivism see Peardon, *The Transition in English Historical Writing*, pp. 103-26.

26   See the abstract of Prichard's "Observations on the Races of People who Inhabit the Northern Regions of Africa". In "Abstracts of Papers, &c Read Before the Philosophical and Literary Society". The paper was read on 25 May 1825.

27   Prichard, *Researches into the Physical History of Mankind*, 3rd ed., 1: 173-74; see also *ibid.*, 1st ed., note on p. 555.

28 Letter to Thomas Hodgkin, 23 June 1838; see also the abstract of Prichard's paper "Observations on the Races of People who Inhabit the Northern Regions of Africa".

29 Eric Hobsbawm, *The Age of Capital 1848-1875* (London: Abacus, 1977 (1975)), p. 38.

30 For Edwards see Antje Sommer, "William Frédéric Edwards, 'Rasse' als Grundlage europäischer Geschichtsdeutung?", p. 372; for Knox see: Robert Knox, *The Races of Men*, 2nd ed. (London: Henry Renshaw, 1862 (1850)), p. 14.

31 John Beddoe, *The Races of Britain. A Contribution to the Anthropology of Western Europe*, 1885. Reprint, intr. David Elliston Allen (London: Hutchinson, 1971), p. 8.

32 Bunsen, "Recent Egyptian Researches", pp. 261, 295. Conybeare considered Prichard as "one of the very ablest men I know". See his letter to W. V. Harcourt from 8 September 1831. In *Gentlemen of Science. Early Correspondence of the British Association for the Advancement of Science*, ed. Jack Morrell, Arnold Thackray (London: Royal Historical Society, 1984), p. 59; [Henry Holland], "Natural History of Man". *Quarterly Review* 86 (1849-50): 1-40; Humboldt, *ΚΟΣΜΟΣ. A General Survey of the Physical Phenomena of the Universe*, trans. Augustin Prichard, 2 vols (London: Baillière, 1845), 1: 386-87; Wiseman, *Twelve Lectures*, 1: 246, 2: 45.

33 Robert Chambers, *Vestiges of the Natural History of Creation*, 12th ed. (Edinburgh, London: Chambers, 1884 (1844)), pp. 335-36.

34 "Dr. Prichard – *Physical History of Mankind*". *Monthly Review* 75 (1814): 127-34, p. 134. See also "Dr. Pritchard [sic] *on the Physical History of Man*". *Annals of Philosophy* 5 (1815): 379-82.

35 "Prichard's *Researches on the Physical History of Man*". *British Critic* n.s., 3 (1815): 292-300, esp. pp. 292-93.

36 "Dr. Prichard – *Physical History of Mankind*". *British Critic*, 3rd s., 7 (1828): 33-61, p. 47.

37 "The Physical History of Man". *North British Review* 4 (1844): 177-201, p. 201.

38 "Physical History of Mankind". *Prospective Review* 3 (1847): 355-69, pp. 355-56.

39 "Ethnology – the Unity of Mankind". *British Quarterly Review* 10 (1849): 408-40, p. 410.

40 "Prichard's *Physical History of Mankind*". *New Quarterly Review* 8 (1846): 95-134, p. 97.

41 "Dr. Prichard *on the Physical History of Mankind*". *British and Foreign Medical Review* 3 (1837): 365-76, p. 376; see also the short notice in *ibid.*, 5 (1838): 543-44.

42 See the notice in *Gentleman's Magazine* n.s., 27 (1847): 398.

43 "Prichard's *Physical History of Mankind*", p. 134.

44 See the notice in *London Medical Gazette* 4 (1847): 248-49.

45 See the notice in *British and Foreign Medical Review* 12 (1841): 519.

46 "Prichard's Natural History of Man". *Dublin Review* 19 (1845): 67-98, p. 68.

47 "Prichard's *Physical History of Mankind*", p. 106 (original emphasis).

48 See the review in *British and Foreign Medical Review* 12 (1841): 519.

49 [William Benjamin Carpenter], "Ethnology or the Science of Races". *Edinburgh Review* 88 (1848): 429-87, p. 440; [Henry Holland], "Natural History of Man", p. 24; see also the article in the *British Quarterly Review*, pp. 413-14.

50 "Prichard's *Physical History of Mankind*", pp. 123, 134; see also the review in *Prospective Review*, p. 362.

51 [Carpenter], "Ethnology or the Science of Races", p. 460.

52 "Prichard's *Physical History of Mankind*", p. 126.

53 See the article in the *North British Review*, pp. 189-90.

54 *Ibid.*, p. 190.

55 "Prichard's *Physical History of Mankind*", p. 130 (original emphasis).

56 [William Robert Grove], "Natural History of Man". *Blackwood's Magazine* 56 (1844): 312-30, p. 313.

57 "Prichard's *Physical History of Mankind*", note on pp. 132-33. The editors of the *New Quarterly* added a footnote to an article on Prichard, distancing themselves from the polygenist leanings of the reviewer.

58 Julien-Joseph Virey, *Histoire naturelle du genre humain*, 2nd ed., 3 vols (Paris: Crochard, 1824), 1: 431-33. (This is a thoroughly revised version of the first edition published in 1800.)

59 William Frédéric Edwards, *Des caractères physiologiques des races humaines considérés dans leurs rapports avec l'histoire: Lettre à Amédée Thierry* (Paris: Compère jeune, 1829), p. 35.

60 Gustave d'Eichthal, "Mémoire sur l'anthropologie ou de l'histoire naturelle de l'homme". Procès-verbal de la séance du 26 mai 1843, *Mémoires de la société ethnologique* 2 (1845): xxxvii-xl, p. xxxviii. D'Eichthal came from a wealthy family, entertained a correspondence with John Stuart Mill and, in the 1830s, became a Saint-Simonian.

61 See Michael Banton, *Racial Theories*, p. 47. Banton did not indicate the source of this quotation. I am much obliged to Michael Biddiss who has found it in the second edition of the *Essai*. See Gobineau, *Essai sur l'inégalité des races humaines*, 2nd ed., 2 vols (Paris: Firmin Didot, 1884), 1: xiv. By contrast, in the first edition Gobineau quoted Prichard as a source of anthropological information:

Gobineau, *Essai sur l'inégalité des races humaines*, 4 vols (Paris: Firmin Didot, 1853-55), 1: 13, 84, 90, 116-18, 184, 290, 371.

62 Pierre Paul Broca, "La linguistique et l'anthropologie". *Bulletins de la société d'anthropologie de Paris* 3 (1862): 264-319, p. 279; quoted from: Bynum, "Time's Noblest Offspring", p. 399. See also Broca, *On the Phenomena of Hybridity in the Genus Homo*, ed. C. Carter Blake (London: Anthropological Society of London, 1864), pp. 2-7.

63 A. de Quatrefages, *Histoire générale des races humaines. Introduction a l'étude des races humaines,* 2 vols (Paris: A. Hennuyer, 1887-89), 1: vii.

64 Wilhelm von Humboldt, August Wilhelm Schlegel, *Briefwechsel,* p. 162 (Humboldt's letter to Schlegel of 21 June 1823).

65 *Memoir of Baron Bunsen,* 1: 477, 482; 2: 134. Throughout the *Memoir* Prichard's name is misspelled as "Pritchard".

66 *Memoir of Baron Bunsen,* 2: 257.

67 Bunsen, "Recent Egyptian Researches", p. 286.

68 *Memoir of Baron Bunsen,* 2: 143.

69 Prichard, *Naturgeschichte des Menschengeschlechts,* trans. R. Wagner, J. G. F. Will, 4 vols (Leipzig: Leopold Voß, 1840-48).

70 For Müller see Joan Leopold, "Ethnic Stereotypes in Linguistics: the Case of Friedrich Max Müller (1847-51)". In *Papers in the History of Linguistics,* ed. Hans Aarsleff *et al.,* pp. 501-12. For Bunsen see Helmut Bobzin, "Christian Carl Josias von Bunsen und sein Beitrag zum Studium der orientalischen Sprachen". In *Universeller Geist und guter Europäer,* ed.

71 Max Müller, *Lectures on the Science of Language,* 3rd ed. (London: Longman *et al.,* 1862 (1861)), p. 11.

72 *Ibid.,* p. 333.

73 Van Amringe does not figure in any of the standard bibliographical dictionaries. His only other publication is a work on *The Nature and Origin of Heat and the Forces of the Universe* (1869).

74 William Frederick van Amringe, *An Investigation of the Theories of the Natural History of Man, by Lawrence, Prichard, and Others Founded Upon Animal Analogies: and an Outline of a New Natural History of Man, Founded Upon History, Anatomy, Physiology, and Human Analogies* (New York: Baker and Scribner, 1848), pp. 229, 317-18, 360.

75 *Ibid.,* pp. 395, 713-14.

76 *Ibid.,* p. 311.

77 *Ibid.,* pp. 217, 713-14.

78 Josiah Clark Nott, George R. Gliddon *et al., Types of Mankind: or, Ethnological Researches, Based Upon the Ancient Monuments, Paintings, Sculptures, and Crania of Races, and Upon Their Natural, Geographical, Philological, and Biblical History: Illustrated by Selections*

from the Inedited Papers of Samuel George Morton, M.D., and by Additional Contributions from Prof. L. Agassiz, W. Usher, and Prof. H. S. Patterson (London: Trübner; Philadelphia: Lippincott, Gambo, 1854). Nott also provided an Appendix to the partial translation of Gobineau's *Essai* published at Philadelphia in 1856.

79 Henry S. Patterson, "Memoir of the Life and Scientific Labors of Samuel George Morton". In *Types of Mankind*, pp. xvii-lvii, see p. xliii.

80 Nott, Gliddon, *Types of Mankind*, p. 54.

81 *Ibid.*, p. 55. They grossly exaggerated Prichard's scientific critique of the Scriptures.

82 *Ibid.*, p. 56.

83 *Ibid.*, pp. 63, 74, 67.

84 *Ibid.*, p. 247.

85 *Ibid.*, p. 229.

86 *Ibid.*, pp. 88-89.

87 Douglas Lorimer has stressed that Victorian racism in the latter half of the nineteenth century must not be referred to anatomy alone, for such a view would amount to underestimating "the potency and ubiquitous character of racism within the culture". See Lorimer, "Science and the Secularization of Victorian Images of Race". In *Victorian Science in Context*, ed. Bernard Lightman (Chicago: University of Chicago Press, 1997), pp. 212-35. For a contrary view see, e.g., Graham Richards, *"Race", Racism and Psychology. Towards a Reflexive History* (London: Routledge, 1997), pp. 8, 14.

88 Nott, Gliddon, *Types of Mankind*, p. 96.

89 Robert Gordon Latham, *Man and his Migrations* (London: John van Voorst, 1851), p. 248. Cf. also *idem, Natural History of the Varieties of Man* (London: John van Voorst, 1850), p. 565.

90 Latham, *Man and his Migrations*, pp. 145, 218-19, 225, 248, the quotation is from p. 249. For a somewhat different interpretation see Carol MacCormack, "Medicine and Anthropology". In *Companion Encyclopedia of the History of Medicine*, ed. W. F. Bynum, Roy Porter, 2 vols (London: Routledge, 1993), 2: 1436-48, p. 1429.

91 Latham, *Natural History*, pp. 14, 120. Unlike Nott and Gliddon, however, he ranged them together with black peoples under the heading "Atlantidae" (Latham's other principal classification groups were "Mongolidae" and "Iapetidae").

92 *Idem, Man and his Migrations*, p. 183.

93 *Ibid.*, p. 150.

94 *Idem, Natural History*, pp. 517, 555-57; see also his *Man and his Migrations*, p. 97. He held that "differences should only be attributed to so independent and so impalpable a force as *race* when all other

things are equal". See *ibid.*, p. 204 (original emphasis).

95 Of course, Prichard would mention "the pure race of the Euskaldunes" or "Brahmans of high and pure caste". But these designations were simply descriptive, he did not believe that "purity of race" had any other ethnological significance; see his *Researches*, 3rd ed., 3: 48; 4: 237.

96 Latham, *Natural History*, p. 517.

97 According to Symonds, Prichard distinguished the Caucasian, Negro, and Mongol varieties of man. Symonds entirely ignored the fact that, in the third edition of the *Researches*, Prichard had distanced himself vehemently from this classification. See Symonds, *Some Account*, p. 17.

98 Prichard, *Researches*, 3rd ed., 1: 281-82. Henry Mayhew, *London Labour and the London Poor...*, 3 vols (London: George Woodfall and Sons, 1851), 1: 1.

99 "Anthropological Review". *Journal of the Anthropological Society of London* 6 (1868): i-cxcvii, p. cxi.

100 On the contrary, in 1843 Prichard wrote a letter to the barrister and amateur ethnologist, Arthur James Johnes, thanking him for the present of Johnes's recent publication: "Philological Proofs of the Original Unity and Recent Origin of the Human Race" (1843). See Letter to Johnes, 24 July 1843. Crossley papers, autograph collection, vol. 3, Manchester Central Library. In this letter Prichard endorsed Johnes's monogenism, adding that "every foreigner who takes the question in hand or alludes to it whether he be German, French or American, decides peremptorily on the otherside [sic], or takes it as a thing granted and almost self evident that there are many distinct human races".

101 Quatrefages, *Histoire générale des races humaines*, 1: 10.

102 Otherwise Woodrow Wilson could hardly have referred Bagehot's views of society to Prichard's teachings. Cf. Nancy Stepan, "Biology and Degeneration: Races and Proper Places", p. 186.

103 Stocking, *Victorian Anthropology*, p. 65.

104 Daniel Wilson, *The Archaeology and Prehistoric Annals of Scotland* (Edinburgh: Sutherland and Knox; London: Simpkin, Marshall, and Co., 1851), pp. 161, 180, 204, 248.

105 Alfred Russel Wallace, *My Life: A Record of Events and Opinions*, 2 vols (London: Chapman & Hall, 1905), 2: 255. Cf. Stocking, *Victorian Anthropology*, p. 97.

106 John Ferguson McLennan, "Hill Tribes in India". *North British Review* 38 (1863): 392-422. Quoted in Stocking, *Victorian Anthropology*, pp. 165-66. For McLennan, see Stocking, *After Tylor. British Social*

Anthropology 1888-1951 (London: Athlone, 1996), pp. 47ff.

107 John Beddoe, *The Races of Britain*, p. xvi.

108 But see his use of Prichard's term "Allophylian", *ibid.*, p. 29.

109 Wilson, *The Archaeology and Prehistoric Annals of Scotland*, p. 161.

110 Cf. the definition given in the *OED*, vol. 1. The term was variously used as a racial and a linguistic category. Max Müller, for example, remarked that Prichard had used "Allophylian" for what he himself had called "Turanian". See F. Max Müller, *The Science of Language founded on Lectures delivered at the Royal Institution in 1861 and 1863*, 2 vols (London: Longmans, Green, and Co., 1891), 1: 397.

111 Stocking, *Victorian Anthropology*, p. 158.

112 Cf. Margaret Hodgen, *The Doctrine of Survivals: A Chapter in the History of Scientific Method in the Study of Man* (London: Allenson & Co., 1936).

113 Cf. Chapter 7 above. For Prichard's notion of "corruption" see his *Egyptian Mythology*, p. 297.

114 Stocking, "The Ethnographer's Magic: Fieldwork in British Anthropology from Tylor to Malinowski". In *idem, The Ethnographer's Magic and Other Essays in the History of Anthropology* (Madison, Wisc.: University of Wisconsin Press, 1992), pp. 12-59, see p. 17.

115 Stocking, *Victorian Anthropology*, p. 79. Stocking tells the history of anthropology as a struggle of "paradigmatic traditions": the Prichardian "biblical" or "ethnological" paradigm being superseded by the "developmental" or "evolutionist", and the "polygenetic" or "physical anthropological" paradigm. See, e.g., his "Paradigmatic Traditions in the History of Anthropology". In *idem, The Ethnographer's Magic*, pp. 342-61, esp. p. 348.

116 Stocking, *Victorian Anthropology*, p. 52.

117 *Idem, After Tylor*, p. 80; *idem, Victorian Anthropology*, p. 248. Evolutionary ethnology was easily reconciled to racial thinking, provided it was assumed that some "races" approached civilization more quickly than others.

118 Stocking, *After Tylor*, p. 15.

119 *Ibid.*, p. 128.

120 For Lang, see *ibid.*, p. 59. For Codrington, see Robert Henry Codrington, "Religious Beliefs and Practices in Melanesia". *Journal of the Anthropological Institute* 10 (1881): 261-316, p. 312; quoted in Stocking, *After Tylor*, p. 42.

121 John Lubbock, *The Origin of Civilisation and the Primitive Condition of Man*, 5th rev. ed. (London: Longmans, Green, and Co., 1889 (1870)), p. xxii.

122 E. B. Tylor, "Anthropology". In *Encyclopaedia Britannica*, ed.
     Thomas Spencer Baines, William Robertson Smith, 9th ed., 24 vols
     (Edinburgh: A. & C. Black, 1875-89), vol. 1. Exceptions were to be
     found, but only outside the field. Thus Max Müller deemed
     Prichard's *Researches* "unparalleled in ethnology". See Müller, *My
     Autobiography*, p. 205.

123 Daniel Hack Tuke on Prichard, *DNB*, vol. 46.

124 In Darwin's early writings Prichard is mentioned only once; see
     Charles Darwin, *Metaphysics, Materialism, and the Evolution of the
     Mind. Early Writings of Charles Darwin*, ed. Paul H. Barrett
     (Chicago: University of Chicago Press, 1980 (1974)), p. 193.
     Darwin wrote: "female genital organs. – make abstract on this
     subject from Lawrence, Blumenbach & Prichard". Darwin's remark
     might have referred to the "Hottentot Venus", dissected by Cuvier.
     Although Prichard did not enlarge on the topic of "reproductive
     organs" he mentioned the results of Cuvier's dissection; see Prichard,
     Researches, 3rd ed., vol. 1, note on p. 326.

125 Stocking, *Victorian Anthropology*, p. 158; *idem, After Tylor*, p. 47.

126 Cf. Eric T. Carlson, Norman Dain, "The Meaning of Moral
     Insanity". *Bulletin for the History of Medicine* 36 (1962): 130-40, pp.
     137-39.

127 Klaus-Peter Koepping, *Adolf Bastian and the Psychic Unity of Mankind.
     The Foundations of Anthropology in Nineteenth Century Germany* (St
     Lucia: University of Queensland Press, 1983), p. 12. For nineteenth-
     century German anthropology, see George W. Stocking Jr, ed.,
     *Volksgeist as Method and Ethic. Essays on Boasian Ethnography and the
     German Anthropological Tradition, History of Anthropology* 8 (Madison,
     Wisc.: University of Wisconsin Press, 1996).

128 Sonu Shamdasani, "C. G. Jung and the Making of Modern
     Psychology" (Ph.D. diss., University College London, 1996), pp.
     440-41. For Bastian's reference to Prichard see Koepping, *Adolf
     Bastian*, p. 109. For Bastian's humanist folk psychology see Matti
     Bunzl, "Franz Boas and the Humboldtian Tradition. From Volksgeist
     and *Nationalcharakter* to an Anthropological Concept of Culture".
     In *Volksgeist as Method and Ethic*, ed. George W. Stocking Jr, pp. 17-
     78, esp. pp. 43-73.

129 See note 80 in Chapter 5 above.

130 Müller, *My Autobiography*, p. 205.

Bibliography

Manuscript Sources

"A List of Subscribers and Donations to Bristol Infirmary 1761-1805".
MS. 35893 (21), Bristol Public Record Office.

"Abstracts of Papers, & c Read Before the Philosophical & Literary Society
Annexed to the Bristol Institution. Beginning with the Paper
Read at the Evening Meeting on 6th January 1825". Compiled
by the Philosophical and Literary Society. MS. B 12361, Bristol
Central Library.

BORTHWICK, J., "Notes from A Course of Lectures on Moral Philosophy.
Delivered by Dugald Stewart Esq. 1806-7", pp. 365-66. MS.
Gen. 843. Special Collections, Edinburgh University Library.

Contract. MS. 5535 (50), Bristol Public Record Office.

ESTLIN, JOHN B., "On Philosophical Necessity". In "Records of the Royal
Medical Society of Edinburgh" 57 (1807-8): 387-418.

Matriculation Indexes. MS. Da 35, Edinburgh University Library, Special
Collections.

PRICHARD, JAMES COWLES, "Of the Varieties of the Human Race". In
"Records of the Royal Medical Society of Edinburgh" 58 (1807-8):
87-134.

————, letter to John Rose Hale, 6 April 1815. MS. 15385 (f.3),
National Library, Edinburgh.

————, "Observations on the Races of People who Inhabit the Northern
Regions of Africa". Paper read on 25 May 1825. In "Abstracts of
Papers, &c Read Before the Philosophical & Literary Society
Annexed to the Bristol Institution. Beginning With the Paper
Read at the Evening Meeting on 6th January 1825". Compiled
by the Philosophical and Literary Society. MS. B 12361, Bristol
Central Library.

————, letter to Thomas Hodgkin, 23 June 1838. Mss. Brit. Emp., S.18,
press mark C. 122/51, Hodgkin Papers, Rhodes House, Oxford.

————, letter to Rudolph Wagner, 30 April 1841. MS. R. Wagner 6,
Nachlaß Rudolph Wagner, Göttinger Universitätsbibliothek,
Manuskriptabteilung.

————, letter to Robert Peel, December 1842. MS. 40512, f. 93, Peel

Papers, vol. 3411, British Library, Manuscript Dept.

————, letter to Arthur James Johnes, 24 July 1843. Crossley papers, autograph collection, vol. 3, Manchester Central Library.

————, letter to William Buckland, 8 March 1845. MS. BU. 241 111, Royal Society of London.

————, Prichard Papers, Royal Geographical Society, London.

Prospectus of a College for Classical and Scientific Education, to be Established in or near the City of Bristol, s.l., s.d., MS. B 23363, Bristol Central Library.

"Records of the Royal Medical Society of Edinburgh" 57 (1807-8): 387-418, Archives of the Royal Medical Society of Edinburgh.

SMITH, RICHARD, "Manuscript Memoirs". MS. 35893 (36) k. i., Bristol Public Record Office.

THATCHER, J., "What is the Most Plausible Theory of Generation?" in "Records of the Royal Medical Society of Edinburgh" 56 (1806-7): 250-65.

"Wernerian Society Minutes". 2 vols, Edinburgh, 1808-30. MS. Dc. 2.55-56, Edinburgh University Library.

PUBLISHED SOURCES

Anonymous Reviews of Prichard

ANON., "Dr. Prichard – *Physical History of Mankind"* . *Monthly Review* 75 (1814): 127-34.

ANON., "Dr. Pritchard [sic] *on the Physical History of Man"* . *Annals of Philosophy* 5 (1815): 379-82.

ANON., "Prichard's *Researches on the Physical History of Man"*. *British Critic* n.s., 3 (1815): 292-300.

ANON., "Prichard *on the Egyptian Mythology"*. *Monthly Review,* 2d s., 92 (1820): 225-42.

ANON., "Prichard's *Analysis of Egyptian Mythology"* . *British Critic,* 2nd s., 14 (1820): 55-69.

ANON., "Dr. Prichard – *Physical History of Mankind"* . *British Critic,* 3rd s., 7 (1828): 33-61.

ANON., "Physical Evidences of the Characteristics of Ancient Races Among the Moderns". *Fraser's Magazine* 6 (1832): 673-79.

ANON., "Meeting of the Provincial Medical Association, 3. Anniversary Meeting, Oxford, July 23, 1835". *Lancet,* Pt. 2 (1834-35): 553.

ANON., "Dr. Prichard *on the Physical History of Mankind'*. *British and Foreign Medical Review* 3 (1837): 365-76.

ANON., "Prichard's Retrospect Address". *Transactions of the Provincial Medical and Surgical Association* 4 (1837): 159-60.

ANON., notice in *British and Foreign Medical Review* 12 (1841): 519.

ANON., "Dr. Prichard's *Natural History of Man*". *British and Foreign Medical Review* 13 (1842): 522.

ANON., "Prichard *on the Natural History of Man*". *British and Foreign Medical Review* 15 (1843): 180-83.

ANON., "The Physical History of Man". *North British Review* 4 (1844): 177-201.

ANON., "Prichard's Natural History of Man". *Dublin Review* 19 (1845): 67-98.

ANON., "Prichard's *Physical History of Mankind*". *New Quarterly Review* 8 (1846): 95-134.

ANON., notice in *Gentleman's Magazine* n.s., 27 (1847): 398.

ANON., notice in *London Medical Gazette* 4 (1847): 248-49.

ANON., "Physical History of Mankind". *Prospective Review* 3 (1847): 355-69.

ANON., "Ethnology – The Unity of Mankind". "Report of the Seventeenth Meeting of the British Association for the Advancement of Science, Held at Oxford, in June, 1847". *British Quarterly Review* 10 (1849): 408-40.

Other Anonymous Items

ANON., "Abstract of the Proceedings of the Medical Section of the Meeting of the British Association for the Advancement of Science held at Bristol, in August, 1836". *British and Foreign Medical Review* 2 (1836): 594-601.

ANON., "Anthropological Review". *Journal of the Anthropological Society of London* 6 (1868): i-cxcvii.

ANON., *Description of the Egyptian Tomb, Discovered by G. Belzoni* (London: John Murray, 1821).

ANON., "Natural History of the Human Race". *Monthly Review* n.s., 3 (1826): 505-15.

ANON., "Obituary of John Bishop Estlin". *Bristol Mirror,* 16 June 1855.

ANON., "Obituary of Thomas Hancock", *London Medical Gazette* 8 (1849): 790.

ANON., "On the Life, Character, Opinions, and Cerebral Development, of Rajah Rammohun Roy", *Phrenological Journal* 8 (1832-34): 577-603.

ANON., review of Ramohun Roy's *Translation of an Abridgement of the Vedant. Monthly Review* 2nd s., 92 (1820): 173-77.

ANON., review of the 7th edition of the *Encyclopaedia Britannica. The Friends' Monthly Magazine* 1, no. XII, tenth month (1831).

ANON., "The Natural History of the Varieties of Man". *Prospective Review* 6 (1850): 449-58.

ANON., "Townsend *on the Character of Moses as an Historian*". *British*

Review 6 (1815): 26-50.

ANON., "Zimmerman's [sic] *Geographical History of Man*". *Monthly Review* 80 (1789): 678-90.

PUBLISHED SOURCES

AARSLEFF, HANS, *The Study of Language in England, 1780-1860* (Minneapolis: University of Minnesota Press, 1983 (1967)).

AARSLEFF, HANS and LOUIS G. KELLY, HANS-JOSEF NIEDEREHE, eds, *Papers in the History of Linguistics, Studies in the History of the Language Sciences* 38 (Amsterdam: J. Benjamins, 1987).

ADRADOS, FRANCISCO R., "Bopp's Image of Indo-European and Some Recent Interpretations". In *Bopp-Symposium*, ed. Reinhard Sternemann, pp. 5-14.

ALFORD, HENRY, "The Bristol Infirmary in My Student Days, 1822-1828". *Bristol Medico-Chirurgical Journal* 8 (1890): 165-91.

ALTSCHULE, MARK D., "The Concept of Civilization as a Social Evil in the Writings of Mid-Nineteenth Century Psychiatrists". In *idem*, *Essays in the History of Psychiatry*, 2nd rev. ed. (New York, London: Grune & Stratton, 1965): 119-39.

AMRINGE, WILLIAM FREDERICK VAN, *An Investigation of the Theories of the Natural History of Man, by Lawrence, Prichard, and Others Founded Upon Animal Analogies: and an Outline of a New Natural History of Man, Founded Upon History, Anatomy, Physiology, and Human Analogies* (New York: Baker and Scribner, 1848).

ANNESLEY, GEORGE, *The Rise of Modern Egypt. A Century and a Half of Egyptian History 1798-1957* (Edinburgh: The Pentland Press, 1994).

APPEL, TOBY, *The Cuvier-Geoffroy Debate: French Biology in the Decades before Darwin* (Oxford: Oxford University Press, 1987).

ARENS, HANS, *Sprachwissenschaft. Der Gang ihrer Entwicklung von der Antike bis zur Gegenwart*, 2nd enl. ed. (Freiburg, München: Karl Alber, 1969).

ARNOLD, THOMAS, *Introductory Lectures on Modern History* (Oxford: John Henry Parker, 1842).

ARX, JEFFREY PAUL VON, *Progress and Pessimism. Religion, Politics, and History in Late Nineteenth Century Britain* (Cambridge, Mass.: Harvard University Press, 1985).

ASSMANN, JAN, *Monotheismus und Kosmotheismus. Ägyptische Formen eines 'Denkens des Einen' und ihre europäische Rezeptionsgeschichte* (Heidelberg: C. Winter, 1993).

———, *Moses the Egyptian. The Memory of Egypt in Western Monotheism*

Bibliography

(Cambridge, Mass.: Harvard University Press, 1997).

AUDOUIN, JEAN VICTOR *et al.*, *Le règne animal distribué d'après son organisation*, 3rd ed., 22 vols (Paris: Fortin, Masson, 1836-49).

AUGSTEIN, H. F.,

――――, "Introduction". In *eadem*, ed., *Race. The Origins of an Idea, 1760-1850* (Bristol: Thoemmes Press, 1996), pp. ix-xxxiii.

――――, "James C. Prichard's Views of Mankind. An Anthropologist Between the Enlightenment and the Victorian Age" (Ph.D. diss., University College London, 1996).

――――, entry for James Cowles Prichard, *New DNB*, forthcoming.

――――, "Paradise On Mount Caucasus – How Physiologists Envisioned 'The Origins Of Mankind: A Contribution To The Prehistory Of Racial Theory'". In *Race, Science and Medicine: Racial Categories and the Production of Medical Knowledge circa 1700-1960*, ed. Waltraud Ernst, Bernard Harris (London: Routledge, forthcoming).

AZARA, FÉLIX DE, *Voyages dans l'Amérique Méridionale, depuis 1781-1801*, 4 vols (Paris: printed for Dentu, 1809).

BANTON, MICHAEL, *Racial Theories* (Cambridge: Cambridge University Press, 1987).

BARFOOT, MICHAEL, "James Gregory (1753-1821) and Scottish Scientific Metaphysics. 1750-1800" (Ph.D. diss., University of Edinburgh, 1983).

[BARROW, JOHN], "Belzoni's *Operations and Discoveries in Egypt*". *Quarterly Review* 24 (1820-21): 139-69.

BARZUN, JACQUES, *Race: A Study in Superstition*, rev. ed. (New York: Harper and Row, 1965).

BECK, HANNO, *Carl Ritter. Genius der Geographie* (Berlin: Dietrich Reimer Verlag, 1979).

――――, "Carl Ritter als Geograph". In *Carl Ritter – Geltung und Deutung*, ed. Karl Lenz, pp. 13-36.

BEDDOE, JOHN, *The Races of Britain. A Contribution to the Anthropology of Western Europe*, 1885. Reprint, intr. David Elliston Allen (London: Hutchinson, 1971).

BENDYSHE, THOMAS, ed., *The Anthropological Treatises of Blumenbach and Hunter* (London: Green, Longman, Roberts, and Green, 1865).

BÉNÉZIT, E., ed., *Dictionnaire des peintres, sculpteurs, dessinateurs et graveurs*, 10 vols (Paris: Gründ, 1976).

BENICHOU, C. and CLAUDE BLANCKAERT, eds, *Julien-Joseph Virey: Naturaliste et Anthropologue* (Paris: Vrin, 1988).

BERNAL, MARTIN, *Black Athena. The Afroasiatic Roots of Classical Civilization*, 2 vols (London: Vintage, 1991 (1987)).

255

Bibliography

BERRIOS, GERMAN E., *The History of Mental Symptoms. Descriptive Psychopathology Since the Nineteenth Century* (Cambridge: Cambridge University Press, 1996).

BEWELL, ALAN, "'On the Banks of the South Sea': Botany and Sexual Controversy in the Late Eighteenth Century". In *Visions of Empire*, ed. David Philip Miller *et al.*, pp. 173-93.

BEYER, ARNO, *Deutsche Einflüsse auf die englische Sprachwissenschaft im 19. Jahrhundert* (Göppingen: Kümmerle, 1981).

BIDDISS, MICHAEL D., *Father of Racist Ideology. The Social and Political Thought of Count Gobineau* (London: Weidenfeld and Nicolson, 1970).

————, ed., *Images of Race* (Leicester: Leicester University Press, 1979).

————, "Arthur de Gobineau (1816-1882) and the Illusions of Progress". In *Rediscoveries*, ed. John A. Hall (Oxford: Clarendon Press, 1986), pp. 27-45.

BITTERLI, URS, "Auch Amerikaner sind Menschen. Das Erscheinungsbild des Indianers in Reiseberichten und kulturhistorischen Darstellungen vom 16. bis 18. Jahrhundert". In *Die Natur des Menschen*, ed. Gunter Mann *et al.*, pp. 15-29.

BLANCKAERT, CLAUDE, "'Les vicissitudes de l'angle facial' et les débuts de la craniométrie (1765-1875)". *Révue de synthèse* 108 (1987): 417-53.

————, "On the Origins of French Ethnology. William Edwards and the Doctrine of Race". In *Bones, Bodies, Behavior. Essays on Biological Anthropology, History of Anthropology* 5, ed. George W. Stocking (Madison: The University of Wisconsin Press, 1988), pp. 20-55.

BLUMENBACH, JOHANN FRIEDRICH, *Beyträge zur Naturgeschichte*, 2 vols (Göttingen: J. C. Dieterich, 1790-1811). Trans. *Contributions to Natural History* (1790-1811). In Thomas Bendyshe, ed., *The Anthropological Treatises of Blumenbach and Hunter*, pp. 277-340.

————, *Handbuch der Naturgeschichte*, 4th enl. ed. (Göttingen: J. C. Dieterich, 1791).

————, "Observations on Some *Egyptian* Mummies Opened in *London*". *Philosophical Transactions* 84 (1794): 177-95.

————, *De generis humani varietate nativa*, 1795. In *The Anthropological Treatises of Blumenbach and Hunter*, ed. Thomas Bendyshe, pp. 67-276.

————, *A Short System of Comparative Anatomy*, trans. William Lawrence (London: Longman, Hurst, Rees, Orme, 1807 (1805)).

————, *The Institutions of Physiology*, trans. John Elliotson, 2nd ed. (London: printed by Bensley for E. Cox, 1817 (1810, German orig. 1798)).

BOBZIN, HARTMUT, "Christian Carl Josias von Bunsen und sein Beitrag zum Studium orientalischer Sprachen". In *Universeller Geist und guter Europäer. Christian Carl Josias von Bunsen 1791-1860. Beiträge zu Leben und Werk des "gelehrten Diplomaten"*, ed. H.-R. Ruppel (Korbach: Wilhelm Bing, 1991), pp. 81-102.

BODENHEIMER, F. S., "Zimmermann's *Specimen Zoologiae Geographicae Quadrupedum*, a Remarkable Zoogeographical Publication at the End of the Eighteenth Century". *Archives internationales d'histoire des sciences* 8 (1955): 351-57.

BOLT, CHRISTINE, *Victorian Attitudes to Race* (London: Routledge and Kegan Paul, 1971).

BOPP, FRANZ, *Die Celtischen Sprachen in ihrem Verhältnisse zum Sanskrit, Zend, Griechischen, Lateinischen, Germanischen, Litthauischen und Slawischen* (Berlin: Dümmler, 1839).

BOWLER, PETER J., "Bonnet and Buffon: Theories on Generation and the Problem of Species". *Journal of the History of Biology* 6 (1973): 259-81.

———, *The Fontana History of the Environmental Sciences* (London: Fontana Press, 1992).

BRADLEY, IAN, *The Call to Seriousness: the Evangelical Impact on the Victorians* (London: Cape, 1976).

BREUER, EDWARD, *The Limits of the Enlightenment. Jews, Germans, and the Eighteenth-Century Study of Scripture* (Cambridge, Mass.: Harvard University Press, 1996).

BRISTOL INSTITUTION, *Proceedings of the Annual Meeting, Held February 8, 1827* (Bristol: J. Mills, 1827).

The Bristol Poll... (Bristol: J. Wansbrough, 1833).

BROBERG, GUNNAR, "Homo Sapiens: Linnaeus's Classification of Man". In *Linnaeus: The Man and his Work*, ed. T. Frängsmyr (Berkeley: University of California Press, 1983), pp. 156-94.

BROCA, PIERRE PAUL, "La linguistique et l'anthropologie". *Bulletins de la société d'anthropologie de Paris* 3 (1862): 264-319.

———, *On the Phenomena of Hybridity in the Genus Homo*, ed. C. Carter Blake (London: Anthropological Society of London, 1864).

BROOKE, JOHN HEDLEY, *Science and Religion. Some Historical Perspectives* (Cambridge: Cambridge University Press, 1991).

BROWNE, JANET, *The Secular Ark. Studies in the Historiography of Biogeography* (New Haven: Yale University Press, 1983).

BRUCE, JAMES, *Travels to Discover the Source of the Nile in the Years 1768, 1769, 1770, 1771, 1772, and 1773*, 3rd ed., 8 vols, ed. Alexander Murray (Edinburgh: A. Constable, Manners & Miller, 1813).

BRYANT, JACOB, *A New System; or an Analysis of Ancient Mythology Wherein an Attempt is Made to Divest Tradition of Fable and to Reduce the Truth to its Original Purity*, 3 vols (London: T. Payne, 1774-76).

BUFFON, GEORGES-LOUIS LECLERC, COMTE DE, *Natural History, General and Particular*, trans. William Smellie, 9 vols (Edinburgh: printed for William Creech, 1780 (1749ff.)).

BUNSEN, CHRISTIAN CARL JOSIAS VON, "On the Results of the Recent Egyptian Researches in Reference to Asiatic and African Ethnology, and the Classification of Languages." In Christian Carl Josias Bunsen, Charles Meyer, Max Müller, *Three Linguistic Dissertations. Read at the Meeting of the British Association in Oxford* (from the *Report of the British Association for the Advancement of Science* for 1847) (London: Richard and John E. Taylor, 1848), pp. 254-99.

————, *A Memoir of Baron Bunsen*, ed. Frances Bunsen, 2 vols (London: Longmans, Green, and Co., 1868).

BUNZL, MATTI, "Franz Boas and the Humboldtian Tradition. From Volksgeist and *Nationalcharakter* to an Anthropological Concept of Culture". In *Volksgeist as Method and Ethic*, ed. George W. Stocking Jr, pp. 17- 78.

BURCKHARDT JR, R. W., "Lamarck, Evolution and the Politics of Science". *Journal of the History of Biology* 3 (1970): 275-98.

————, *The Spirit of System: Lamarck and Evolutionary Biology* (Cambridge, Mass.: Harvard University Press, 1977).

BURROW, JOHN, *Evolution and Society. A Study in Victorian Social Theory* (Cambridge: Cambridge University Press, 1966).

————, "The Uses of Philology in Victorian England". In *Ideas and Institutions of Victorian England. Essays in Honour of George Kitson Clark*, ed. Robert Robson (London: Bell, 1967), 180-204.

————, *A Liberal Descent, Victorian Historians and the English Past* (Cambridge: Cambridge University Press, 1981).

BUSH, GRAHAM, *Bristol and its Municipal Government, 1820-1850* (Bristol: printed for the Record Society, 1976).

BÜTTNER, MANFRED, "Zur Beziehung zwischen Geographie, Theologie und Philosophie im Denken Carl Ritters". In *Carl Ritter – Geltung und Deutung*, ed. Karl Lenz, pp. 75-91.

BYNUM, W. F., "Time's Noblest Offspring: The Problem of Man in the British Natural Historical Sciences, 1800-1863" (Ph.D. diss., University of Cambridge, 1974).

————, "The Great Chain of Being After Forty Years: An Appraisal". *History of Science* 13 (1975): 1-28.

————, "Varieties of Cartesian Experience in Early Nineteenth Century Neurophysiology". In *Philosophical Dimensions of the Neuro-*

Medical Sciences, ed. S. F. Spicker, H. T. Engelhardt (Dordrecht: Reidel, 1976), pp. 15-33.

————, "The Cardinal's Brother: Francis Newman, Victorian Bourgeois". In *Enlightenment, Passion and Modernity: Essays in Honor of Peter Gay*, ed. M. Micale, R. Dietle (Palo Alto: Stanford University Press, 1999).

CANNON, GARLAND, *Oriental Jones: A Biography* (London: Indian Council for Cultural Relations, 1964).

————, "Sir William Jones and Applied Linguistics". In *Papers in the History of Linguistics*, ed. Hans Aarsleff *et al.*, pp. 379-89.

CANNON, SUSAN F., *Science in Culture: The Early Victorian Period* (New York: Dawson and Science History Publications, 1978).

————, "Humboldtian Science". In *eadem, Science in Culture*, pp. 73-110.

————, "The Cambridge Network". In *eadem, Science in Culture*, pp. 29-71.

CARLSON, ERIC T. and NORMAN DAIN, "The Meaning of Moral Insanity". *Bulletin of the History of Medicine* 36 (1962): 130-40.

CARPENTER, LANT, *A Review of the Labours, Opinions, and Character of Rajah Rammohun Roy; in a Discourse, on Occasion of his Death, Delivered in Lewin's Mead Chapel, Bristol...* (London: R. Hunter, 1833).

[CARPENTER, WILLIAM BENJAMIN], "Ethnology or the Science of Races". *Edinburgh Review* 88 (1848): 429-87.

CAVALLI-SFORZA, L. LUCA and PAOLO MENOZZI, ALBERTO PIAZZA, *The History and Geography of Human Genes* (Princeton: Princeton University Press, 1994).

CERAM, C. W., *Gods, Graves and Scholars in Documents* (London: Thames and Hudson, 1965).

CHADWICK, OWEN, *The Secularization of the European Mind in the Nineteenth Century* (Cambridge: Cambridge University Press, 1975).

CHAMBERLIN, J. EDWARD and SANDER L. GILMAN, eds., *Degeneration. The Dark Side of Progress* (New York: Columbia University Press, 1985).

CHAMBERS, ROBERT, *Vestiges of the Natural History of Creation*, 12th ed. (Edinburgh, London: Chambers, 1884 (1844)).

CHAMPOLLION, JEAN-FRANÇOIS, *Lettre à M. Dacier, Secrétaire Perpétuel de l'Académie royale des inscriptions et belles-lettres, relative à l'alphabet des hiéroglyphes phonétiques...* (Paris: Firmin Didot, 1822).

CHAMPOLLION-FIGEAC, JEAN-JACQUES, *L'univers. Histoire et déscription de tous les peuples anciennes. Egypte ancienne* (Paris: Firmin Didot, 1839).

CLARK, MICHAEL, "'Morbid Introspection', Unsoundness of Mind, and British Psychological Medicine, c. 1830-1900". In *The Anatomy of Madness*, ed. W. F. Bynum, Roy Porter, Michael Shepherd, 3 vols (London, vols 1 and 2: Tavistock; vol. 3: Routledge, 1985-88).

CLARKE, EDWIN and L. S. JACYNA, *Nineteenth-Century Origins of Neuroscientific Concepts* (Berkeley: University of California Press, 1987).

CODRINGTON, ROBERT HENRY, "Religious Beliefs and Practices in Melanesia". *Journal of the Anthropological Institute* 10 (1881): 261-316.

COFFIN, JEAN-CHRISTOPHE, "Is Modern Civilization Sick? The Response of Alienists in Mid-Nineteenth Century France". In *Proceedings of the 1st European Congress on the History of Psychiatry and Mental Health Care*, ed. Leonie de Goei, Joost Vijselaar (Rotterdam: Erasmus, 1993), pp. 267-75.

COHN, NORMAN, *Noah's Flood. The Genesis Story of Western Thought* (New Haven: Yale University Press, 1996).

COOTER, ROGER, *The Cultural Meaning of Popular Science. Phrenology and the Organization of Consent in Nineteenth-Century Britain* (Cambridge: Cambridge University Press, 1984).

CORSI, PIETRO, *Science and Religion: Baden Powell and the Anglican Debate 1800-1860* (Cambridge: Cambridge University Press, 1988).

COWLING, MARY, *The Artist as Anthropologist. The Representation of Type and Character in Victorian Art* (Cambridge: Cambridge University Press, 1989).

CRABBS, JACK A., *The Writing of History in Nineteenth-Century Egypt. A Study in National Transformation* (Cairo: The American University in Cairo Press, 1984).

CRICHTON, ALEXANDER, *An Inquiry into the Nature and Origin of Mental Derangement, Comprehending a Concise System of the Physiology and Pathology of the Human Mind and a History of the Passions and their Effects*, 2 vols (London: T. Cadell Jr and W. Davies, 1798).

CROSS, S. J., "John Hunter, the Animal Oeconomy, and Late Eighteenth Century Physiological Discourse". *Studies in the History of Biology* 5 (1981): 1-110.

CULL, RICHARD, "Short Biographical Notice of the Author". In Prichard, *The Natural History of Man*, 4 ed., 2 vols, ed. Edwin Nossis (London: Balliéré, 1855), vre. 1, pp. xxi-xxiv

CULLER, A. DWIGHT, *The Victorian Mirror of History* (New Haven, London: Yale University Press, 1985).

CUNNINGHAM, ANDREW and NICHOLAS JARDINE, eds, *Romanticism and the*

Sciences (Cambridge: Cambridge University Press, 1990).

CUVIER, GEORGES, *Recherches sur les ossemens fossiles de quadrupèdes où l'on rétablit des caractères de plusieurs espèces d'animaux que les révolutions du globe paroissent avoir détruites*, 4 vols (Paris: Deterville, 1812).

———, *Discours sur les révolutions de la surface du globe, et sur les changemens qu'elles ont produits dans le règne animal*, 3rd rev. ed. (Paris: G. Dufour and Editions d'Ocagne, 1825 (1812)).

DALE, PETER ALLAN, *The Victorian Critic and the Idea of History* (Cambridge, Mass.: Harvard University Press, 1977).

DANIEL, GLYN, *The Idea of Prehistory* (Harmondsworth: Penguin, 1964 (1962)).

———, *The Origins and Growth of Archaeology* (Harmondsworth: Penguin, 1967).

DARWIN, CHARLES, *Voyage of the Beagle. Journal of Researches*, 1839, ed. Janet Browne, Michael Neve (Harmondsworth: Penguin Books, 1989).

———, *Metaphysics, Materialism, and the Evolution of the Mind. Early Writings of Charles Darwin*, ed. Paul H. Barrett (Chicago: University of Chicago Press, 1980 (1974)).

DARWIN, ERASMUS, *Zoonomia or, the Laws of Organic Life*, 2 vols (London: printed for J. Johnson, 1794-96).

DASGUPTA, B. N., *The Life and Times of Rajah Ramohun Roy* (New Delhi: Ambika, 1980).

DEMANDT, ALEXANDER, *Der Fall Roms. Die Auflösung des römischen Reiches im Urteil der Nachwelt* (München: Beck, 1984).

DESMOND, ADRIAN, *Archetypes and Ancestors. Palaeontology in Victorian London 1850-1875* (London: Blond and Briggs, 1982).

———, *The Politics of Evolution. Morphology, Medicine, and Reform in Radical London* (Chicago: University of Chicago Press, 1992 (1989)).

DESMOULINS, LOUIS-ANTOINE, *Histoire naturelle des races humaines ... d'après des recherches spéciales d'antiquités, de physiologie, d'anatomie et de zoologie* (Paris: Treuttel, 1826).

DETELBACH, MICHAEL, "Humboldtian Science". In *Cultures of Natural History*, ed. N. Jardine *et al.*, pp. 287-304.

Dictionary of National Biography, ed. Leslie Stephen, Sidney Lee, 63 vols (London: Smith, Elder & Co., 1885-1900).

DIEFFENBACH, LORENZ, *Celtica I. Sprachliche Documente zur Geschichte der Kelten; zugleich als Beitrag zur Sprachforschung überhaupt* (Stuttgart: Imle & Liesching, 1839).

DONALDSON, JOHN WILLIAM, *The New Cratylus, or Contributions Towards a*

More Accurate Knowledge of the Greek Language (Cambridge: J. and J. J. Deighton, 1839).

DÖRNER, KLAUS, *Bürger und Irre*, 2nd rev. ed. (Frankfurt: Syndikat/EVA, 1984).

DOUGHERTY, FRANK W. P., "Buffons Bedeutung für die Entwicklung des anthropologischen Denkens im Deutschland der zweiten Hälfte des 18. Jahrhunderts". In *Die Natur des Menschen*, ed. Gunter Mann *et al.*, pp. 221-79.

———, "Christoph Meiners und Johann Friedrich Blumenbach im Streit um den Begriff der Menschenrasse". In *Die Natur des Menschen*, ed. Gunter Mann *et al.*, pp. 89-111.

———, "Johann Friedrich Blumenbach und Samuel Thomas Soemmerring: Eine Auseinandersetzung in anthropologischer Hinsicht". In *Samuel Thomas Soemmerring und die Gelehrten der Goethezeit*, ed. Gunter Mann, Jost Benedum, Werner Kümmel (Stuttgart: Gustav Fischer, 1988), pp. 35-56.

DUCHET, MICHÈLE, *Anthropologie et histoire au siècle des lumières. Buffon, Voltaire, Rousseau, Helvétius, Diderot* (Paris: F. Maspéro, 1971).

DYCK, JOACHIM, *Athen und Jerusalem. Die Tradition der argumentativen Verknüpfung von Bibel und Poesie im 17. und 18. Jahrhundert* (München: Beck, 1977).

EARLE, PLINY, *Institutions for the Insane in Prussia, Austria and Germany* (New York: Wood, 1854).

EDWARDS, WILLIAM FRÉDÉRIC, *Des caractères physiologiques des races humaines considérés dans leurs rapports avec l'histoire: Lettre à Amédée Thierry* (Paris: Compère jeune, 1829).

———, *De l'influence des agents physiques sur la vie (1824): On the Influence of Physical Agents on Life*, trans. T. Hodgkin, W. Fisher (London: printed for S. Highley, 1832).

———, "Fragments d'un mémoire sur les Gaëls". *Mémoires de la société ethnologique* 2 (1845): 13-47.

EICHTAHL, GUSTAVE D', "Mémoire sur l'anthropologie ou de l'histoire naturelle de l'homme". Procès-verbal de la séance du 26 mai 1843, *Mémoires de la société ethnologique* 2 (1845): xxxvii-xl.

EIGEN, JOEL PETER, *Witnessing Insanity: Madness and Mad-Doctors in the English Court* (New Haven: Yale University Press, 1995).

EMCH-DÉRIAZ, ANTOINETTE, "The Non-Naturals Made Easy". In *The Popularization of Medicine 1650-1850*, ed. Roy Porter (London: Routledge, 1992), pp. 134-59.

Encyclopaedia Britannica, ed. Robert Cox, Thomas Stewart Traill, 6th ed., 20 vols (Edinburgh: A. Constable & Co., 1823).

Encyclopaedia Britannica, ed. Thomas Spencer Baines, William Robertson

Smith, 9th ed., 24 vols (Edinburgh: A. & C. Black, 1875-89).

Encyclopaedia Britannica, ed. Hugh Chisholm, 11th ed., 29 vols (Cambridge: Cambridge University Press, 1911).

ESQUIROL, JEAN ETIENNE DOMINIQUE, *Des Passions, considérées comme causes, symptômes et moyens curatifs de l'aliénation mentale* (Paris: Didot Jeune, AN XIV [1805]).

————, "Monomanie". In *idem, Des maladies mentales considérées sous les rapports médical, hygiénique et médico-légal*, 2 vols (Paris: J.-B. Baillière, 1838).

EVANS, ARTHUR WILLIAM, *Warburton and the Warburtonians. A Study in Some Eighteenth-Century Controversies* (Oxford: Oxford University Press, 1932).

F. E...S [sic], ANDREW HORN, JAMES COWLES PRICHARD, "On the Cosmogony of Moses". *The Philosophical Magazine* 46 (1815): 285-92; 47 (1816): 9-11, 110-17, 241-43, 258-63, 339-44, 346-48, 431-34; 48 (1816): 18-22, 111-17, 201, 276-78, 300.

FAGAN, BRYAN M., *The Rape of the Nile. Tomb Robbers, Tourists, and Archaeologists* (New York: Charles Scribner's Sons, 1975).

FARBER, PAUL L., "Buffon and the Concept of Species". *Journal of the History of Biology* 5 (1982): 259-84.

FELDMAN, BURTON and ROBERT D. RICHARDSON, *The Rise of Modern Mythology 1680-1860* (Bloomington: Indiana University Press, 1972).

FINK, KARL J., "Storm and Stress Anthropology". *History of the Human Sciences* 6 (1993): 51-71.

FONTANA, BIANCAMARIA, *Rethinking the Politics of Commercial Society: the Edinburgh Review 1802-1832* (Cambridge: Cambridge University Press, 1985).

FORBES, DUNCAN, *The Liberal Anglican Idea of History* (Cambridge: Cambridge University Press, 1952).

FORBES, J. and A. TWEEDIE, J. CONOLLY, eds, *The Cyclopaedia of Practical Medicine*, 4 vols (London: Sherwood, Gilbert, Piper, 1833-35).

FOUCAULT, MICHEL, *The Order of Things. An Archaeology of the Human Sciences* (London: Tavistock, 1970 (1966)).

FOX, CHRISTOPHER and ROY PORTER, ROBERT WOKLER, eds., *Inventing Human Science. Eighteenth-Century Domains* (Berkeley: University of California Press, 1995).

GALL, FRANZ JOSEPH and GASPAR [sic] SPURZHEIM, *Anatomie et physiologie du système nerveux en général, et du cerveau en particulier, avec des observations sur la possibilité de reconnoître plusieurs dispositions intellectuelles et morales de l'homme et des animaux, par la configuration de leurs têtes*, 5 vols (Paris: printed by F. Schoell for the Bibliothèque Grècque-Latine-Allemande, 1810-19).

[GARNETT, RICHARD], "Prichard *on the Celtic Languages*". *Quarterly Review* 57 (1836): 80-110.

GEISS, IMMANUEL, *Geschichte des Rassismus* (Frankfurt am Main: Suhrkamp Verlag, 1988).

GELDBACH, ERICH, *Der gelehrte Diplomat. Zum Wirken Christian Carl Josias Bunsens* (Leiden: E. J. Brill, 1980).

GIBBON, EDWARD, *Memoirs of My Life*, ed. Georges A. Bonnard (London: Nelson, 1966).

GILLISPIE, CHARLES COULSTON, *Genesis and Geology. A Study in the Relations of Scientific Thought, Natural Theology, and Social Opinion in Great Britain, 1790-1850* (Cambridge, Mass.: Harvard University Press, 1969 (1951)).

————, ed., *Dictionary of Scientific Biography*, 14 vols (New York: Charles Scribner's Sons, 1970-76).

————, *Science and Polity in France at the End of the Old Regime* (Princeton: Princeton University Press, 1980).

GILMAN, STUART C., "Political Theory and Degeneration: From Left to Right, from Up to Down". In *Degeneration. The Dark Side of Progress*, ed. J. Edward Chamberlin *et al.*, pp. 165-98.

GOBINEAU, ARTHUR DE, *Essai sur l'inégalité des races humaines*, 4 vols (Paris: Firmin Didot, 1853-55).

————, *Essai sur l'inégalité des races humaines*, 2nd ed., 2 vols (Paris: Firmin Didot, 1884).

GOLDSTEIN, JAN, *Console and Classify. The French Psychiatric Profession in the Nineteenth Century* (Cambridge: Cambridge University Press, 1987).

GÖRG, MANFRED, *Die Beziehungen zwischen dem alten Israel und Ägypten. Von den Anfängen bis zum Exil* (Darmstadt: Wissenschaftliche Buchgesellschaft, 1997).

GOSSMAN, LIONEL, "Augustin Thierry and Liberal Historiography". *History and Theory*, Beiheft 15 (1976): 3-83.

GRAY, J. E. GRAY and THOMAS HODGKIN, J. C. PRICHARD, *Queries Respecting the Human Race, to be Addressed to Travellers and Others, Drawn up by a Committee of the British Association for the Advancement of Science, Appointed in 1838* (London: Richard and John E. Taylor, 1841).

GREGORY, FREDERICK, "Kant's Influence on Natural Scientists in the German Romantic Period". In *New Trends in the History of Science. Proceedings of a Conference held at the University of Utrecht*, ed. Robert Visser *et al.* (Amsterdam: Rodopi, 1989), pp. 53-66.

Bibliography

GROSS, MARTIN L., "The Lessened Focus of Feeling: A Transformation in French Physiology in the Early Nineteenth Century". *Journal of the History of Biology* 12 (1979): 231-71.

[GROVE, WILLIAM ROBERT], "Natural History of Man". *Blackwood's Magazine* 56 (1844): 312-30.

GUERRA, FRANCISCO, "Felix de Azara". In *Dictionary of Scientific Biography*, ed. C. C. Gillispie, 1: 351-52.

GUTCH, JOHN MATHEW, *Observations or Notes Upon the Writings of the Ancients Upon the Materials which they Used, and Upon the Introduction of the Art of Printing; Being Four Papers Read Before the Philosophical and Literary Society, Annexed to the Bristol Institution, at their Evening Meetings in 1827* (Bristol: J. M. Gutch, 1827).

HALE, MATTHEW, *The Primitive Origination of Mankind, Considered and Examined According to the Light of Nature* (London: printed for William Shrowsbery, 1672).

HAMILTON, WILLIAM, *Remarks on Several Parts of Turkey. Part I. Ægyptiaca, or some Account of the Antient and Modern State of Egypt, as Obtained in the Years 1801, 1802* (London: printed for T. Payne, Cadell and Davies, 1809).

HANCOCK, THOMAS, *Essay on Instinct and Its Physical and Moral Relations* (London: William Phillips, George Yard *et al.*; Edinburgh: W. & C. Tait, 1824).

HARE, EDWARD, "The History of 'Nervous Disorders' from 1600 to 1840, and a Comparison with Modern Views". *British Journal of Psychiatry* 159 (1991): 37-45.

HARRISON, J. M., "The Crowd of Bristol 1790-1835" (Ph.D. diss., University of Cambridge, 1983).

HARRISON, ROSS, *Bentham* (London: Routledge, Kegan Paul, 1983).

HARTWICH, WOLF-DANIEL, *Die Sendung Moses* (München: Wilhelm Fink Verlag, 1997).

HASLAM, JOHN, *Medical Jurisprudence as it Relates to Insanity, According to the Law of England* (London: C. Hunter, 1817).

HENRIQUES, URSULA R. Q., *Before the Welfare State: Social Administration in Early Industrial Britain* (London: Longmans, 1979).

HERBERT, SANDRA, "Between Genesis and Geology: Darwin and Some Contemporaries in the 1820s and 1830s". In *Religion and Irreligion in Victorian Society. Essays in honor of R. K. Webb*, ed. R. W. Davis, R. J. Helmstadter (London, New York: Routledge, 1992), pp. 68-84.

HERDER, JOHANN GOTTFRIED, *Ideen zur Geschichte der Menschheit*, 3 parts, ed. Julian Schmidt, 1784-91 (Leipzig: Brockhaus, 1869).

HERVEY, NICHOLAS, "The Lunacy Commission 1845-60, with Special Reference to the Implementation of Policy in Kent and Surrey" (Ph.D. diss., Bristol University, 1987).

HILTON, BOYD, *The Age of Atonement. The Influence of Evangelicalism on Social and Economic Thought, 1785-1865, 2nd ed.* (Oxford: Oxford University Press, 1991 (1988)).

HOBSBAWM, ERIC, *The Age of Capital 1848-1875* (London: Abacus, 1977 (1975)).

HODGEN, MARGARET, *The Doctrine of Survivals: A Chapter in the History of Scientific Method in the Study of Man* (London: Allenson & Co., 1936).

HODGKIN, THOMAS, "Biographical Notice of Dr. Prichard". *British Foreign and Medical Review* 27 (1849): 550-59.

———, "Obituary of Dr. Prichard". *Journal of the Ethnological Society of London* 2 (1848-50): 182-207.

HOENIGSWALD, HENRY M. and LINDA F. WIENER, eds, *Biological Metaphor and Cladistic Classification: An Interdisciplinary Perspective* (Philadelphia: University of Pennsylvania Press, 1987).

[HOLLAND, HENRY], "Natural History of Man". *Quarterly Review* 86 (1849-50): 1-40.

HOME, HENRY, LORD KAMES, *Sketches of the History of Man*, 2nd ed., 4 vols (Edinburgh: printed for W. Creech, 1788).

HORSMAN, REGINALD, "Origins of Racial Anglo-Saxonism in Great Britain Before 1850". *Journal of the History of Ideas* 37 (1976): 387-410.

HUDSON, NICHOLAS, "From 'Nation' to 'Race': The Origin of Racial Classification in Eighteenth-Century Thought". *Eighteenth-Century Studies* 29 (1996): 247-64.

HUMBOLDT, ALEXANDER VON, *ΚΟΣΜΟΣ. A General Survey of the Physical Phenomena of the Universe*, trans. Augustin Prichard, 2 vols (London: Baillière, 1845).

———, *Briefe an Christian Carl Josias Freiherr von Bunsen* (Leipzig: Brockhaus, 1869).

HUMBOLDT, WILHELM VON, *Prüfung der Untersuchungen über die Urbewohner Hispaniens vermittelst der Vaskischen* [sic] *Sprache* (Berlin: Dümmler, 1821).

———, *Über die Verschiedenheit des menschlichen Sprachbaus und ihren Einfluß auf die geistige Entwickelung des Menschengeschlechts*, 1836 (London: Routledge, Thoemmes, 1995).

——— and AUGUST WILHELM SCHLEGEL, *Briefwechsel*, ed. Albert Leitzmann, introd. B. Delbrück (Halle: Max Niemeyer, 1908).

HUME, DAVID, "Of National Characters". In *idem, The Philosophical Works*, 4 vols, ed. Thomas H. Green, Thomas H. Grose, 1882-86.

Reprint (Aalen: Scientia Verlag, 1964), 3: 244-58.

HUNTER, JOHN, "Observations Tending to Show That the Wolf, Jackal, and Dog, are all of the Same Species" (1787-1789). In *The Works of John Hunter*, ed. James F. Palmer, annotated by Richard Owen, 4 vols (London: Longman, Rees, Orme, Brown, Green, and Longman, 1837), 4: 319-30.

IGGERS, GEORG C., *The German Conception of History: The National Tradition of Historical Thought from Herder to the Present* (Middletown, Conn.: Wesleyan University Press, 1968).

ISICHEI, ELISABETH, *Victorian Quakers* (London: Oxford University Press, 1970).

IVERSEN, ERIK, *The Myth of Egypt and its Hieroglyphs in European Tradition*, 2nd ed. (Princeton: Princeton University Press, 1993).

JACOBI, CARL WIGAND MAXIMILIAN, *Sammlungen für die Heilkunde der Gemüthskrankheiten* (Elberfeld: Schönian'sche Buchhandlung, 1830).

JACOBSON, MATTHEW FRYE, *Whiteness of a Different Color. European Immigrants and the Alchemy of Race* (Cambridge, Mass.: Harvard University Press).

JACYNA, L. S., "Somatic Theories of Mind and the Interests of Medicine in Britain, 1850-1879". *Medical History* 26 (1982): 233-58.

————, *Philosophic Whigs. Medicine, Science and Citizenship in Edinburgh, 1789-1848* (London, New York: Routledge, 1994).

JAMES, LAWRENCE, *The Rise and Fall of the British Empire* (London: Little, Brown and Co., 1994).

JAMES, SIMON, "The Ancient Celts, Discovery or Invention?" *British Museum Magazine* 28 (1997): 18-23.

JARDINE, N. and J. A. SECORD, E. C. SPARY, eds, *Cultures of Natural History* (Cambridge: Cambridge University Press, 1995).

JAY, ELISABETH, *The Religion of the Heart. Anglican Evangelicalism and the Nineteenth Century Novel* (Oxford: Clarendon Press, 1979).

JENKINS, IAN, "'Contemporary Minds'. Sir William Hamilton's Affair with Antiquity". In *Vases & Volcanoes*, ed. Ian Jenkins, Kim Sloan (London: British Museum Press, 1996), pp. 40-64.

JENKYNS, RICHARD, *The Victorians and Ancient Greece* (Oxford: Blackwell, 1980).

JESPERSEN, OTTO, *Language. Its Nature, Development and Origins* (London: Allen & Unwin, 1949 (1922)).

JONES, GRETA, *Social Darwinism in English Thought: The Interaction Between Biological and Social Theory* (Brighton: Harvester Press, 1980).

JONES, SIR WILLIAM, "Discourse the Ninth on the Origin and Families of

Nations, delivered 23 February, 1792". In *idem, Discourses Delivered at the Asiatick Society 1785-1792*, ed. Roy Harris (London: Routledge, Thoemmes, 1993), pp. 185-204.

———, "On the Gods of Greece, Italy, and India". In *idem, Works*, 6 vols (London: G. G. and J. Robinson, 1799), 1: 229-80.

KAPLONY-HECKEL, URSULA, "Bunsen – der erste deutsche Herold der Ägyptologie". In *Der gelehrte Diplomat*, ed. Erich Geldbach, pp. 64-83.

KASS, AMALIE M. and EDWARD H. KASS, *Perfecting the World. The Life and Times of Dr. Thomas Hodgkin 1798-1866* (Boston: Harcourt Brace Jovanovich, 1988).

KENNEDY, VANS, *Researches into the Origin and Affinity of the Principal Languages of Asia and Europe* (London: Longman, Rees, Orme, Brown and Green, 1828).

KENRICK, JOHN, An Essay on Primeval History (London: B. Fellowes, 1846.

KITCHING, JOHN, "Lecture on Moral Insanity". *British Medical Journal* 1 (1857): 334-36, 389-91, 453-56.

KLAPROTH, JULIUS, "Observations sur les racines des langues sémitiques". In Andreas Adolf de Merian, *Principes de l'étude comparative des langues* (Paris: Schubart, Heideloff; Leipzig: Ponthieu, Michelsen, 1828), pp. 209-40.

KLIGER, SAMUEL, *The Goths in England. A Study in Seventeenth and Eighteenth Century Thought* (Cambridge, Mass.: Harvard University Press, 1952).

KNIGHT, THOMAS ANDREW, "On the Economy of Bees...". *Philosophical Transactions* 97 (1807): 234-44.

———, "On the Hereditary Instinctive Propensities of Animals...". *Philosophical Transactions* 127 (1837): 365-69.

KNOX, ROBERT, *The Races of Men*, 2nd ed. (London: Henry Renshaw, 1862 (1850)).

KOEPPING, KLAUS-PETER, *Adolf Bastian and the Psychic Unity of Mankind. The Foundations of Anthropology in Nineteenth Century Germany* (St Lucia: University of Queensland Press, 1983).

KOERNER, E. F. KONRAD, *Practicing Linguistic Historiography: Selected Essays* (Amsterdam: J. Benjamins, 1989).

———, "Friedrich Schlegel and the Emergence of Historical Comparative Grammar". In *Koerner, Practicing Linguistic Historiography*, pp. 269-90.

———, "Toward a Historiography of Linguistics. 19th and 20th Century Paradigms". In *idem, Practicing Linguistic Historiography*, pp. 21-54.

Bibliography

KOERNER, LISBET, "Purposes of Linnaean Travel: A Preliminary Research Report". In *Visions of Empire*, ed. David Philip Miller *et al.*, pp. 117-52.

KOLLER, ARMIN HAJMAN, *The Theory of Environment, an Outline of the History of the Idea of Milieu, and its Present Status* (Menasha: University of Chicago Press, 1918).

KREMER, PETER, "Carl Ritters Einstellung zu den Afrikanern, Grundlagen für eine philanthropisch orientierte Afrikaforschung". In *Carl Ritter – Geltung und Deutung*, ed. Karl Lenz, pp. 127-54.

LAIRD, M. A., ed., *Bishop Heber in Northern India. Selections from Heber's Journal* (Cambridge: Cambridge University Press, 1971).

LARSON, JAMES L., *Reason and Experience. The Representation of Natural Order in the Work of Carl von Linné* (Berkeley: University of California Press, 1971).

LATHAM, ROBERT GORDON, *Natural History of the Varieties of Man* (London: John van Voorst, 1850).

————, *Man and his Migrations* (London: John van Voorst, 1851).

LATIMER, JOHN, *The Annals of Bristol*, 3 vols, 1887-1902 (Bath: Kingsmead Reprints, 1970).

LAWRENCE, CHRISTOPHER, "Medicine as Culture: Edinburgh and the Scottish Enlightenment" (Ph.D. diss., University College London, 1984).

————, "The Edinburgh Medical School and the End of the 'Old Thing' 1790-1830". *History of Universities* 7 (1988): 259-86.

LEHMANN, WILLIAM, *Henry Home, Lord Kames, and the Scottish Enlightenment: A Study in National Character and in the History of Ideas* (The Hague: M. Nijhoff, 1971).

LEIGH, DENIS, "James Cowles Prichard, M. D., 1786-1848". *Proceedings of the Royal Society of Medicine* 48 (1955): 586-90.

LEMAHIEU, D. L., *The Mind of William Paley. A Philosopher and his Age* (Lincoln: University of Nebraska Press, 1976).

LÉMONON, MICHEL, "L'idée de race et les écrivains français de la première moitié du xixe siècle". *Die neueren Sprachen* 69 (1970): 283-92.

LENERS, RUTH, *Geschichtsschreibung der Romantik im Spannungsfeld von historischem Roman und Drama. Studie zu Augustin Thierry und dem historischen Theater seiner Zeit*, Bonner romanistische Arbeiten 23 (Frankfurt, Bern: Peter Lange, 1987).

LENOIR, TIMOTHY, "Generational Factors in the Origin of *Romantische Naturphilosophie*". *Journal of the History of Biology* 11 (1978): 57-100.

————, *The Strategy of Life, Teleology and Mechanics in Nineteenth Century German Biology* (Dordrecht: Reidel, 1982).

269

LENZ, KARL, ed., *Carl Ritter – Geltung und Deutung. Beiträge des Symposiums anläßlich der Wiederkehr des 200. Geburtstages von Carl Ritter November 1979 in Berlin (West)* (Berlin: Dietrich Reimer Verlag, 1981).

LEOPOLD, JOAN, "British Applications of the Aryan Theory of Race to India, 1850-1870". *English Historical Review* 89 (1974): 578-603.

————, "Ethnic Stereotypes in Linguistics: the Case of Friedrich Max Müller (1847-51)". In *Papers in the History of Linguistics*, ed. Hans Aarsleff *et al.*, pp. 501-12.

LEVENTHAL, ROBERT S., "Language Theory, the Institution of Philology and the State: the Emergence of Philological Discourse 1770-1810". In *Papers in the History of Linguistics*, ed. Hans Aarsleff *et al.*, pp. 349-63.

LEVERE, TREVOR H., *Poetry Realized in Nature. Samuel Taylor Coleridge and Early Nineteenth-Century Science* (Cambridge: Cambridge University Press, 1982).

LINDEN, MARETA, *Untersuchungen zum Anthropologiebegriff des 18. Jahrhunderts* (Bern: Herbert Lang, 1976).

LISHMAN, WILLIAM A., *Organic Psychiatry* (Oxford: Blackwell, 1990).

LITTLE, BRYAN, *The City and County of Bristol. A Study in Atlantic Civilisation* (London: Werner Laurie, 1954).

LIVINGSTONE, DAVID, "Human Acclimatization: Perspectives on a Contested Field of Enquiry in Science, Medicine and Geography". *History of Science* 25 (1987): 359-94.

LOCKE, JOHN, *Philosophical Works*, 2 vols, ed. J. A. St. John (London: George Bell and Sons, 1905-8).

LORIMER, DOUGLAS, "Science and the Secularization of Victorian Images of Race". In *Victorian Science in Context*, ed. Bernard Lightman (Chicago: University of Chicago Press, 1997), pp. 212-35.

LUBBOCK, JOHN, *The Origin of Civilisation and the Primitive Condition of Man*, 5th ed. (London: Longmans, Green and Co., 1889 (1870)).

MacCORMACK, CAROL, "Medicine and Anthropology". In *Companion Encyclopedia of the History of Medicine*, ed. W. F. Bynum, Roy Porter, 2 vols (London: Routledge, 1993), 2: 1436-48.

MacDOUGALL, HUGH A., *Racial Myth in English History. Trojans, Teutons, and Anglo-Saxons* (Montreal: Harvest House, 1982).

MACKAY, DAVID, *In the Wake of Cook: Exploration, Science & Empire, 1780-1801* (London: Croom Helm, 1985).

————, "Agents of Empire: The Banksian Collectors and Evaluation of New Lands". In *Visions of Empire*, ed. David Philip Miller *et al.*, pp. 38-57.

MALTHUS, THOMAS ROBERT, *An Essay on the Principle of Population: A View of Its Past and Present Effects on Human Happiness, With an Inquiry Into Our Prospects Respecting the Future Removal of the Evils which it Occasions*, 2nd ed. (London: J. Johnson, 1803 (1798)).

MANN, GUNTER and JOST BENEDUM, WERNER F. KÜMMEL, eds, *Die Natur des Menschen. Probleme der physischen Anthropologie und Rassenkunde (1750-1850)* (Stuttgart: Gustav Fischer, 1990).

MANUEL, FRANK E., *The Eighteenth Century Confronts the Gods* (Cambridge, Mass.: Harvard University Press, 1959).

MARSHALL, PETER, *Bristol and the Abolition of Slavery* (Bristol: printed for the Historical Association, 1973).

MATTHEWS, WILLIAM, "The Egyptians in Scotland: The Political History of a Myth". In *Viator, Medieval and Renaissance Studies* 1 (Berkeley, Los Angeles: University of California Press, 1970), pp. 289-306.

MAYHEW, HENRY, *London Labour and the London Poor...*, 3 vols (London: George Woodfall and Sons, 1851).

MAYR, ERNST, *The Growth of Biological Thought. Diversity, Evolution, and Inheritance* (Cambridge, Mass.: The Belknap Press of Harvard University Press, 1982).

MAZZOLINI, RENATO G., "Anatomische Untersuchungen über die Haut der Schwarzen (1700-1800)". In *Die Natur des Menschen*, ed. Gunter Mann *et al.*, pp. 169-87.

————, "Il colore della pelle e l'origine ell'antropologia fisica". In *L'Epopea delle soperte*, ed. Renzo Zorzi (Florence: Leo S. Olschki, 1994), pp. 227-39.

MCLAUGHLIN, PETER, *Kant's Critique of Teleology in Biological Explanation* (Lewiston: E. Mellen Press, 1991).

MCLENNAN, JOHN FERGUSON, "Hill Tribes in India". *North British Review* 38 (1863): 392-422.

MEE, JON, *Dangerous Enthusiasm. William Blake and the Culture of Radicalism in the 1790s* (Oxford: Clarendon Press, 1992).

MEEK, RONALD, *Social Science and the Ignoble Savage* (Cambridge: Cambridge University Press, 1976).

MEIJER, MIRIAM CLAUDE, *The Anthropology of Petrus Camper* (Ann Arbor, Mich: UMI Dissertation Services, 1991).

MEINERS, CHRISTOPH, *Verschiedenheiten der Menschennaturen (die verschiedenen Menschenarten) in Asien und den Südländern, in den Ostindischen und Südseeinseln, nebst einer historischen Vergleichung der vormahligen und gegenwärtigen Bewohner dieser Continente und Eylande*, 3 vols (Tübingen: J. G. Cotta, 1811-15).

MEYER, HEINRICH, *The Age of the World. A Chapter in the History of Enlightenment* (Allentown, Pa.: Muhlenberg College, 1951).

271

MICHAELIS, JOHN DAVID, *Commentaries on the Laws of Moses*, trans. Alexander Smith, 4 vols (London: Rivington, Longman, Hurst, Rees, Orme, and Brown, 1814).

MILES, ROBERT, *Racism* (London: Routledge, 1989).

MILL, JOHN STUART and JEREMY BENTHAM, *Utilitarianism and Other Essays*, ed. Alan Ryan (London: Penguin, 1987).

———, "Coleridge". In J. S. Mill, Jeremy Bentham, *Utilitarianism and Other Essays*, pp. 177-226.

———, "Whewell on Moral Philosophy". In J. S. Mill, Jeremy Bentham, *Utilitarianism and Other Essays*, pp. 228-70.

MILLER, DAVID PHILIP, "Introduction". In *Visions of Empire*, ed. David Philip Miller *et al.*, pp. 1-18.

MILLER, DAVID PHILIP and PETER HANNS REILL, eds, *Visions of Empire. Voyages, Botany, and Representation of Nature* (Cambridge: Cambridge University Press, 1996).

MOMIGLIANO, ARNOLDO, "Ancient History and the Antiquarian". In *idem*, *The Classical Foundations of Modern Historiography* (Berkeley, Los Angeles: University of California Press, 1990).

MORRELL, JACK B., "Professors Robison and Playfair, and the Theophobia Gallica: Natural Philosophy, Religion and Politics in Edinburgh, 1789-1815". *Notes and Records of the Royal Society of London* 26 (1971): 43-63.

MORRELL, JACK B. and ARNOLD THACKRAY, *Gentlemen of Science. Early Years of the British Association for the Advancement of Science* (Oxford: Clarendon Press, 1981).

———, eds, *Gentlemen of Science. Early Correspondence of the British Association for the Advancement of Science* (London: Royal Historical Society, 1984).

MORTON, SAMUEL GEORGE, "Hybridity in Animals and Plants, Considered in Reference to the Question of the Unity of Species". *Edinburgh New Philosophical Journal* 43 (1847): 262-87.

MÜLLER, F. MAX, *Lectures on the Science of Language*, 3rd ed. (London: Longman *et al.*, 1862 (1861)).

———, *The Science of Language founded on Lectures delivered at the Royal Institution in 1861 and 1863*, 2 vols (London: Longmans, Green, and Co., 1891).

———, *My Autobiography. A Fragment* (London: Longmans *et al.*, 1901).

MÜLLER, JOHANNES VON, *An Universal History in Twenty-Four Books*, trans. J. C. Prichard, William Tothill, 3 vols (London: Longman, Hurt, Rees, Orme, and Brown, 1818).

MÜLLER, K. E., "Carl Ritter und die kulturhistorische Völkerkunde". *Padeuma* 11 (1965): 24-57.

Bibliography

NASSE, CHRISTIAN FRIEDRICH, "Ueber die Benennung und die vorläufige Eintheilung des psychischen Krankseyns". *Zeitschrift für psychische Ärzte* 1 (1818): 1-48.

NEVE, MICHAEL, "Natural Philosophy, Medicine and the Culture of Science in Provincial England: The Case of Bristol, 1780-1850, and Bath, 1750-1820" (Ph.D. diss., University College London, 1984).

————, "Orthodoxy and Fringe: Medicine in Late Georgian Bristol". In *Medical Fringe and Medical Orthodoxy 1750-1850*, ed. W. F. Bynum, Roy Porter (London: Croom Helm, 1987), pp. 40-55.

NEWMAN, FRANCIS WILLIAM, *Lectures on Logic, or on the Science of Evidence Generally Embracing Both Demonstrative and Probable Reasonings, With the Doctrine of Causation. Delivered at Bristol College in the Year 1836* (Oxford: J. H. Parker; London: J. G. and F. Rivington, 1838).

————, *Phases of Faith; or, Passages from the History of my Creed* (London: John Chapman, 1850).

NEWSOME, DAVID, *Two Classes of Men. Platonism & English Romantic Thought* (London: John Murray, 1974).

NICOLSON, MALCOLM, "Alexander von Humboldt, Humboldtian Science and the Origins of the Study of Vegetation". *History of Science* 25 (1987): 167-94.

NOORDEN, WERNER VON, *Der Kliniker Christian Friedrich Nasse 1778-1851* (Jena: G. Fischer, 1929).

NORTH, J. D., "Chronology and the Age of the World". In *Cosmology, History, and Theology*, ed. W. Yourgrau, A. D. Breck (New York: Dover; London: Constable, 1977), pp. 307-33.

NOTT, JOSIAH CLARK and GEORGE R. GLIDDON et al., *Types of Mankind: or, Ethnological Researches, Based Upon the Ancient Monuments, Paintings, Sculptures, and Crania of Races, and Upon Their Natural, Geographical, Philological, and Biblical History: Illustrated by Selections from the Inedited Papers of Samuel George Morton, M.D., and by Additional Contributions from Prof. L. Agassiz, W. Usher, and Prof. H. S. Patterson* (London: Trübner; Philadelphia: Lippincott, Gambo, 1854).

NOWEL, INGRID, "Das Leben von Giovanni Battista Belzoni". Introd. to G. Belzoni, *Entdeckungs-Reisen in Ägypten 1815-1819* (Köln: DuMont, 1982), pp. 11-17.

ODOM, HERBERT, "Prichard, James Cowles". In *Dictionary of Scientific Biography*, ed. C. C. Gillispie, 11: 136-38.

OEHLER-KLEIN, SIGRID, *Die Schädellehre Franz Joseph Galls in Literatur und Kritik des 19. Jahrhunderts, Soemmerring Forschungen* 8 (Stuttgart: Gustav Fischer Verlag, 1990).

OLENDER, MAURICE, *Les langues du paradis. Aryens et Sémites: un couple providentiel* (Paris: Gallimard, Le Seuil, 1989).

OLSON, RICHARD, *Scottish Philosophy and British Physics 1750-1880. A Study in the Foundations of the Victorian Scientific Style* (Princeton: Princeton University Press, 1975).

OSPOVAT, DOV, *The Development of Darwin's Theory. Natural History, Natural Theology & Natural Selection 1838-1859* (Cambridge: Cambridge University Press, 1981).

OWEN, A. L., *The Famous Druids. A Survey of Three Centuries of English Literature on the Druids* (Oxford: Clarendon Press, 1962).

The Oxford English Dictionary, ed. J. A. Simpson, E. S. C. Weiner, 2nd ed., 20 vols (Oxford: Clarendon Press, 1989).

PALTER, ROBERT, "Hume and Prejudice". *Hume Studies* 21 (1995): 3-23.

PANAGL, OSWALD, "Figurative Elemente in der Wissenschaftssprache von Franz BOPP". In *Bopp-Symposium*, ed. Reinhard Sternemann, pp. 195-207.

PATTERSON, HENRY S., "Memoir of the Life and Scientific Labors of Samuel George Morton". In *Types of Mankind*, ed. J. C. Nott *et al.*, pp. xvii-lvii.

PEACOCK, T. L., *The Novels*, ed. David Garnett (London: Rupert Hart-Davis, 1948).

PEARDON, THOMAS PRESTON, *The Transition in English Historical Writing, 1760-1830* (New York: Columbia University Press, 1933).

PEDERSEN, HOLGER, *Linguistic Science in the Nineteenth Century*, trans. J. W. Spargo (Cambridge: Cambridge University Press, 1931).

The Penny Cyclopaedia, ed. The Society for the Diffusion of Useful Knowledge, 27 vols (London: Charles Knight and Co., 1833-43).

PICTET, ADOLPHE, *De l'affinité des langues celtiques avec le sanscrit* (Paris: Benjamin Duprat, 1837).

PINEL, PHILIPPE, *A Treatise on Insanity*, trans. D. D. Davis (Sheffield: Cadell and Davies, 1806).

PINKERTON, JOHN, *Dissertation on the Origin and Progress of the Scythians or Goths, being an Introduction to the Ancient and Modern History of Europe* (London: John Nichols, 1787).

PLEWE, ERNST, "Carl Ritter. Von der Kompendien- zur Problemgeographie". In *Carl Ritter – Geltung und Deutung*, ed. Karl Lenz, pp. 37-53.

POCOCK, J. G. A., *The Ancient Constitution and the Feudal Law. A Study in English Historical Thought in the Seventeenth Century*, rev. ed. (Cambridge: Cambridge University Press, 1987 (1957)).

POLIAKOV, LÉON, *Le mythe Aryen. Essai sur les sources du racisme et des*

nationalismes, rev. ed. (Bruxelles: Editions Complexe, 1987
(1971)).

POPKIN, RICHARD H., "The Philosophical Bases of Modern Racism". In
*Philosophy and the Civilizing Arts. Essays Presented to H. W.
Schneider,* ed. Craig Walton, John P. Anton (Athens, Ohio: Ohio
University Press, 1974), pp. 126-65.

PORTER, ROY, *The Making of Geology. Earth Science in Britain 1660-1815*
(Cambridge: Cambridge University Press, 1977).

————, *Mind-Forg'd Manacles. A History of Madness in England from the
Restoration to the Regency* (London: Athlone Press, 1987).

POTTS, ALEX, *Flesh and the Ideal. Winckelmann and the Origins of Art
History* (New Haven: Yale University Press, 1994).

POULTON, E. B., "A Remarkable Anticipation of Modern Views on
Evolution". In *idem, Essays on Evolution* (Oxford: Clarendon,
1908).

POYNTER, J. R., *Society and Pauperism. English Ideas on Poor Relief, 1795-
1834* (London: Routledge, 1969).

PREYER, ROBERT, "Bunsen and the Anglo-American Literary Community
in Rome". In *Der gelehrte Diplomat,* ed. Erich Geldbach, pp. 35-
44.

PRICHARD, JAMES COWLES,

————, *Disputatio inauguralis de generis humani varietate* (Edinburgh:
Abernethy and Walker, 1808).

————, *Researches into the Physical History of Man,* 1813. Reprint, ed.
George W. Stocking Jr (Chicago: University of Chicago Press,
1973).

————, "Remarks on the Older Floetz Strata of England". *Annals of
Philosophy* 6 (1815): 20-26.

————, *An Analysis of the Egyptian Mythology: To which is Subjoined a
Critical Examination of the Remains of Egyptian Chronology*
(London: John and Arthur Arch, 1819).

————, *A History of the Epidemic Fever, Which Prevailed in Bristol, During
the Years 1817, 1818, and 1819; Founded on Reports of St. Peter's
Hospital and the Bristol Infirmary* (London: John and Arthur
Arch, 1820).

————, *A Treatise on Diseases of the Nervous System, Part the First:
Comprising Convulsive and Maniacal Affections* (London: Thomas
and George Underwood, 1822).

————, "Beobachtungen über die Beziehung des Gedächtnisses zum
Gehirn". *Zeitschrift für die Anthropologie* 7 (1824): 243-50.

————, *Researches into the Physical History of Mankind,* 2nd ed., 2 vols
(London: John and Arthur Arch, 1826).

————, *A Review of the Doctrine of a Vital Principle, as Maintained by Some Writers on Physiology with Observations on the Causes of Physical & Animal Life* (London: John and Arthur Arch, 1829).

————, "Horae Africanae". *The Friends' Monthly Magazine* 2, no. 13 (1830): 737-38.

————, *The Eastern Origin of the Celtic Nations Proved by a Comparison of Their Dialects With the Sanskrit, Greek, Latin, and Teutonic Languages, Forming a Supplement to Researches into the Physical History of Mankind* (Oxford: S. Collingwood, 1831).

————, "Insanity". In *The Cyclopaedia of Practical Medicine*, ed. J. Forbes *et al.*, 2: 10-32, 847-75.

————, "Soundness and Unsoundness of Mind". In *The Cyclopaedia of Practical Medicine*, ed. J. Forbes *et al.*, 4: 39-55.

————, "Temperament". In *Cyclopaedia of Practical Medicine*, ed. J. Forbes *et al.*, 4: 159-74.

————, "Remarks on the Application of Philological and Physical Researches to the History of the Human Species". In *Report of the First and Second Meetings of the British Association for the Advancement of Science; at York in 1831, and at Oxford in 1832* (London: John Murray, 1833), pp. 529-44.

————, *A Treatise on Insanity, and Other Disorders Affecting the Mind* (London: Sherwood, 1835).

————, "An Address, Delivered at the Third Anniversary Meeting of the Provincial Medical and Surgical Association, July 23rd, 1835". *The Transactions of the Provincial Medical and Surgical Association*, 4 (1836), 1-54.

————, *Researches into the Physical History of Mankind*, 3rd ed., 3 vols (London: Sherwood, Gilbert, Piper, 1836-47).

————, "Abstract of a Comparative Review of Philological and Physical Researches, as Applied to the History of the Human Species". *Edinburgh New Philosophical Journal* 26 (1838): 308-26.

————, "Letter to Dr Hodgkin". *Extracts from the Papers and Proceedings of the Aborigines Protection Society* 1, no. 2 (1839): 56-58.

————, "On the Extinction of Human Races". *Edinburgh New Philosophical Journal* 28 (1839-40): 166-70.

————, "A Clinical Lecture Delivered to the Pupils of the Bristol Infirmary". *London Medical Gazette* n.s., 1 (1840-41): 8-13.

————, "Insanity". In *The Library of Medicine*, ed. Alexander Tweedie, 8 vols (London: Whittaker and Co., 1840-42), 2: 102-42.

————, *Naturgeschichte des Menschengeschlechts*, trans. R. Wagner, J. G. F. Will, 4 vols (Leipzig: Leopold Voß, 1840-48).

————, *On the Different Forms of Insanity, in Relation to Jurisprudence.*

Designed for the Use of Persons Concerned in Legal Questions Regarding Unsoundness of Mind (London: H. Baillière, 1842).

————, *The Natural History of Man* (London: H. Baillière, 1843).

————, *Histoire naturelle de l'homme*, trans. F. D. Roulin, (Paris: J.-B. Baillière, 1843).

————, "Observations on the Connexions of Insanity with Diseases in the Organs of Physical Life". *Provincial Medical and Surgical Journal* 7 (1844): 323-24.

————, "On the Relations of Ethnology to Other Branches of Knowledge" (Anniversary Address delivered at the Anniversary Meeting, 22. 6. 1847, of the Ethnological Society). *Journal of the Ethnological Society of London* 1 (1848): 301-29.

————, "On the Recent Progress of Ethnology" (Anniversary Address for 1848 to the Ethnological Society of London). *Edinburgh New Philosophical Journal* 46 (1848): 53-72.

————, "Ethnology". In *A Manual of Scientific Enquiry Prepared for the Use of Her Majesty's Navy and Adapted for Travellers in General*, ed. John Herschel (London: John Murray, 1849), p. 424.

————, *The Natural History of Man* 4. ed., 2 vols, ed. Edwin Norris (London: Baillière, 1855).

————, *Manual of Ethnology, Extract from the Admiralty Manual of Scientific Enquiry* (London: W. Clowes and Sons, 1859).

QUATREFAGES, A. DE, *Histoire générale des races humaines. Introduction à l'étude des races humaines, 2 vols* (Paris: A. Hennuyer, 1887-89).

QUERNER, HANS, "Christoph Girtanner und die Anwendung des Kantischen Prinzips in der Bestimmung des Menschen". In *Die Natur des Menschen*, ed. Gunter Mann *et al.*, pp. 123-36.

RAISTRICK, ARTHUR, *Quakers in Science and Industry* (London: Bannisdale Press, 1950).

REDGRAVE, SAMUEL, *A Dictionary of Artists of the English School* (London: Longmans, Green and Co., 1874).

REHBOCK, PHILIP F., *The Philosophical Naturalists. Themes in Early Nineteenth-Century British Biology* (Madison: The University of Wisconsin Press, 1983).

RICHARDS, GRAHAM, *"Race", Racism and Psychology. Towards a Reflexive History* (London: Routledge, 1997).

RISSE, GUENTER B., *Hospital Life in Enlightenment Scotland* (Cambridge: Cambridge University Press, 1986).

RITTER, CARL, *Die Vorhalle Europäischer Völkergeschichten vor Herodotus, um den Kaukasus und an den Gestaden des Pontus, eine Abhandlung zur Alterthumskunde* (Berlin: G. Reimer, 1820).

————, *Die Erdkunde im Verhältniß zur Natur und zur Geschichte des*

Menschen, oder allgemeine vergleichende Geographie, 7 vols
(Berlin: G. Reimer, 1832-43).

ROGER, JACQUES, *Les sciences de la vie dans la pensée française du XVIIIe
siècle* (Paris: Armand Colin, 1963).

————, *Buffon* (Ithaca: Cornell University Press, 1997 (1989)).

ROSENFELD, LOUIS, *Thomas Hodgkin. Morbid Anatomist and Social Activist*
(Lanham, Md.: Madison Books, 1992).

ROSNER, LISA, *Medical Education in the Age of Improvement. Edinburgh
Students and Apprentices, 1760-1826* (Edinburgh: Edinburgh
University Press, 1991).

ROSSI, PAOLO, *The Dark Abyss of Time,* trans. Lydia G. Cochrane (Chicago:
University of Chicago Press, 1984).

ROULIN, FRANÇOIS DÉSIRÉ, "Mémoire sur quelques changemens observés
dans les animaux domestiques transportés de l'ancien monde dans
le nouveau continent, lue à l'Académie Royale des Sciences le 29.
Sept. 1828". *Annales des sciences naturelles* 16 (1829): 16-34.

ROUSE, MARTIN L., "The Bible Pedigree of the Nations of the World".
*Journal of the Transactions of The Victoria Institute, or,
Philosophical Society of Great Britain* 38 (1906): 123-50.

ROUSSEAU, JEAN, "Les trois méthodes de la comparaison chez Wilhelm von
Humboldt". In *Papers in the History of Linguistics,* ed. Hans
Aarsleff *et al.,* pp. 461-64.

RUDOLPHI, CARL ASMUND, *Beyträge zur Anthropologie und allgemeinen
Naturgeschichte* (Berlin: Königliche Akademie der
Wissenschaften, 1842).

RUDWICK, MARTIN, *Scenes from Deep time. Early Pictorial Representations of
the Prehistoric World* (Chicago: University of Chicago Press, 1992).

RUPKE, NICOLAAS A., *The Great Chain of History. William Buckland and the
English School of Geology (1814-1849)* (Oxford: Clarendon Press,
1983).

————, *Richard Owen. Victorian Naturalist* (New Haven: Yale University
Press, 1994).

RUSSELL, NICHOLAS, *Like Engend'ring Like: Heredity and Animal Breeding
in Early Modern England* (Cambridge: Cambridge University
Press, 1986).

SAINT-HILAIRE, ETIENNE GEOFFROY, *"Rapport fait à l'Académie des Sciences
sur un mémoire de M. Roulin...".* *Annales des sciences naturelles* 16
(1829): 34-44.

SAUNDERS, JANET, "Quarantining the Weak-Minded: Psychiatric Definitions
of Degeneracy and the Late-Victorian Asylum". In *The Anatomy
of Madness,* ed. W. F. Bynum, *et al.,* 3: 273-96.

SCHAFFER, SIMON, "Visions of Empire: Afterword". In *Visions of Empire,* ed. David Philip Miller *et al.*, pp. 335-52.

SCHIEBINGER, LONDA, *Nature's Body. Gender in the Making of Modern Science* (Boston: Beacon Press, 1993).

SCHLEGEL, AUGUST WILHELM, "De l'origine des Hindous". *Transactions of the Royal Society of Literature of the United Kingdom* 2 (1834): 405-46.

————, "Vorrede". In Prichard, *Darstellung der Aegyptischen Mythologie verbunden mit einer kritischen Untersuchung der Ueberbleibsel der Aegyptischen Chronologie*, trans. L. Haymann (Bonn: Eduard Weber, 1837), pp. i-xxxiv.

SCHLEGEL, FRIEDRICH, *Ueber die Sprache und Weisheit der Indier: Ein Beitrag zur Begründung der Alterthumskunde*, 1808, ed. E. F. Konrad Koerner (Amsterdam: J. Benjamins, 1977).

SCHOFIELD, ROBERT E., *Mechanism and Materialism: British Natural Philosophy in an Age of Reason* (Princeton: Princeton University Press, 1970).

SCHWAB, RAYMOND, *La renaissance Orientale* (Paris: Payot, 1950).

SCULL, ANDREW, "Was Insanity Increasing?" In *idem, Social Order/Mental Disorder. Anglo-American Psychiatry in Historical Perspective* (London: Routledge, 1989), pp. 239-49.

————, *The Most Solitary of Afflictions. Madness and Society in Britain, 1700-1900* (New Haven: Yale University Press, 1993).

SHACKLETON, ROBERT, "The Evolution of Montesquieu's Theory of Climate", *Revue internationale de philosophie* 9 (1955): 317-29.

SHAFFER, E. S., *"Kubla Khan" and the Fall of Jerusalem. The Mythological School in Biblical Criticism and Secular Literature 1770-1880* (Cambridge: Cambridge University Press, 1975).

SHAMDASANI, SONU, "C. G. Jung and the Making of Modern Psychology" (Ph.D. diss., University College London, 1996).

SHAPIN, STEVEN, "Homo Phrenologicus: Anthropological Perspectives on an Historical Problem". In *Natural Order. Historic Studies of Scientific Culture*, ed. Barry Barnes, Steven Shapin (Beverly Hills: Sage, 1979), pp. 41-72.

SIEGERT, HANS, "Zur Geschichte der Begriffe 'Arier' and 'arisch.'" *Wörter und Sachen* n.s., 4 (1941-42): 84-99.

SLOAN, PHILLIP R., "Buffon, German Biology, and the Historical Interpretation of Biological Species". *The British Journal for the History of Science* 12 (1979): 109-53.

————, "From Logical Universals to Historical Individuals: Buffon's Concept of Biological Species". In *Histoire du concept d'espèce dans les sciences de la vie*, ed. J. L. Fischer, J. Roger (Paris: Fond. Singer-Polignac, 1986), pp. 101-40.

SLOTKIN, JAMES SYDNEY, ed., *Readings in Early Anthropology* (London: Methuen, 1965).

SMEND, RUDOLF, *Epochen der Bibelkritik* (München: Chr. Kaiser Verlag, 1991).

————, "Aufgeklärte Bemühungen um das Gesetz. Johann David Michaelis 'Mosaisches Recht'". In *idem, Epochen der Bibelkritik*, pp. 63-73.

————, "Lowth in Deutschland". In *idem, Epochen der Bibelkritik*, pp. 43-62.

SMITH, MUNRO, *A History of the Bristol Royal Infirmary* (Bristol: J. W. Arrowsmith, 1917).

SMITH, ROGER, *Trial by Medicine. Insanity and Responsibility in Victorian Trials* (Edinburgh: Edinburgh University Press, 1981).

SNYDER, E. D., *The Celtic Revival in English Literature, 1760-1800* (Cambridge, Mass.: Harvard University Press, 1923).

SOMMER, ANTJE, "William Frédéric Edwards, 'Rasse' als Grundlage europäischer Geschichtsdeutung?" In *Die Natur des Menschen*, ed. Gunter Mann *et al.*, pp. 365-409.

SOUTHALL, ISABEL, *Memorials of the Prichards of Almeley and Their Descendants* (Birmingham, 1901).

SPARN, WALTER, "Vernünftiges Christentum. Über die geschichtliche Aufgabe der theologischen Aufklärung im 18. Jh. in Deutschland". In *Wissenschaften im Zeitalter der Aufklärung*, ed. Rudolf Vierhaus (Göttingen: Vandenhoeck & Ruprecht, 1985), pp. 18-57.

STAGL, JUSTIN, *A History of Curiosity. The Theory of Travel 1550-1800* (Chur: Harwood Academic Publishers, 1995).

STEPAN, NANCY, *The Idea of Race in Science: Great Britain 1800-1960* (London: Macmillan, 1982).

————, "Biology and Degeneration: Races and Proper Places". In *Degeneration. The Dark Side of Progress*, ed. J. Edward Chamberlin *et al.*, pp. 97-120.

STERNEMANN, REINHARD, *Bopp-Symposium 1992 der Humboldt-Universität zu Berlin. Akten der Konferenz vom 24. 3.-26. 3. 1992, aus Anlaß von Franz Bopps 200-jährigem Geburtstag am 14. 9. 1991* (Heidelberg: Winter, 1993).

STOCKING JR, GEORGE W.,

————, "From Chronology to Ethnology. James Cowles Prichard and British Anthropology. 1800-1850". Introduction to Prichard, *Researches into the Physical History of Man*, 1813, pp. ix-cx.

————, *Victorian Anthropology* (New York: Free Press, 1987).

————, ed., *The Ethnographer's Magic and Other Essays in the History of*

Anthropology (Madison, Wis.: University of Wisconsin Press, 1992).

————, "The Ethnographer's Magic: Fieldwork in British Anthropology from Tylor to Malinowski". In *idem, The Ethnographer's Magic*, pp. 12-59.

————, "Paradigmatic Traditions in the History of Anthropology". In *idem, The Ethnographer's Magic*, pp. 342-61.

————, *After Tylor. British Social Anthropology 1888-1951* (London: Athlone, 1996).

————, ed., *Volksgeist as Method and Ethic. Essays on Boasian Ethnography and the German Anthropological Tradition, History of Anthropology* 8 (Madison, Wisc.: University of Wisconsin Press, 1996).

SUZUKI, AKIHITO, "An Anti-Lockean Enlightenment?: Mind and Body in Early Eighteenth-Century English Medicine". In *Medicine and the Enlightenment*, ed. Roy Porter (Amsterdam: Rodopi, 1994), pp. 226-59.

SWAIN, G., *Le sujet de la folie* (Toulouse: Privat, 1977).

SYMONDS, JOHN ADDINGTON, *Some Account of the Life, Writings, and Character of the Late James Cowles Prichard* (Bristol: Evans & Abbott, 1849).

TEMKIN, OWSEI, *Galenism: Rise and Decline of a Medical Philosophy* (Ithaca: Cornell University Press, 1973).

TOULMIN, STEPHEN and JUNE GOODFIELD, *The Discovery of Time* (Chicago: University of Chicago Press, 1965).

TSIAPERA, MÁRIA, "Organic Metaphor in Early 19th Century Linguistics". In *History and Historiography of Linguistics. Papers from the Fourth International Conference on the History of the Language Sciences, Trier, 24.-28. 8. 1987*, ed. Hans-Josef Niederehe, Konrad Koerner, 2 vols (Amsterdam: J. Benjamins, 1990), 2: 577-87.

TUKE, D. HACK, entry on Prichard in *Dictionary of National Biography*, vol. 46.

————, *Prichard and Symonds in Especial Relation to Mental Science with Chapters on Moral Insanity* (London: Churchill, 1891).

TURNER, FRANK M., *Between Science and Religion: The Reaction to Scientific Naturalism in Late Victorian England* (New Haven, London: Yale University Press, 1974).

————, "The Victorian Conflict Between Science and Religion: A Professional Dimension". *Isis* 69 (1978): 356-76.

————, *Contesting Cultural Authority. Essays in Victorian Intellectual Life* (Cambridge: Cambridge University Press, 1993).

————, "Cultural Apostasy and the Foundations of Victorian Intellectual Life". In *idem, Contesting Cultural Authority*, pp. 38-72.

————, "The Crisis of Faith and the Faith that was Lost". In *idem,*

Contesting Cultural Authority, pp. 73-100.

TYLOR, E. B., "Anthropology". In *Encyclopaedia Britannica*, 9th ed., vol. 1.

VANSITTART, PETER, *In Memory of England. A Novelist's View of History* (London: John Murray, 1998).

VERWEY, GERLOF, *Psychiatry in an Anthropological and Biomedical Context. Philosophical Presuppositions and Implications of German Psychiatry, 1820-1870* (Dordrecht: Reidel, 1984).

VIREY, JULIEN-JOSEPH, *Histoire naturelle du genre humain*, 2nd ed., 3 vols (Paris: Crochard, 1824).

WAAL MALEFIJT, ANNEMARIE DE, *Images of Man. A History of Anthropological Thought* (New York: Alfred A. Knopf, 1974).

WAIT, DANIEL GUILDFORD, *Jewish, Oriental, and Classical Antiquities; Containing Illustrations of the Scriptures, and Classical Records from Oriental Sources* (Cambridge: printed by J. Smith for the University, 1823).

WALKER, NIGEL and SARAH MCCABE, *Crime and Insanity in England*, 2 vols (Edinburgh: Edinburgh University Press, 1973).

WALLACE, ALFRED RUSSEL, *My Life: A Record of Events and Opinions*, 2 vols (London: Chapman & Hall, 1905).

WARBURTON, WILLIAM, *The Divine Legation of Moses demonstrated, on the Principles of a Religious Deist, from the Mission of the Doctrine of a Future State of Reward and Punishment in the Jewish Dispensation*, 2 vols (London: Fletcher Gyles, 1738-41).

WATERMAN, A. M. C., *Revolution, Economics and Religion. Christian Political Economy, 1798-1833* (Cambridge: Cambridge University Press, 1991).

WEINER, DORA, "Mind and Body in the Clinic: Philippe Pinel, Alexander Crichton, Dominique Esquirol, and the Birth of Psychiatry". In *The Languages of Psyche. Mind and Body in Enlightenment Thought*, ed. G. S. Rousseau (Berkeley: University of California Press, 1990), pp. 331-402.

————, "'Le geste de Pinel': The History of a Psychiatric Myth". In *Discovering the History of Psychiatry*, ed. Mark S. Micale, Roy Porter (Oxford: Oxford University Press, 1994), pp. 232-47.

WELLS, KENTWOOD D., "Sir William Lawrence (1783-1867). A Study of Pre-Darwinian Ideas on Heredity and Variation". *Journal of the History of Biology* 4 (1971): 319-61.

WHEWELL, WILLIAM, *History of the Inductive Sciences*, 3 vols (London: J. W. Parker, 1837).

WHITE, CHARLES, *An Account of the Regular Gradation in Man and in Different Animals and Vegetables...* (London: printed for C. Dilly, 1799).

WILLIAMS, ELISABETH A., *The Physical and the Moral, Anthropology, Physiology, and Philosophical Medicine in France, 1750-1850* (Cambridge: Cambridge University Press, 1995).

WILLIAMS, GWYN A., "Romanticism in Wales". In *Romanticism in National Context*, ed. Roy Porter, Mikuláš Teich (Cambridge: Cambridge University Press, 1988), pp. 9-36.

WILLSON, A. LESLIE, *A Mythical Image: The Ideal of India in German Romanticism* (Durham, NC: Duke University Press, 1964).

WISEMAN, NICHOLAS, *Twelve Lectures on the Connexion Between Science and Revealed Religion*, 2 vols (London: Joseph Booker, 1836).

WITHERS, CHARLES W. J., "Geography, Enlightenment and the Paradise Question". In *Geography and the Enlightenment*, ed. Charles W. J. Withers, David Livingstone (Chicago: University of Chicago Press, 1999, forthcoming).

WOKLER, ROBERT, "From *l'homme physique* to *l'homme moral* and back: Towards a History of Enlightenment Anthropology". *History of the Human Sciences* 6 (1993): 121-38.

WOOD, P. B., "The Natural History of Man in the Scottish Enlightenment". *History of Science* 28 (1990): 89-123.

YEO, RICHARD, "William Whewell, Natural Theology and the Philosophy of Science in Mid Nineteenth Century Britain". *Annals of Science* 36 (1979): 493-512.

————, *Defining Science: William Whewell, Natural Knowledge, and Public Debate in Early Victorian Britain* (Cambridge: Cambridge University Press, 1993).

YOUNG, B. W., *Religion and Enlightenment in Eighteenth-Century England. Theological Debate from Locke to Burke* (Oxford: Clarendon Press, 1998).

YOUNG, ROBERT J. C., *Colonial Desire. Hybridity in Theory, Culture and Race* (London: Routledge, 1995).

YOUNG, ROBERT M., *Mind, Brain and Adaptation in the Nineteenth Century* (Oxford: Clarendon Press, 1970).

————, *Darwin's Metaphor: Nature's Place in Victorian Culture* (Cambridge: Cambridge University Press, 1985).

ZACHARASIEWICZ, WALDEMAR, *Die Klimatheorie in der Englischen Literatur und Literaturkritik von der Mitte des 16. bis zum frühen 18. Jahrhundert* (Wien: Braumüller, 1978).

Index

Index